CLINICAL PRACTICE OF ACUPUNCTURE

Second Edition

Prof. Dr. A.L. Agrawal
MBBS, D.Ac., PhD (Ac.)
Fellow of Acupuncture Foundation of Sri Lanka
Fellow of Korea Acupunture Association

Dr. G.N. Sharma
MBBS, M.S., FCIP, M.Ac.F.I., F.Ac.F.I.
Diploma in Applied Psychology

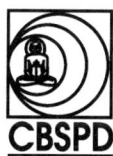

CBSPD

CBS Publishers & Distributors Pvt Ltd

New Delhi • Bengaluru • Chennai • Kochi • Kolkata • Lucknow • Mumbai
Hyderabad • Jharkhand • Nagpur • Patna • Pune • Uttarakhand

Clinical Practice of Acupuncture

ISBN: 978-81-239-0338-5

Second Edition: 1985
Reprint: 1994, 1997, 2000, 2003, 2006, 2009, 2012, 2013, 2014, 2017, 2018, 2019, 2022, 2023, **2025**
First Edition: 1980

Published by **Satish Kumar Jain** and produced by **Varun Jain** for

CBS Publishers & Distributors Pvt Ltd

4819/XI Prahlad Street, 24 Ansari Road, Daryaganj, New Delhi 110 002, India.
Ph: 011-23266838, 23289259   Website: www.cbspd.com
e-mail: delhi@cbspd.com
Corporate Office: 204 FIE, Industrial Area, Patparganj, Delhi 110 092
Ph: 011-4934 4934   Fax: 011-4934 4935
e-mail: publishing@cbspd.com; publicity@cbspd.com

Branches

- **Bengaluru:** Seema House 2975, 17th Cross, KR Road, Banasankari 2nd Stage, Bengaluru 560 070, Karnataka, India
  Ph: +91-80-26771678/79   Fax: +91-80-26771680   e-mail: bangalore@cbspd.com
- **Chennai:** 18/8B, Subbarayan Street, Shenoy Nagar, Chennai 600 030, Tamil Nadu, India
  Ph: +91-44-42032115, 26681266   e-mail: chennai@cbspd.com
- **Kochi:** 42/1325, 1326, Power House Road, Opp KSEB, Power House, Ernakulum Kochi 682 018, Kerala, India
  Ph: +91-484-4059061-65,67   Fax: +91-484-4059065   e-mail: kochi@cbspd.com
- **Kolkata:** 147, Hind Ceramics Compound, 1st Floor, Nilgunj Road, Belghoria, Kolkata-700056, West Bengal, India
  Ph: +033-25633055, 033-25633056   e-mail: kolkata@cbspd.com
- **Lucknow:** Basement, Khushnuma Complex, 7 Meerabai Marg (Behind Jawahar Bhawan), Lucknow-226001, UP, India
  Ph: +0522-4000032   e-mail: tiwari.lucknow@cbspd.com
- **Mumbai:** PWD Shed, Gala no 25/26, Ramchandra Bhatt Marg, Next to JJ Hospital Gate no. 2, Opp. Union Bank of India, Noorbaug, Mumbai-400009, Maharashtra, India
  Ph: 022-66661880/89   e-mail: mumbai@cbspd.com

Representatives

- Hyderabad 0-9885175004   • Jharkhand 0-9811541605   • Nagpur 0-8692091830
- Patna 0-9334159340   • Pune 0-9664372571   • Uttarakhand 0-9716462459

Printed at Mudrak, Noida, UP

To

Prof. Anton Jayasuriya of Sri Lanka whose perpetual guidance, encouragement and help inspired the authors to bring out this book.

The Scholars of acupuncture whose meritorious contributions have provided new dimensions to this ancient art of healing.

The World Health Organization for recognizing acupuncture.

FOREWORD

We are witnessing in the latter half of the twentieth century a surge of interest in the healing art of .acupuncture, mainly due to its potential for minimising human suffering to an extent which has not been hither to possible.

As an alternative to medicine, acupuncture has been recognised as the most futuristic in the field because it is safe, simple, the most economical and the least activating of side effects. Physicians from every school of medicine, Western, Ayurvedic, homeopathic, herbal and Chiropractic, are showing an increasing interest in getting themselves trained in acupuncture for this reason. This incentive has been hightened after the World Health Organization recognised that acupuncture and other traditional healing arts have to be harnessed to the maximum degree as part of its global strategy to provide adequate health care to everyone in the world by the year 2000 A.D.

The authors are medical doctors with vast experience in practising the science of acupuncture who have treated more than twenty thousand patients in India. Dr. A. L. Agrawal was trained in Hong Kong in acupuncture therapy and is keenly associated with various acupuncture societies of the world. Whilst participating in the course of international seminars on acupuncture he has imbibed valuable knowledge.

Dr. G. N. Sharma is a well-known surgeon and an upcoming acupuncture specialist from India. With his wide experience and knowledge in practical field he is also a keen writer on medical topics. He holds great promise for his contribution to this science in medical world.

Our scientific understanding of acupuncture over the last decade has increased significantly due to the work of notable researchers like Chang Hsiang-Tung of the Peoples Republic of China, Ronald Melzack and Bruce Pomeranz of Canada, John Bonica and Robert Becker of the U.S.A., Victor Adamenko and the Kirlians of the U.S.S.R. and numerous others. The horrendous complications produced retrogenically with most modern medicine make it all the more impertative to explore methods like acupuncture which utilise the body's own in-built healing mechanism to cure the ailments.

While a great deal has been written about the traditional theories on acupuncture in West, they are disappointingly vague as to how these theories can be utilised in practice. It would appear that the lack of explicit direction on such points is a major reason for many acupuncture doctors for getting discouraged from probing the traditional methods to any great depth. Such limitations leave much to be desired for research work on acupuncture.

The authors have spared no pains to avoid ambiguities and have wisely refrained from introducing material of doubtful value. Instead they have concentrated on giving a clear explanation on the basic principles and how the clinician could use them in everyday practice. The presentation is remarkable for its elegance of style and clarity of exposition.

It has been a great personal privilege for me to have been associated with Dr. A.L. Agrawal for many years. I have no doubt that this book would be of great help to many others to acquire a clear understanding of the traditional methods for purposes of clinical practice as well as for research.

ANTON JAYASURIYA
Institute of Acupuncture
Colombo South General Hospital
Kalubowila, Sri Lanka

PREFACE TO THE SECOND EDITION

A large number of readers had sent us extremely valuable comments on the first edition of the book in the light of which we decided to revise the text thoroughly and make extensive modifications in the illustrations. A fresh chapter entitled "Stimulation in Acupuncture" has been added to introduce the reader to the various methods of stimulation—both ancient and modern. Photographs and descriptions of latest equipment like laser stimulator, ultrasonic stimulator, etc. have been included in this chapter.

Lebelling of the illustrations has been revised thoroughly and many line illustrations have been redrawn to bring in clarity to the concepts discussed in the text. About 24 fresh clinical photographs have been introduced for the reference of the reader. In addition, certain errors that had crept into the typesetting of the previous edition, have been suitably rectified.

The overwhelming response to the first edition from our readers and friends has enthused the first author to write a number of other books, the final draft of one of which ("Cosmetic Acupuncture") is now ready for publication. The other titles in the series will follow.

The authors are thankful to Mr. Y. N. Arjuna, Editorial Consultant, for the painstaking care taken by him in bringing out this edition of the book.

A. L. Agrawal
G. N. Sharma

PREFACE TO THE FIRST EDITION

The authors have been inspired to write this book from their personal observations of the existing modes and means of healing which entail a lot of complications, reactions, toxicity and what not; and require the patient to move from door to door, from a pathologist to a radiologist and then to another analyst or specialist for innumerable tiring and time consuming investigations. For the patient all these investigations and checkup mean a lot of expenses too. Society now seems to have been fed up with the present procedures of healing that bring in their wake a sense of despair, anxiety and helplessness not to talk of expenses. The modern man seems to be clamouring to cry a halt to all this and demanding some system of setting bodily ailments right which would be easy, understandable, less expensive and less time consuming.

The present panacea to the problems of the patients seems to lie in the age-honoured Chinese system of healing called *Acupuncture*. This system has proved to be an answer to many problems of diagnosis and treatment from the doctors' point of view and exertion and expensiveness from the patients; and has been tested on the touchstone of both. The authors were further encouraged to put in the form of this book the essence of their own study in a simple and easily comprehensible language, as the study revealed the remarkable success of this system in different countries and climes in the recent times. This book is meant to cater to the student and practitioner of the system of acupuncture alike.

Perceptive readers will be exhilirated to find chapters on surface anatomy, basic physiology, living body and electricity which are not the usual features of this kind of books ordinarily available, but the knowledge of which is rudimentary to the making of an acupuncturist. Special endeavour has been made to avoid verbosity and superfluous details. Another salient feature of this book is that a full chapter on diagnostic methods—traditional Chinese methods and modern methods has been included in it. And, as pulse diagnosis is the very crux and nucleus of the acupuncture system of treatment, a full separate chapter has been devoted to it, though in a way pulse diagnosis forms a part of general diagnosis.

If this book in its present form helps the student and practitioner of the art and science of acupuncture ever so little and advances the science in however small a measure, the authors will deem that their efforts have not been in vain; on the contrary they will have the satisfaction that their pains have been enormously rewarded. As it is, this book fulfills a long-cherished desire of the authors to render their iota of service to the suffering humanity.

Any suggestions and advise for the improvement in the form and content of this book would be welcome to the authors.

A.L. AGRAWAL
G. N. SHARMA

ACKNOWLEDGEMENTS

The authors convey their deep sense of greatfulness to Dr. Anton Jayasuriya who has been the inspiration and constant guide behind the making of this book, and, but for whose invaluable help, this book had never been completed.

They also wish to convey their sincere thanks to Dr. Takeshi Sawa of Japan, Dr. Sidney Rose Neil of U.K., Dr. K.L. Tiwari, Dr. H.L. Bansal, Dr. P.S. Deshpande and Dr. S. P. Marda for their scholarly contribution which has greatly enriched the contents of this book.

The authors would also like to convey their deep appreciation for the valuable help rendered in editing the book to Dr. S.R. Julka, Dr. J.P. Banchhor, Dr. Shashi Rustgi, Dr. Mrs. Anjana Bharati and Shri B.S. Parihar of India which has made possible this book to come out in such a fine shape. Our thanks also go to Mr. B.R. Sahu and Mr. R.S. Rai for their pains taken in making the drawings and sketches and also to Mr. V.K. Kothari for helping in the completion of this work.

The authors would be failing in their obligations in not expressing their gratitude to their many friends and members of the Acupuncture Foundation of India, who have encouraged and helped them in all possible ways in the early completion of the book.

CONTENTS

Foreword   *v*
Preface to the Second Edition   *vii*
Preface to the First Edition   *ix*
Acknowledgements   *xi*

1. INTRODUCTION   **1–5**

   What is Acupuncture *1*
   The Story of the Needles *1*
   Myths and Legends *2*
   Nei Jing *2*
   Systemetisation *3*
   The Influence of Taoism *3*
   Pulse Diagnosis *3*
   Westernisation of the Chinese Medicine *3*
   Renascence of Acupuncture *3*
   The Origin of Moxibustion *4*
   The Ancient Philosophy *4*
   The Old Indian Technique *4*
   Future of Acupuncture *4*

2. THEORIES OF ACUPUNCTURE   **6–18**

   Traditional Theories *6*

      The concept of Qi; The principles of Yin and Yang; The network of 'Jing Luo'; The concept of the five elements; The traditional law of energy flow

   Modern Theories *11*

      The neurophysiological basis for acupuncture; Gate control theory of pain; Motor gate theory; The thalamic neuron theory; Hypothesis of excessive meridian energy; The viscero somatic reflex theory; Theory of defence mechanism and tissue regeneration; Theory of hypnosis; Acupuncture meridians and Darwin's theory of evolution;

Embryological theory; The endorphine release theory; The Kyung-rank system; Acu points visualised by Kirlian photography

Effect of Acupuncture *15*
Subjective effects; Objective effects

3. **SURFACE ANATOMY**   **19–31**

Unit of Measurement *19*
The Line and Planes of Reference *19*
Identifying the Land Marks *21*
Front of the neck; Mandible; Orbits; Head; Brain; Face; Upper limb; Back; Scapula; Anterior chest wall; Abdomen; Gluteal region; Lower limb

4. **PHYSIOLOGY OF THE CONTROL OF BODY FUNCTION**   **32–46**

Biological Control Systems *32*
Nervous system; Hormones; Interrelations between neural and humoral control systems; Response of the body to stress and trauma

5. **THE LIVING BODY AND ELECTRICITY**   **47–64**

Electrical Treatment *47*
How electricity flows in the living body; The living body can also store electricity; The power of the electric stimulation is proportional to the density of the current; Negative electricity gives better stimulation using less electricity; What are voltage and current

Electricity as an Element of the Inner Environment of a Living Body *55*
Acidity and Alkalinity; The function of body fluids and ions

6. **ELECTRIC STIMULATOR USED FOR ACUPUNCTURE**   **65–71**

Various Kinds of Therapy by Using Electricity *65*
Basic Description of the Electric Stimulator *66*
General Care on Use *66*
Easily Practicable Trouble Shooting *67*
Basic Knowledge Concerning Electric Stimulation for Acupuncture *68*

7. **STIMULATION IN ACUPUNCTURE**   **72–82**

Types of Stimulation in Acupuncture *72*
Ancient System of Stimulation *72*
Modern methods of Stimulation *76*

8. **METHODS OF DIAGNOSIS**   **83–85**

Modern Diagnostic Methods *83*
The Traditional Chinese Diagnostic Methods *84*
Methods Which Should be Adopted by Practitioners of the Acupuncture in the Modern Times *85*

9. PULSE DIAGNOSIS   86–91

Traditional Pulse Positions   *86*
Methods of Pulse Diagnosis   *87*
Normal Pulse   *89*
     Seasonal variations; What to record in pulse diagnosis; The basic qualities of a pulse; The most important characteristics of the pulses; Number system of pulse readings; Fatal pulses; The characteristics of a good diagnostician; What a traditional Chinese diagnostician does; Readings and interpretations

10. METHODS OF ACUPUNCTURE   92–97

ACUPUNCTURE NEEDLES   92
Various Types of Needles and Their Usage   *92*
     Common needle (filliform needle); Triangular needle (sanlingchen); Seven star needles (Plum-Blossom needle); Press needle; Hidden subdermal needles; Sterilisation of the needles
Technique of Acupuncture   *94*
     Te-chi (taking of vital energy); Direction the needle; Point to point (PP); Types of stimulation; Manipulation of needle; Degree of stimulation; Duration of stimulation
Point Injection Therapy and Embedding Therapy   *97*
     Point injection therapy; Embedding therapy (cat-gut therapy)

11. MOXIBUSTION   98–101

Preparation of the Moxa Wool and Its Use   *98*
Different Methods of Moxibustion   *99*
     Direct moxibustion; Indirect moxibustion

12. COMPLICATIONS AND CONTRA-INDICATIONS OF ACUPUNCTURE   102–104

     Needle dystocia; Bent needle; Broken needles; Fainting; Injury to internal organs; Bleeding; Infection; Forgotten needle
Contra-Indications of Acupuncture   *103*

13. ACUPUNCTURE POINTS   105–116

Nomenclature   *105*
     Meridian points; Extra meridian points; Floating points (Ah-shi points); Jing-Well points; Alarm points; The Back-Shu points; The Mu-front points; The Yuan (source) points; The Luo-connecting points; Dangerous points; Influential points; Distal points; The five Shu points; The confluent points; Tonification points; Sedation points

14. SYSTEMIC DESCRIPTION OF MERIDIANS   117–235

    THE LUNG MERIDIAN   117
    THE LARGE INTESTINE MERIDIAN   124
    THE STOMACH MERIDIAN   134
    THE SPLEEN MERIDIAN   146
    THE HEART MERIDIAN   155
    THE SMALL INTESTINE MERIDIAN   159
    THE URINARY BLADDER MERIDIAN   165
    THE KIDNEY MERIDIAN   181
    THE PERICARDIUM MERIDIAN   189
    THE TRIPLE WARMER MERIDIAN   193
    THE GALL BLADDER MERIDIAN   199
    THE LIVER MERIDIAN   210
    THE GOVERNING VESSELS MERIDIAN   216
    THE CONCEPTIONAL VESSELS MERIDIAN   223
    THE EIGHT EXTRA MERIDIANS   229

15. THE EXTRA-ORDINARY POINTS   236–245

    Extra-Ordinary Points on the Head and Neck   *236*
    Extra-Ordinary Points on the Trunk   *239*
    Extra-Ordinary Points on the Upper Extremity   *241*
    Extra-Ordinary Points on the Lower Extremity   *243*

16. RECENT ACUPUNCTURE POINTS   246–257

    Head and Neck   *246*
    Thorax and Adbomen   *248*
    Upper Limb   *252*
    Lower Limb   *255*

17. AURICULO THERAPY   258–270

    Advantages; Indications; Contraindication; Anatomy of the auricle;
    Auricular area; Nerve supply of the auricle
    Distribution and Description of the Auricular Acupuncture Points   *261*
    Auricular lobule; Tragus (corresponds to nose and pharynx);
    Supratragic (heart and external ear); Anti-tragus (head region);
    Antihelix (trunk); Triangular fossa (deltoid fossa); Crus of helix;
    Helix; Scapha; Cymba conchae; Cavum conchae (thoracic region);
    Cranial Surface of the auricle
    Commonly Used for Auricular Points   *269*
    Rules for the Selection of the Points   *269*
    Procedure

18. SCALP NEEDLING THERAPY   271–277

    Division of the areas; The main indications; Rules for the selection
    of the points; Techniques of manipulation

19. NOSE, HAND AND FOOT ACUPUNCTURE   278-285

NOSE ACUPUNCTURE 278

Description of the Points *278*

  First line; Second line; Third line; Extra points

HAND ACUPUNCTURE 280

FOOT ACUPUNCTURE 282

ACUPUNCTURE THERAPY   287

RULES FOR SELECTION OF THE POINTS   289

20. PSYCHIATRIC DISEASES   291-305

ANXIETY NEUROSIS AND NEUROASTHENIA 291

Treatment of Neuroasthenia *292*

IMPOTENCE 293

INSOMNIA 295

ANOREXIA NERVOSA 296

ADDICTION 296

Drug Addiction *297*

Alcohol Addiction *297*

Smoking *298*

TICS (HABIT SPASMS) 298

NOCTURNAL ENURESIS 300

MENTAL RETARDATION 301

HYSTERIA 302

SCHIZOPHRENIA 304

21. NEUROLOGICAL DISEASES   306-336

HEADACHE 306

Mechanisms of Headache *306*

Differential Diagnosis *306*

Frontal Headache *307*

Temporal Headache *307*

Occipital Headache *308*

Headache at Vertex *308*

MIGRAINE 308

  Insomnia; Headache with loss of appetite and nausea

TRIGEMINAL NEURALGIA 310

Pain in the Region of Ophthalmic Branch *310*

Pain in the Region of Maxillary Branch *311*

Pain in the Region of Mandibular Branch *312*

BELL'S PALSY 312

SQUINT 314

PTOSIS 315

HEMIPLEGIA 316

PARAPLEGIA 318

POLIOMYELITIS 320

WRIST DROP 325

FOOT DROP 326

CEREBRAL PALSY 327
Conditions characterised by spastic weakness of the muscles
Extrapyramidal Disorders *328*
PERIPHERAL NEUROPATHY 328
POSTHERPETIC NEURALGIA 329
DISORDERS OF SPEECH 331
EPILEPSY 333
PARKINSONISM 335

22. MUSCULO-SKELETAL DISEASES   337–353

Rules for the Selection of the Points for Musculo-Skeletal Diseases   *337*
RHEUMATOID ARTHRITIS 338
DE QUERVAIN'S DISEASE 341
CARPAL TUNNEL SYNDROME 342
TENNIS ELBOW 342
GOLFER'S ELBOW (PULLED ELBOW) 343
FROZEN SHOULDER HAND SYNDROME 343
PLANTER FASCITIS 345
ANKYLOSING SPONDYLITIS 346
BACKACHE 347
SCIATICA 348
WRY NECK (TORTICOLLIS) 350
OSTEOARTHRITIS OF THE CERVICAL SPINE 351
MYALGIA CHEST 352

23. SPECIAL SENSE ORGANS   354–371

DISEASES OF THE EYE 354
Myopia *354*
Cataract *355*
Glaucoma *355*
Acute Conjunctivitis *356*
Night Blindness *357*
Optic Neuritis *358*
Detachment of Retina *359*
Color Blindness *360*
Photophobia *360*
Optic Atrophy *361*
DISEASE OF THE EAR 362
Tinnitus *362*
Vertigo *363*
Meniere's Disease *364*
Chronic Suppurative Otitis Media *365*
Deaf-Mutism *365*
DISEASES OF THE NOSE 368
Rhinitis *368*
Epistaxis *369*
DISEASES OF ORAL CAVITY 370
Toothache *370*
Aphthous Ulcers *371*

24. GASTROINTESTINAL DISEASES 373–383

INDIGESTION 373
PAIN IN ABDOMEN 374
PEPTIC ULCER 375
ACUTE APPENDICITIS 377
DIARRHOEA 377
CONSTIPATION 378
PILES 379
CHRONIC CHOLECYSTITIS AND GALLSTONES 380
VIRAL HEPATITIS 381
CIRRHOSIS OF LIVER 382

25. RESPIRATORY DISEASES 384–390

UPPER RESPIRATORY TRACT INFECTION 384
SINUSITIS 385
BRONCHITIS 386
PULMONARY TUBERCULOSIS 388
BRONCHIAL ASTHMA 389

26. CARDIOVASCULAR DISEASES 391–397

CARDIAC NEUROSIS 391
ANGINA PECTORIS 392
MYOCARDIAL INFARCTION 392
PALPITATION 393
HYPERTENSION 394
BURGER'S DISEASE 396

27. UROLOGICAL DISEASES 398-402

RENAL COLIC 398
INCONTINENCE OF URINE 399
RETENTION OF URINE 400
ANURIA 400
OEDEMA 401

28. OBSTETRIC AND GYNAECOLOGICAL DISEASES 403–409

MORNING SICKNESS 403
MALPOSITIONS OF THE FOETUS 403
INFERTILITY 404
AMENORRHOEA 405
IRREGULARITIES OF MENSTRUATION 405
DYSMENORRHOEA 406
LEUCORRHOEA 407
PROLAPSE OF UTERUS 408
MANAGEMENT OF NORMAL DELIVERY 409

29. METABOLIC DISEASES 410–412

OBESITY 410
DIABETES MELLITUS 411

30. SKIN DISEASES   413–417

    ECZEMA 413
    PSORIASIS 414
    ACNE VULGARIS   415
    VITILIGO 416
    ALOPECIA 416

31. MEDICAL EMERGENCIES   418–423

    COMA 418
    SHOCK 419
    HIGH FEVER 420
    HEAT STROKE 421
    TETANUS 422

32. MISCELLANEOUS DISEASES   424–426

    ANAEMIA 424
    ALLERGY 425

ACUPUNCTURE ANAESTHESIA   427

33. INTRODUCTION TO ACUPUNCTURE ANAESTHESIA   429–435

    History *429*
    Advantages of Acupuncture Anaesthesia *429*
    Disadvantages *430*
    Indications *430*
    Contraindications *430*
    MOST COMMONLY USED ACUPUNCTURE POINTS 431
    ESSENTIAL PREANAESTHETIC PROCEDURES AND PREPARATION OF
    THE PATIENT 433
    Premedication *433*
    Procedure *434*
    Application of Different Traditional and Modern Theories   *434*

34. POINTS PRESCRIPTIONS FOR ANAESTHESIA   436–444

    Dental Extraction   *436*
    Operations on the Thorax *440*
    Operation on the Skull and Brain *442*

MAGNETOTHERAPY AND FUTURE OF ACUPUNCTURE   445

35. USE   OF MAGNETOTHERAPY IN ACUPUNCTURE   447–449

36. THE FUTURE OF ACUPUNCTURE IN THE THIRD WORLD   450–457

INDEX   459–464

1

INTRODUCTION

Introduction of acupuncture is the story of the march of traditional Chinese treatment techniques over the past 5000 years. This is such a long period of time that any art of healing which could emerge alive through this period certainly cannot be called an ordinary procedure of needling and stimulation, and it does deserve the attention, interest, research, evaluation and above all a warm welcome by the modern medical world.

Let us listen to the music of the pulses in the Chinese way. The orchestra of the pulses represents the melodies of life. When the sound of music is harsh, the life of the individual is at risk. But we cannot listen to this music by ear. It is through the finger tips that you perceive this melody. The past, present and the future of the melody is known through this music. To talk about this music may sound ridiculous to a westernised mind, and even more absurd may sound the idea of normalising this music through needles. But this procedure has stood the test of time and now there is growing curiosity about acupuncture all over the world. It is gradually becoming acceptable to wider sections of medical men. It stands on the border of east and west and through it the two cultures are blending together.

WHAT IS ACUPUNCTURE

The treatment of various diseases of the body carried out by inserting very fine needles into the specific points of the body is termed *acupuncture*. It is a therapeutic method in medical science. It comprises two parts—to needle and to heat. In Latin, *acus* means needle and *pungue* means pricking. The whole body is endowed with a number of spots— the acupuncture points. These points, when stimulated either by needles or by warming, bring about the cure. The source of needle stimulation can be hand or electricity. The heating is done by burning a kind of herb *Artemisia vulgaris* and the technique is called moxibustion. The two techniques needling and moxibustion can be used separately or in combination.

THE STORY OF THE NEEDLES

In the ancient days when people had no knowledge of metals, the so called needles were actually pointed stones. They were termed as 'bian' (sharp) stones, *Shuo Wen Jie Zi*

1

(analytical dictionary of characters) of the second century explained the word 'bian' as a sharp stone used to prick at the body surface in order to cure diseases. These bian stones used to be of various shapes like a knife, a sword, a needle, etc. In the later years such bian stones were replaced by the needles made of bone or bamboo. In some races (Eskimos, for example) the pointed stones are still being used to cure the diseases. During the Shang Dynasty (16–11 century B.C.), it became possible to manufacture bronze. In the course of evolution, needles of iron, silver or gold came into use.

In an excavation in 1968 of an ancient tomb (113 B.C.) in Maohing, Hebei province, among the relics were found golden and fine silver needles as a witness to the original shape of the ancient needles.

MYTHS AND LEGENDS

How old and worshipped this art of acupuncture is can be imagined from the findings of a recent excavation carried out at Liang-Cheng mountain, Wei-Shan county of Shandong province. The four tablets of Han Dynasty were unearthed on which the carved design of a supernatural being half-man half-bird holding a large needle trying to puncture the body of a patient was found. This is an evidence of the prevailing knowledge of acupuncture in the primitive society.

Another interesting legend pertains to some warriors, wounded by arrows who recovered from their chronic illnesses on account of the acupuncture effects brought about by the arrows. According to the legends, acupuncture and herbal therapy was started by two ancient gods of the Chinese people. They were known as Huang Di and Shen Nung (3737–2697 B.C.), the second and third of the three August emperors, preceded by Fu Hsi, the legendary discoverer of the Pa Kua. The existence of such legendary gods has not been proved. Shen Nung was the creator of herbal therapy. He is respected throughout the Orient, with temples in his honour still standing in places like Hanoi in Vietnam. Each temple possesses three memorials on the main altar, to Fu Hsi, Shen Nung, and Huang Ti. It appears from the history that Huang Di, the yellow emperor, stands next to Fu Hsi and Shen Kung as the father of acupuncture.

NEI JING

It is said in legends that Huang Di took the throne of China from Shen Nung in 2697 B.C. He was a man of great wisdom. He formulated the classic of Chinese medicine and his conclusions and principles of anatomy, medicine and health were written down in the *Nei Jing*, popularly called the Huang Di Nei Jing Su Wen, the yellow emperor's classic of internal medicine. Chi Po, chief minister and physician, helped him in accomplishing this task. The book is written in two parts. The first part, known as Su Wen or simple questions, contains the principles of medicine and the theory of the universe as it relates to the human health. Acupuncture is described in the second part known as Ling Shu, or magic gate. This deals with the prevention and cure of illness and the actual ways an acupuncturist may adopt to achieve this.

As medical theory, the descriptions in Nei Jing were far ahead of times. The circulation of the blood in blood vessels was well-described which was discovered in the West thousands of years later. Nei Jing was again compiled later by Wang Ping of Tang Dynasty. It has always received the favour of China's emperors, and long before the Sung version, about 49 editions of Nei Jing had already came into the medical field.

SYSTEMETISATION

The acupuncture points were first systemetically described during the Tsin Dynasty (A.D. 25(–420) and about 349 basic acupuncture points and about 649 in all were listed on the human body. In the Tang Dynasty (A.D. 618–907) a strong need was felt to start an acupuncture centre and a special department was established at the Imperial medical college of China. During A.D. 960–1297 acupuncture was further systemetised and it was not untill 1026, that acupuncture was officially recognised and an official manual was compiled in this regard. It contained the description of 657 total acupuncture points (including 354 basic points). The human body model made of bronze for the teaching purpose was also made in the same year.

THE INFLUENCE OF TAOISM

It was in the Han Dynasty that the spread of Taoism throughout China led to the systematisation of the acupuncture and herbal medicine. Taoism taught theories of Yin and Yang as the basis of proper living. It reached its peak between the third and the seventh centuries. During this period doctors discovered effective cures for serious ailments. The most eminent physician of the Taoist era was Ko Kung, who was born in Kiangsu province.

PULSE DIAGNOSIS

Huang Fu-Mi (215-282 A.D.) wrote a book called Chia Ching on moxibustion and acupuncture. Curiously enough while the teachings of Shun, the famous contemporary physician, were disregarded, acupuncture continued to flourish amongst the clinicians.

Wang Shu wrote Ne-Jing, a treatise on pulse diagnosis, at the very end of the Han era. This book was later translated into Arabic, Persian, Tibetan, Japanese and the art migrated to the Middle East and Europe. Two books were published in Germany in the Seventeenth Century--one in 1682 at Frankfurt and the other in 1686 at Nuremberg.

WESTERNISATION OF THE CHINESE MEDICINE

During the Ming Dynasty (1368-1644) China had started using the knowledge of western medicine while acupuncture, China's own art, was becoming popular in the western Europe. During both the Ching Dynasty (1644-1911) and the nationalist China (1911-1949) acupuncture lost favour of the rulers and it remained suppressed with little or no progress at all.

Chiang Kai-Shek and the Kuomingtang also popularised and favoured western medicine. The Chinese doctors started studying western medical theory and technique. Many Chinese doctors who studied the western medicine, had no real desire to give up their ancient healing art of acupuncture and moxibustion but they did not want to take the risk of being labelled as communists and showed no ostensible interest.

RENASCENCE OF ACUPUNCTURE

After the dawn of the Peoples Republic of China in 1949, the development of traditional culture was associated with patriotism and national pride and thus acupuncture also became cynosure of medical science. More recent developments took place in 1958. Many different methods of treatment were developed such as the needling of hands, nose, ears, face and head, the needling with long fine needles, hot needles, warm needles and the injection of distilled water into certain points, an instrument for detecting the points and a glass figure marked with acupuncture points were made.

In the same year, acupuncture anaesthesia was first successfully carried out and a few operations were performed. Of course, this came after a long experimental period of trial and error. Today acupuncture anaesthesia is extensively used in many hospitals of China.

In 1970, when China opened her doors to the West again, acupuncture started achieving new heights. An ever increasing number of medical practitioners in the various countries started studying and experimenting on the subject seriously. Today many medical institutions have recognised it as a method of therapy and numerous achievements have been registered.

THE ORIGIN OF MOXIBUSTION

Moxibustion originated in northern China. As this region is mountainous and frequently attacked by piercing cold winds, and surrounded by scathing, in the primitive races, when people used to warm themselves with fire, they accidently discovered that applying heat to or scorching the abdominal region at night relieved the symptoms of abdominal pain, distension and fullness. Based on these observations hot pressings and moxibustion method were developed and used for the treatment of illness and pain.

THE ANCIENT PHILOSOPHY

The ancient philosophic theory of the five elements and the concept of Yin and Yang has been extensively used since the spring and autumn period (770–467 B.C.) of Chinese history. The theory of meridians and Luo connection and flow of 'Qi' through them is the nucleus of the theory of acupuncture. Two types of forces are believed to exist; life essence and semen. The life essence of latter heaven helps in the formation of life energy which is known as 'Qi' and nourishes the child after birth. Each and every act of the universe is brought about by 'Qi' which functions by bi-polarity. The whole universe is polarised into two opposite forces, positive and negative, and the system of meridians, pulses, organs, mother and son law, husband and wife law, day and night law are the examples of this concept.

The whole world is divided into five elements—wood, fire, earth, metal and water—which transform into one another and this process is perpetual.

THE OLD INDIAN TECHNIQUE

In India burn marks of counter-irritation are often found on the bodies of villagers. Red hot iron rods are put on the body for treating diseases and surprisingly many of these marks are located on the classical acupuncture points. Pricking the auricle is also done by some old styled practitioners for curing asthma. A hole is made and some ring is worn on that point. This point coincides with the soothing asthma point of auricular therapy.

FUTURE OF ACUPUNCTURE

In the light of modern medical science, the mechanism by which it operates is not properly understood, although many theories have been enunciated. Scholars have tried to explain the success of acupuncture on the neurophysiological basis, hypnosis, and the Darwinian theory of evolution. The outstanding contributions have come from Ronald Melzack and Anton Jayasuriya who put forward the gate control theory of pain relief and motor gate theory of late motor recovery. Kirlian photography too has unveiled new dimension for the research in the field.

Only future would be able to tell us what heights this method of curing human disease will rise to. If safety, inexpensiveness, convenience, ease of learning and practising, and a high percentage of success are any augury, a bright and glorious status awaits this ancient art of healing.

2
THEORIES OF ACUPUNCTURE

An understanding of the fundamentals is the basic necessity for practising any science of healing. Starting the treatment without having a clear concept of the subject leads not only to the failure of the treatment but sometimes be hazardous. Although a lot of literature is pouring in every day and new theories of acupuncture are being enunciated, none of them fully explain the age-old, traditional concepts of the Chinese acupuncture. Tremendous efforts are being made to explain the Chinese theories in the light of the modern medical science to search its relations with the various known anatomical pathways, physiological principles and biochemical changes. The prodigality of the theories is an evidence of the paucity of the concrete explanation on the subject. Nevertheless the efforts are not futile. Scholars have discovered many correlations between them, these perpetual endeavours of the medical men will certainly unveil the hidden secrets of the amazing science of acupuncture. In order to have a clear concept of the subject, it is worthwhile to discuss the traditional Chinese theories first and the modern theories later.

TRADITIONAL THEORIES

The Concept of Qi

The concept of '*Qi*' or '*Chi*' (pronounced as Chee) is some vital motivating force in the body which burns as a fuel all over one's life. It has neither been established by any science in any particular fashion nor has it been assessed in any other way. It is only to be experienced and appreciated. The modern medical science because of its over-systemetisation is silent about it. But in the history of many old medical disciplines it forms the fundamental concept of the whole system.

In the Indian philosophy it is known as *Prana*. Yogis call it *Prana Vayu*. As long as *Prana* or *Prana Vayu* exists in the body, the heart beats, the brain works, the lungs breathe and the whole organism stays as a living miracle. No one has seen this *Prana* but the concept is age old and unchallenged.

The principle of *Prana* and *Prana Vayu* is quite similar to the traditional Chinese concept of '*Qi*' or the energy of life. '*Qi*' is universal and present at all times in different forms. In the body it permeates all living cells and tissues. It is the invisible force responsible for all the movements of life. True '*Qi*' comes from the heaven and manifests as a living soul during birth.

6

It is the main working force behind all the events of the life and controls the functioning of the main acts of the organ and systems of the body. Whether it is the breathing and gaseous exchange at the level of the lungs, digestion and absorption in the intestines or multiplication of the germinal epithelium in the reproductive organs, it is the manifestation of the '*Qi*'. It permeates all living cells and circulates rhythmically in the body and a constant process of the transformation of air, food and water into the '*Qi*' takes place throughout one's life.

The Principles of Yin and Yang

The Yin and Yang are the two aspects of the '*Qi*' energy. According to the Yellow emperors classic of internal medicine the principle of Yin and Yang is the basic principle of the entire universe. Good health is the state of energy balance between these two and its upsetting results in a disease. They function as two opposite poles, negative and positive and are complementary to each other. There are perpetual vibrations between them. Yang stands for male, sun, heaven, sharp, clean, up, motion, strength, warmth, dispersion, destruction and all that is positive. Yin stands for female, moon, earth, dirty, down, quietitude, cold, chronic, peace, harmony, endurance, debility, weakness and all that is negative.

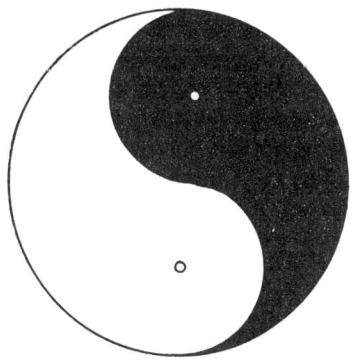

In the ancient Chinese literature the concept of Yin and Yang is usually depicted in the form of the so called 'Chinese Monad'. It is represented by a closed circle divided into two equal halves by a sinus curve. Two different colours are used, usually red for Yang and blue or green for Yin. In each half of the circle there is a small circle of the opposite colour and opposite sense indicating the bud of Yin sleeping in the bosom of Yang while the bud of Yang sleeps in the bosom of Yin (Fig. 2.1).

It is further believed that Yin is active within and acts as a guardian of Yang. Yang is active on the surface and functions as a regulator of Yin. Yin stores up essence and Yang protects it.

Fig. 2.1   Symbol of yin and yang (Chinese monad).

The Network of 'Jing Luo'

The routes through which '*Qi*' flows in the body are known as meridians or channels. In Chinese they are termed as *Jing Luo* (*Jing*—Path, *Luo*—Connection).

Meridians running vertically from below upwards or above downwards are the main meridians and traditionally termed as Jing. There are twelve paired main meridians and 8 extra ordinary meridians. The collateral connections that link the main meridians together are called Luo.

Twelve paired meridians originate from the internal viscera of the body and are named according to the concerned organ. The viscera are divided into two categories—solid or Zang organs, hollow or Fu organs. Zang organs store the '*Qi*' while Fu organs discharge it. The meridians originating from Zang organs are negative (*Yin*) and those originating from Fu organs are positive (*Yang*) in polarity. These *Yin* and *Yang* meridians are linked (Luo—connected) by collaterals.

To converse the polarity of Yang and Yin each organ contains a part of both the principles in variable proportions.

			Yin		Yang	
Main	Paired	Arm	Lung	(L)	Large Intestine	(LI)
			Pericardium	(P)	Triple Warmer (Sanjiao)	(TW) (SJ)
			Heart	(H)	Small Intestine	(SI)
		Leg	Spleen	(Sp)	Stomach	(St)
			Liver	(Liv)	Gall Bladder	(GB)
			Kidney	(K)	Urinary Bladder	(UB)
Extraordinary	Unpaired		Conceptional Vessel	(CV)	Ren Mai	(Ren)
			Governing Vessel	(GV)	Du Mai	(DU)
			Belt Vessel		Dai Mai	
			Vital Vessel		Chong Mai	
	Paired		Yang Ankle Vessel		Yang Chiao Mai	
			Yin Ankle Vessel		Yin Chiao Mai	
			Yang Regulating Vessel		Yang Wei Mai	
			Yin Regulating Vessel		Yin Wei Mai	

For the health and well-being of the body and mind, there must be sufficient and equal energy in each of these meridians.

The Concept of the Five Elements

According to the traditional Chinese concept the whole universe is divided into five elements. These are not the old Greek elements nor do they belong to the periodic table of modern physical science. Further, the names of the elements do not signify exactly the same material in the strict, literary sense. The five elements exist in the heaven and the same elements exist on the earth. In the living body they symbolise the internal organs and their cycles explain the phenomenon of nature. Fire symbolises heart, small intestine, pericardium and triple warmer; earth symbolises stomach and spleen; metal stands for lung and large intestine; water symbolises kidney and urinary bladder, and wood represents liver and gall bladder. We know that each one of these organs possesses its own meridian, these elements symbolise those particular meridians too.

These five elements are constantly transformed into one another and there are two cycles of events in this process of transformation—creative and destructive (Fig. 2.2).

Use of the concept of five elements in practical application of acupuncture is on the basis of correlation and representation of the organs given below.

The Traditional Law of Energy Flow

While flowing in the meridians 'Qi' obeys certain definite rules in respect of the direction, time and side of the body. The knowledge of this flow is essential for selecting the meridian and acupuncture points, time of therapy and the side of the body.

	Luo Connecting	
	Yin	Yang
Fire		
Major	Heart	Small Intestine
Minor	Pericardium	Triple Warmer
Earth	Spleen	Stomach
Metal	Lung	Large Intestine
Water	Kidney	Urinary Bladder
Wood	Liver	Gall Bladder

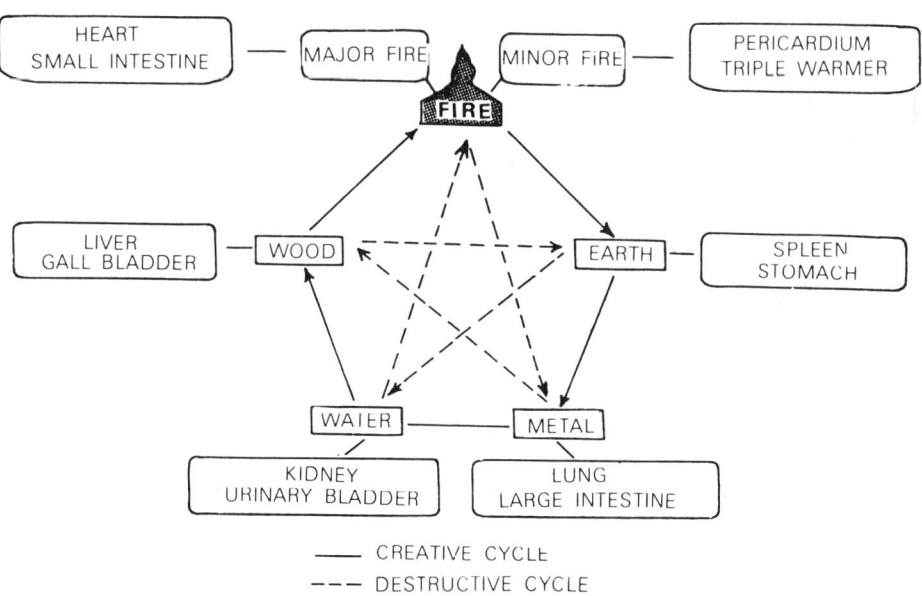

——— CREATIVE CYCLE
- - - DESTRUCTIVE CYCLE

Fig. 2.2 Concepts of five elements.

Mother and Son Law

'Qi' always flows from mother to the son. For the proper feeding (flow) the mother should be well nourished herself and the child should be strong enough to receive. In the flow of energy the son becomes the mother of the following meridian after receiving the energy and in turn the recipient organ again becomes the mother of the next following organ. Thus:

     Liver is the mother of heart.

     Heart is the mother of spleen.

     Spleen is the mother of lung.

     Kidney is the mother of liver.

     Lung is the mother of kidney.

Husband-wife law

Husband dominates the wife, Yang dominates Yin and left wrist pulse dominates right wrist pulse. Organs related to the husband are small intestine, heart, gall bladder, liver, urinary bladder and kidney while those related to the wife are large intestine, lung, stomach, spleen, triple warmer and pericardium.

In normal balanced rhythm left wrist pulse should be slightly stronger than the right wrist pulse.

The mid-day mid-night law and organ clock

This law describes the relationship between the organs receiving maximum flow of energy at the opposite times. The organ clock shows the circulation of vital energy through various organs and meridians in relation to time (Fig. 2.3). Study of this law is helpful in deciding the time of treatment of a disease in order to obtain maximum benefit.

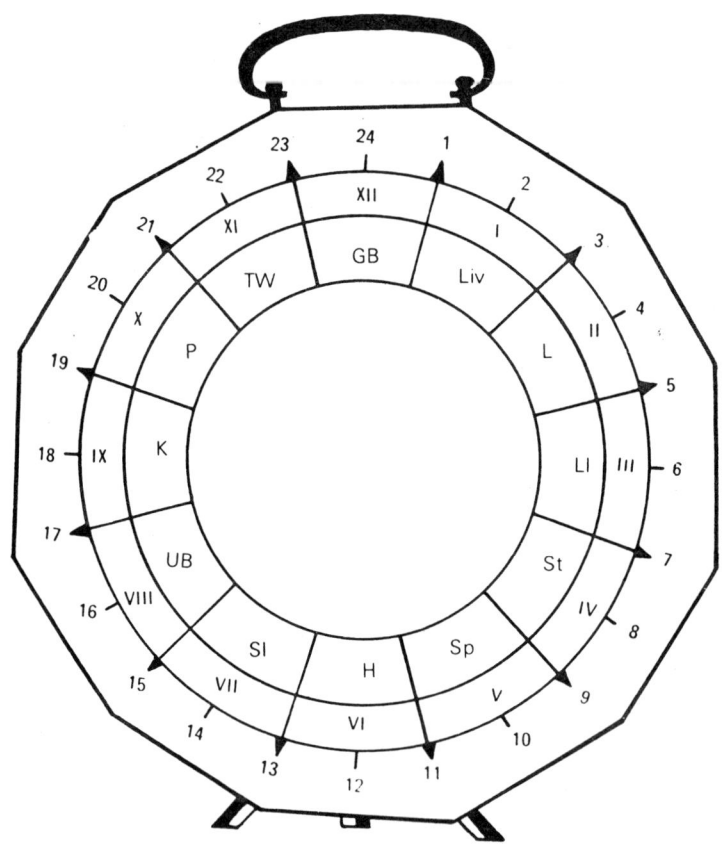

Fig. 2.3   Organ Clock—Liv liver, L lung, LI large intestine, St stomach,
Sp spleen, SI small intestine, UB urinary bladder, K kidney,
P pericardium, TW triple warmer, GB gall bladder.

MODERN THEORIES

The Neurophysiological Basis for Acupuncture

Whatever the meridian and 'Qi' may be or imply, nervous system and nerve impulses must be involved in realising the acupuncture effect (Chang). If an acupuncture point is pre-anaesthetised with a drug, subsequent needling will produce no acupuncture effect. This effect indicates that acupuncture produces its effect through mediation of nerve (Ling and Clive, 1977).

Autonomic nervous system also appears to play an important role in the working of acupuncture (Ionescu-Tirgoviste, 1973; Smith and Kenyon, 1973; Looney, 1974). Ling and Clive (1977) have proved a direct involvement of the autonomic nervous system in an experiment on a cat. By applying electrical stimulation at Ququan (Live-8) in the cat, they observed potential changes at the hypothalamus, the control centre of the autonomic nervous system. By applying acupuncture (electrical stimulation) at Zusanli (St-36) in a rat, Lee observed significant decrease in blood velocity after 10 minutes of stimulation of sympathetic nerve controlling vasoconstriction.

Sensation and control of activities in the internal organs are regarded as the translations of message carried by nerve impulses in the sensory nerves and in the autonomic nerves in the coding of which the pattern and mean frequency are the two major components. If the message could be altered before or on reaching the destination (the brain or the organ) the sensation would be changed. The physical mechanism involved is that the message of nerve impulse can be altered by external means (Ling and Clive, 1977) and acupuncture works by altering neural coding (Chang) by electrical and thermal intervention. This coding alteration is interpreted on the basis of dipole theory (Wei). According to the dipole theory, excitation phenomena—electrical, thermal and optical—are considered to be the macroscopic manifestations of quantum transmission of electric dipoles at the surface of nerve membrane (Wei, 1971, 1972, 1974). Other important observations reported by various research workers are listed below.

1. Through repetitive stimulation of the nervous system, unused or little used nerve circuits could possibly become effective after degeneration of other previously functional nerve pathways (Illis, 1973).

2. Sprouting of new synapses from nearby intact nerve fibres is also observed explaining the synaptic changes (Illis, 1973).

3. There is a re-establishment of transmission and the dynamic changes at the synaptic level of the central nervous system (Cook, 1973, 1974).

4. Medial reticular formation of the mid-brain contains pain reacting cells and it appears to play a role in producing acupuncture analgesia (Shanghai, 1973).

5. There is an inhibitory interaction in the thalamus between the incoming impulses from the points of acupuncture and the site of pain (Chang, 1973).

6. Segmental relations exist between the point of needling and the point where the pain threshold is most remarkably raised.

7. The local muscular activity during acupuncture is believed to be a reflex activity rather than a direct result of mechanical irritation by the needle.

8. There exists a specific positive correlation between certain chemical synaptic transmitters such as 5 hydroxy tryptamine and the pain relieving effect of acupuncture.

Gate Control Theory of Pain

This theory explains the physiology of pain. All pain impulses are first controlled and modulated in the substantia gelationosa (first functional gate) of the spinal cord before they travel up through the opposite spino-thalamic tracts (second functional gate). When they reach cerebral cortex, the patient feels pain (Ronald, Melzack and Wall, 1965). The existence of two more functional gates has been suggested (Wald, 1972), paraventricular and the contralateral neuclei of the thalamus and the medial reticular formation of the mid-brain also work as functional gates. By the stimulation of the acupuncture point, the over-crowding of the impulses occurs at the functional gates and they are blocked from proceeding further. This raises the pain threshold and analgesia occurs.

Motor Gate Theory

Jayasuriya and Fernando (1977) have explained the phenomenon of late motor recovery by the 'motor gate theory'

According to the theory the functional motor gates situated in the spinal cord are blocked in pathological conditions and acupuncture re-opens them.

The motor gate comprises the following:

1. Efferent pathway: Axons arise from anterior horn cells going to the motor end-plates.
2. Renshaw cells situated in the ventro-lateral part of the ventral horn of grey matter.
3. Cajal cells situated in the intermediate nucleus of Cajal. These are in synaptic connection with anterior horn cells (inhibitory type).
4. Afferent pathway.
5. Synaptic connections with Renshaw cells: Efferents give synaptic connections to Renshaw cells, which are excitatory in nature. Renshaw cells in turn have axons which effect synaptic connections back with the anterior horn cells.

Functions of the Gate

Hyperactivity of the cells automatically leads to an increase in the inhibitory effect exerted on them by the Renshaw and Cajal cells including a return to more normal levels of activity. Under normal circumstances the gates situated between the anterior horn and Renshaw cells and anterior horn and Cajal cells are open.

When a derangement occurs in the central nervous system the motor gate is liable to become pathologically closed (blocked).

Gate opening by Acupuncture

When an acupuncture needle is inserted into a selected acupuncture point (many of which coincide with the motor points of muscles, Gunn et al., 1976) the afferent barrage so generated is potentially capable of acting on the anterior horn cells through the intermediate cells of Cajal.

The Thalamic Neuron Theory (Lee, 1977, 1978)

The salient points of the hypothesis are:

1. In conjunction with any pathological process a focus of abnormal activities is set up in the brain.
2. Stimulating the nerve cells of this focus via peripheral stimulation such as acupuncture can normalise the activity of those abnormal cells, usually by repeated stimulations similar to the process of habituation or conditioning.

3. There is a homunculus or neuronal representation of a miniature human body in the central nervous system which is the master control of all physiological functions and this particular homunculus probably resides in the thalamus.

4. This homunculus assumes the posture of a fetus with its large head buried in the pelvic region and its hands and feet crowded around the face. The hands and feet cross over to the contralateral sides as in a fetus.

5. Along these neuronal chains are functionally discrete groups of neurones which represent the acupuncture loci in the periphery. These groups of neurons representing the acupuncture points, function like regional managers. Each neuronal group processes information from the areas within its sphere of influence and can also exert a powerful effect on these areas.

This hypothesis gives an explanation of many acupuncture principles and help to relate clinical symptoms with the treatment parts and their effect. But the fact remains that it is still an unproven hypothesis.

Hypothesis of Excessive Meridian Energy (Gordon and Butler, 1974)

On excess of Yin or Yang depending to which group the organ belongs, nature endeavours to dissipate the excess energy by channelling it through the meridians to the skin surface. This creates a hot spot which overflows the tiny treatment point, not uncommonly disbursing through the surface of the skin to a sizable area. It is possible for this excess energy, in addition to effecting the underlying muscles to flow into another meridian and pass on some of this excess energy through its treatment points.

The Viscero Somatic Reflex Theory

According to Felix Mann (1972) acupuncture functions through a reflex which he calls as cutaneo-visceral reflex. Ishikawa (1949, 1962) also postulated the existence of visceral somatic reflexes. Their hypothesis is mostly based on the observation of referred pain felt at the distal parts of the body in the diseases of the viscera (e.g. backache in the diseases of stomach, shoulder pain in cardiac diseases) and relief obtained in the original ailment by stimulating the point of referred pain.

Theory of Defence Mechanism and Tissue Regeneration

Defence, immunity and tissue regeneration mechanisms are postulated to be triggered by tissue injury products resulting from microinjuries by acupuncture with or without needles, manipulation or electrical stimulation. This happens initially through the activation of the neuro-endocrine system and later through the reticulo-endothelial system (Cracium, 1973).

Stimulations applied on the surface of the body act upon the body's own defence mechanisms and produce quantities of ACTH, cortisone or any other humoral substances that are appropriate to the stimulations; and in many instances, the humoral substances produced in this manner provide a biological defence against diseases in general, infections as well as non-infections, including the degenerative diseases (Selye, 1950).

Platt (1974) has observed the release of serotonin (5HT) histamine bound electrostatically to endogenous heparin bradykinin, slow reacting substances (SSS-A) and possibly other products as yet unidentified.

Theory of Hypnosis

According to Kroger (1972) acupuncture works through hypnosis. He has operated many cases under hypnosis.   However, the points against this hypothesis are as follows:

1. All the cases where acupuncture is successful do not possess hypnotisability (Shibutani, 1973).
2. If acupuncture point is infiltrated with xylocaine, the distal anaesthetic effect does not occur (Lee, 1974).
3. Acupuncture effects blood pressure (Less, 1974).
4. Acupuncture produces leucocytosis (Brown, 1974).
5. Hypnosis produces increases in delta and theta wave activity and a significant decrease in the alpha and beta wave activity.

Acupuncture at placebo acupuncture points produced no significant effect on EEG, where as electro acupuncture at specific loci produced significant attenuation of the delta and theta waves (Ulett, 1974).

Acupuncture Meridians and Darwin's Theory of Evolution (Lee, 1978)

Some scholars have tried to explain the concept of Yin and Yang in the light of Darwin's theory of evolution.   Yang in Chinese means Sun and Yin shade or the lack of Sun.   The side that is exposed to Sun is Yang and the side that is shaded from the Sun is Yin, if man gives up his erect posture and walks on four limbs.   Therefore what seems to be an arbitrary system of Yin and Yang classification of meridians can actually find logic in the more primitive forms of life that came to exist on the planet earth long before man set foot on this world.

Embryological Theory

The way in which classical meridians are arranged suggests the possibility of embryological relationship between the viscera, meridians and their Luo connections (Felix Mann, 1972).

Three germinal layers of the embryo are represented as follows:

Ectoderm   1. Lung meridian
                2. Large Intestine meridian
                3. Stomach meridian
                4. Spleen meridian
Endoderm   1. Heart meridian
                2. Small intestine meridian
                3. Urinary bladder meridian
                4. Kidney meridian
Mesoderm   1. Pericardium meridian
                2. Triple Warmer meridian
                3. Gall bladder meridian
                4. Liver meridian

The same possibility is suggested by the observation of acupuncture effects on the embryologically related organs.   For example, needling of the kidney meridian not only effects the kidney but organs which are developmentally related to it such as the ovary, uterus and fallopian tubes.

The Endorphine Release Theory

Pomeranz (1976) has suggested the theory of endorphine release through sensory receptors lying deep in the muscle.   Endorphine is a naturally occurring neuropeptide and possesses natural pain killing properties.

The Kyungrank System

Korean scholars (Kum Bong Han and his team) have shown the existence of an integrated system of ducts, entirely independent of the vascular, lymphatic, blood and nervous systems. They call this the Kyungrank system. During their experiments they injected a radio-isotope into an acupuncture point. They could watch the flow of the fluid from acupuncture point on the skin inwards and then finally outwards again. The flow of the fluid coincided with the paths of meridians.

Acu points visualised by Kirlian photography

Kirlian photography is a Soviet invention made back in 1939 by S. D. Kirlian and V. Kirlian. In this technique living beings are observed and photographed under high frequency and high voltage electrical fields.

It is thought that all living things have both a physical body and an energy body. This energy body is seen as a halo or aura in Kirlian photographs. Gaikin (1953) of Leningrad observed energy flare on the acu points in Kirlian photographs. Wei (1975) has observed evoked potential changes at the thalamus, the corticospinal tract and posterior hypothalamus, but no changes on the sensory cortices in the cat. It is suggested (Wei and Gaikin) that energy flare in the Kirlian photographs gives an indication of 'Qi' under acupuncture, but Wouter W. Vander Schaar (1976) finds Kirlian photography unreliable as the pictures in that are not reproducible.

EFFECT OF ACUPUNCTURE

When a needle is inserted on the acupuncture points of the body, it leads to various types of subjective and objective effects. The subjective and objective effects were known to the traditional acupuncturists since the very beginning but they did not have any proper explanation for them. These effects were continuously observed by them and the whole of the acupuncture treatment was based on various objective effects such as analgesia and sedation.

During needling, as the subjective effects are felt by the patient alone, they cannot be scientifically explained and sustained. However, they are the physiological changes incidental to acupuncture and the changes themselves constitute the very basis of acupuncture.

Subjective Effects

When a needle is passed on an acupuncture point the following sensations are experienced by the patient:

1. Pain

   Whenever any needle or a sharp instrument is penetrated in the body, pain is the first sensation experienced by the patient.

2. Numbness

   When a needle is accurately passed on the acupuncture point a feeling of numbness along the meridian is experienced by the patient.

3. Soreness

   A feeling of soreness is experienced by the patient.

4. Heaviness

   Sometimes the patient feels the part of needling is becoming heavy. This feeling is generally found in the extremities.

5. Distension

The patient feels some things moving from the place of needling along and upto the end of the meridian.

A combination of more than two types of feelings indicates that the needles have been accurately placed and energy is stimulated properly.

In Chinese description this is known as taking of T-chi (vital energy).

Objective Effects

1. Analgesia

Acupuncture has a pain-relieving effect, probably due to over-crowding of the motor gates with stimuli and on this basis acupuncture anaesthesia too has been explained.

2. Sedation

Acupuncture on certain points brings tranquility and sedation.

3. Immunity improvement

By acupuncture immunity improves and it probably works through some defence mechanism.

4. Homeostasis

5. Motor recovery

The basis of motor recovery is given while discussing the theories and all the objective symptoms have been explained on scientific basis.

References

1. Acupuncture anaesthesia coordination group of Shanghai College of Traditional Chinese Medicine, Shanghai Normal College and Shu Ku-ang Hospital of Shanghai College of Traditional Chinese Medicine, Shanghai: The rule of the mid-brain reticular formation in acupuncture anaesthesia. *Chinese Medical Journal*, 3: 136-138, 1973.

2. Acupuncture Anaesthesia Research Unit, People's Hospital HSU YI Country, Kiangsu: Electrophysiological study of spinal reflexes under acupuncture anaesthesia. *Chinese Medical Journal*, 3: 139-143, 1973.

3. Brown, M.D. et al.: The effect of acupuncture on white blood cell counts. *Am. J. Chin Med*, 4: 383-398 1974.

4. Chein, E. Y. and M.A.K. Shapiro. A mini-symposium on acupuncture, *American Medical Association Journal*, 227 (11), 1122, March 11, 1974.

5. Chang, Hsiang-tang,: Integrative action of thalamus in the process of acupuncture for analgesia. *Scientia Sinica*, 16, 25-60, 1973.

6. Cook, A.V.: Regeneration in the central nervous system, *Lancet*, June 23, 1442-1443.

7. Cook, A.V.: Electrical stimulation of the spinal cord. *Lancet*, May 4, 1974, 869-1443.

8. Cracium, T. Toma: Central nervous reactions after acupuncture. *Am. J. Acupuncture*, 1 : 61-66, 1973.

9 Cracium, T. Toma and Turdesu: Neuro-modifications after acupuncture. *Am. J. Acupuncture*.

10. Donald A. Berman: Acupuncture– hypnosis or reality. *Am. J. Acupuncture*, 4 (4), 1976.

11. Edmund, Y.N. Chein, M.D.: Neurological mechanism in the recovery of motor and sensory functions by acupuncture. *Am. J. Acupuncture*, 3, March 1975, pp. 69-70.

12. Fujii. M.: Responses to acupuncture and moxibustion, *J. Osaka Medical Society*, 26 : 11-19, 1929 (JAPAN).

13. Gunn, C.C., Ditchburn, F.G. et al.: Acupuncture loci. A Proposal for their classification according to their relationship to know neural structures. *Am. J. Chin. Med.*, 4 (2), 1976, 183-195.

14. Gordon, L. and Butler D.C. : Hypothesis of excessive meridian energy. *Am. J. Acupuncture*, **2**, 1974. July-Sept. 210-211.

15. Hirromaru Ogata : Simplified energetic concepts of classical Chinese acupuncture. *Am. J. Acupuncture*, **6** (3), July-Sept., 1978.

16. Harman V. Elatt : Defence mobilization and tissue regeneration theory. *Am. J. Acupuncture*, **2** July-Sept. 1974 : 167-174.

17. Ishikawa, H. : The law of centripetal double innervation and viscero somatic reflex. *J. Autonomic Nervous System* 1.1.4, 1948-1949 (In Japanese).

18. Ishikawa, T. : Electrodermal points and cutaneo-visceral reflex. *Ilagku-Shoin*, 1962 (In Japanese).

19. Ionescu-Tirgoviste, C. : Theory of mechanism of action in acupuncture. *Am. J. Acupuncture*, **1**, 193, 1973.

20. Illis, L.S. : Regeneration in the central nervous system, *Lancet*, May 12, 1973, 1035-37.

21. Illis, L.S. : *Brain* 96 (1), 47-60, 1973.

22. Jayasuriya, A. Fernando, F. : *Principles and Practice of Scientific Acupuncture*. Lake House Investment Ltd., 42 Ramanayaka Nawatha, Colombo-2, Sri-Lanka, 1977, 69-71, 237.

23. Jayasuriya, A., Fernando, F. : The motor gate theory—A neurophysiological model to explain the phenomenon of late motor recovery following use of acupuncture in paralytic conditions. *Am. J. Acupuncture*, **6** (3), July-Sept.,1978.

24. Kroegar, W.S. : The scientific rationale for acupuncture anaesthesia. *Psychosomatics*, **14** : 191, 1973.

25. Kroegar, W.S. Steinberg, J. : *Childbirth and hypnosis*, Doubleday & Co., New York, 1971.

26. Kroegar, W.S. : Hypnosis and acupuncture, *Journal of American Medical Association*, **20** : 1012-1013, 1972.

27. Kirlian, S.D. and Kh. Kirlian : Photography and visual observations by means of high frequency currents. *J. Sci and Applied Photography and Cinematography*, **6**, 1961, 397-403.

28. Lee. T-sun Nin : Thalamic neuron theory : A hypothesis concerning pain and acupuncture. Medical Hypothesis, 3, 113-121, 1977.

29. Lee T-sun Nin : The Thalamic neuron theory and classical acupuncture. *Am. J. Acupuncture*, **6** (4), Oct.-Dec., 1978.

30. Lee T-sun Nin : A Treatise on acupuncture meridians. *Am. J. Acupuncture*, **6** (4), Oct. Dec., 1978. pp. 283-288.

31. Lee, D.D. : Cardiovascular effects of acupuncture on anaesthesised dogs. *Am. J. Chin. Med.*, **3** : 271-282, 1974.

32. Ling, Y. Wei, and Clive Hodson, Transmission and acupuncture, **5** (1), January-March 1977. PP. 69-83.

33. Lee, et al. : A study of electrical stimulation of acupuncture locus. TausAnil [(St-36) on mesenteric microcirculation. *Am. J. Chin. Med.*, **2**, 53-66, 1974.

34. Looney, G.L. : Autonomic theory of acupuncture. *A. U. Chin. Med.* **2**, 332-333, 1974.

35. Salet, B. and Ulett, G. et al. : Hypno and acupuncture analgesic—A neurophysiologic reality. Presented at the First World Congress of Biological Psychiatry, Buenos Aires, Sept. 1974.

36. Shibutani, K. : Evaluation of the therapeutic effect of acupuncture. Presented at the National Institute of Health Conference of Acupuncture, Bathesda, Md., Feb. 1973.

37. Shanghai Institute of Physiology, Shanghai : Electrical response to nocuous stimulation and its inhibition in nucleus centralis lateralis of thalamus in rabbits. *Chinese Medical Journal*, 131-135, 1973.

38. Smith, A.D. and D.H. Kenyon : Acupuncture and ATP. How they may be related, *A. M. J. Chin. Med.*, 1, 91-97, 1973.

39. Selye, H. : *Physiology and Pathology of Exposure to Strain*. Acta, Inc., Montreal, 1950. *The Strain of Life*. Wilshire Book Company, North Jolly Wood, Calif.

40. Seichi, S. : Hematological data before and after acupuncture and moxibustion. *J. Kyoto Univ. Medical College*, **100**, 1925, (In Japanese).

41. Tolbert J. Small : *Am. J. Acupuncture*, **2**, April-June, 1974 : 77-87.

42. Vaciav Kajdos : Theoretical principles of Chinese medicine, *Am. J. Acupuncture*, **1**, July-Sept. 1973, 89-92.

43. Wei L.Y. : Dipole theory of heat production and absorption in nerve axon. *Biophys J.*, **12**, 1159-1170, 1972.

44. Wei L.Y. : Dipole mechanisms of electrical, optical and thermal energy transduction in nerve membrane. *Ann. N.Y. Acad. Sci.*, **277**, 285-293, 1974.

45. Wouter W. Vander Schasr : Validity of Kirlian photography relating to organ pathology diagnosis and acupuncture. *Am. J. Acupuncture*, **4** (3), July-Sept. 1976, 252-256.

46. Wei, L.Y. : Molecular mechanisms of nerve excitation and conduction. *Bull. Math. Biophys*, **31**, 39-58, 1969.

47. Wei, L.Y. : Quantum theory of nerve excitation. *Bull. Math. Biophys.*, **33**, 187-194, 1971.

48. Wei, L.Y. : Quantum theory of time varying stimulation in nerve. *Bull. Math. Biol.*, **35**, 359-374, 1973.

49. Wei, L.Y. : Possible origin of action potential and birefringence change in nerve axon. *Bull. Math. Biophys.*, **33**, 521-537, 1971.

50. Wei, L.Y. : Brain response and Kirlian photography of the cat under acupuncture. *Am. J. Acupuncture*, **3**, (3), July-Sept. 1975.

51. Tiller, W.A. : Some physical characteristics of acupuncture points and meridians. Transcript of acupuncture Symposium. *Stanford University*, June 1972. The Academy of Parasychology and Medicine, 30-69.

3

SURFACE ANATOMY

Success of the acupuncture treatment lies not only in the correct prescription but also in the exact localisation of the point while needling. Proper knowledge of the important surface anatomical landmarks on the human body is essential for locating the points with highest possible accuracy, and every acupuncturist ambitious of becoming master of the magic of the needles must know the art of localising the points. In this chapter, an attempt has been made to equip the student with a broad knowledge of the surface anatomy required for locating the acupuncture points with accuracy. Care has been taken to avoid all unnecessary details not required for the purpose and the description is restricted to the landmarks of the acupuncture interest only.

UNIT OF MEASUREMENT

Unit of the measuring system used by an acupuncturist is t-sun or cun and it is expressed as a 'unit' in proportion to the patient's body itself. One t-sun is defined as the distance between the palmar creases over the proximal and distal interphalangeal joints of the middle finger of the patient. Breadth of the thumb at its interphalangeal joint is also considered as one t-sun. The combined breadth of the index and middle or the ring and little fingers is 1.5 t-sun. The combined breadth of the four fingers held adjoining is 3 t-sun, the measurement being taken at the level of the proximal interphalangeal joint of the little finger (Fig. 3.1). One Fen is equal to 0.1 t-sun and eight t-suns make one Fu. Because t-sun, Fen and Fu are the terms used in relation to the patient's own body, the acupuncturist must first compare his t-sun against the patient's and make proper adjustments in measurements before localising the points on the patient's body.

THE LINES AND PLANES OF REFERENCE

Anterior and posterior midlines : When the patient is standing straight, with the eyes in front chin pointing forwards, arms by the sides of the body, palms directed forward, both the patella looking in front and both feet kept together, the anterior midline of body passing from the centre of the forehead, root of the nose, centre of the sternum,

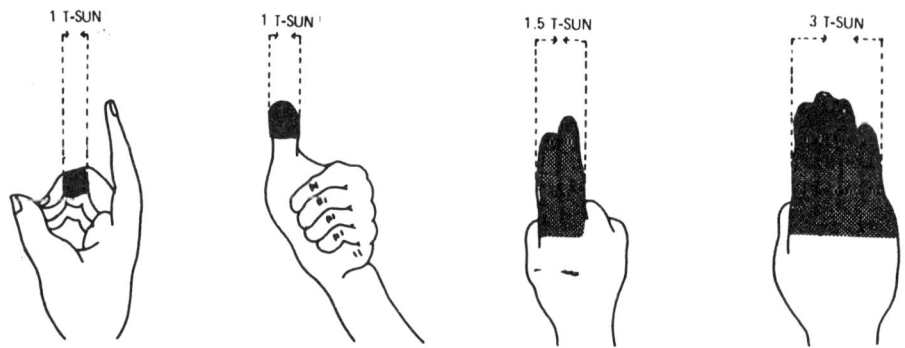

Fig. 3.1 Unit of measurement.

umbilicus and is called as the anterior midline of the body. The posterior midline passing from the centre of the back of the head through all the spinous processes to the centre of the tip of the coccyx is called as the posterior midline of the body. The points nearer the midlines are medial in relation to the points which are away from the midlines and are lateral. On the upper limb, the points on the inner side of the limb near the body surface are the inner, medial or ulnar in position while those on the outer part are outer, lateral or radial in position.

2. The mid-clavicular line : Commonly used as a reference, extends downwards from the midpoint of the clavicle, just medial to the nipple.

3. The nipple line : It lies lateral to the mid-clavicular line and passes through the centre of the nipple.

4. Axillary lines :
    Anterior axillary line : It is drawn downwards from the anterior axillary fold.
    Mid-axillary line : It lies midway between the anterior and posterior axillary lines.
    Posterior axillary line : It is drawn downwards from the posterior axillary fold.

5. Natural hair lines : These lines though taken as land marks, are not the fixed lines because of the variations in the normal distribution of the hair on the heads of the individuals. The anterior limit of the hairs on the scalp is termed as anterior hair line. Posterior is termed as the posterior hair line and the lateral is termed as the lateral hair line. The distance between the anterior hair line and posterior hair line is 12 t-suns. Anterior hair line to mid-eyebrow point (glabella) is 3 t-suns.

6. Skin creases and folds : The skin creases and folds are obvious from their appearance and relation to the particular joint or area.
    The most commonly referred folds and skin creases are as follows :
    (a) Gluteal fold : At the junction of the buttock with the back of the thigh.
    (b) Popliteal creases : On the back of the knee joint, placed transversely on the popliteal surface.
    (c) Elbow crease : In front of the elbow joint, transversely placed, extending from one epicondyle to another. It becomes more prominent on bending the elbow.
    (d) Distal wrist crease : It is transversely placed distal most crease on the front of the wrist joint (at the junction of the wrist with the hand).
    The distance between cubital crease to wrist crease is 12 t-suns (Fig. 3.2).

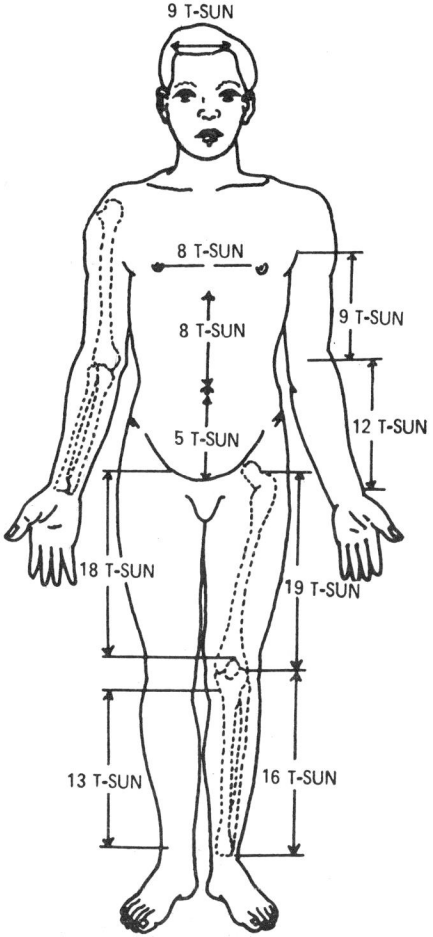

Fig. 3.2 Proportional unit of measurement.

IDENTIFYING THE LAND MARKS

Front of the Neck

The clavicles are the horizontally placed bones between the front of the neck and front of the chest. They are two in number, and both can be felt and seen. Put your right index finger in the groove between the two clavicles in the midline. This is the suprasternal notch and on both sides of it are the sternoclavicular joints. Turn your face to the left side against the resistance of the palm of your own left hand. You will find a vertically placed muscle running upwards on the right side. Run your finger along this muscle. Your finger will feel another bony point on the upper end of the muscle behind the ear. The muscle is sternocleidomastoid and this bone is the tip of the mastoid process (Fig. 3.3). Repeat the same procedure on the other side. Now come back to the suprasternal notch and start palpating the neck in the midline from below upwards and identify in sequence, the rings of the trachea, the arch of the cricoid cartilage, the anterior border of the thyroid cartilage, the body of the hyoid bone submental region and the chin (Fig. 3.4).

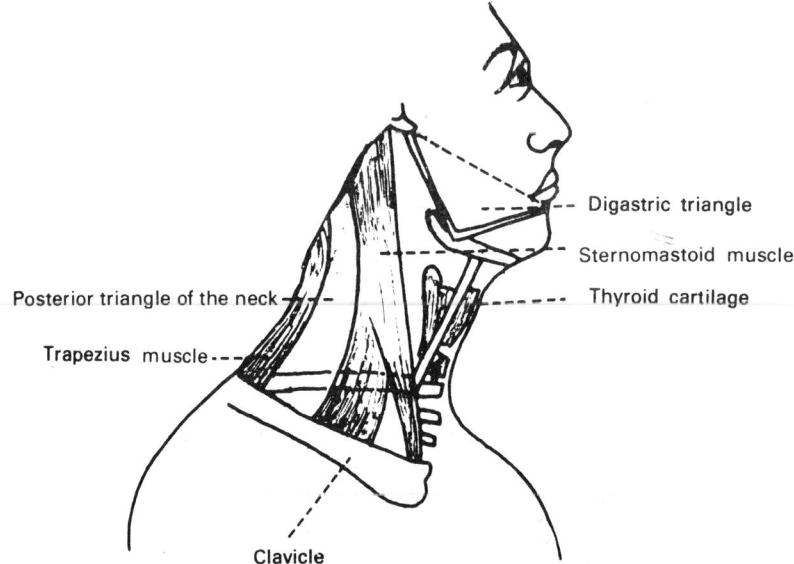

Fig. 3.3 Surface land marks on side of the neck.

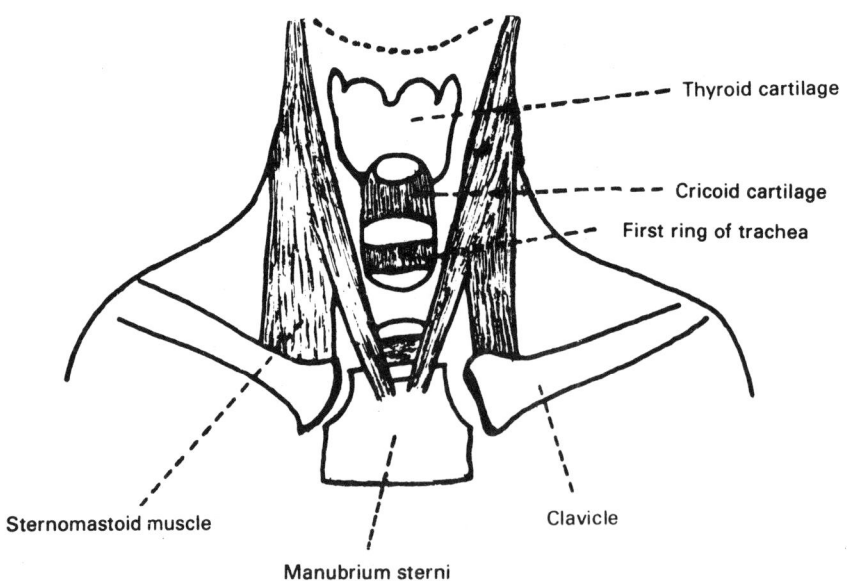

Fig. 3.4 Surface land marks of front of the neck.

Mandible

Run your finger from the chin towards the mastoid process known to you already and identify in sequence, the lower border of the mandible, angle of the mandible and the ramus of the mandible. The ramus is covered with a thick muscle called the masseter that can be felt contracting when the jaws are clenched. The head of the mandible is in front of the tragus. Place your finger in front of your own tragus, and open your mouth. The head of the mandible is felt gliding in the temperomandibular joint. Identify the mental foramen an inch and a half from the midline and midway between the gum and the lower border of the mandible. Now observe the area of the neck bounded by the lower border of the mandible, imaginary line connecting the angle of the mandible to the mastoid process, anterior midline of the neck and the anterior border of the sternocleidomastoid muscle. This is the anterior triangle of neck (Fig. 3.5).

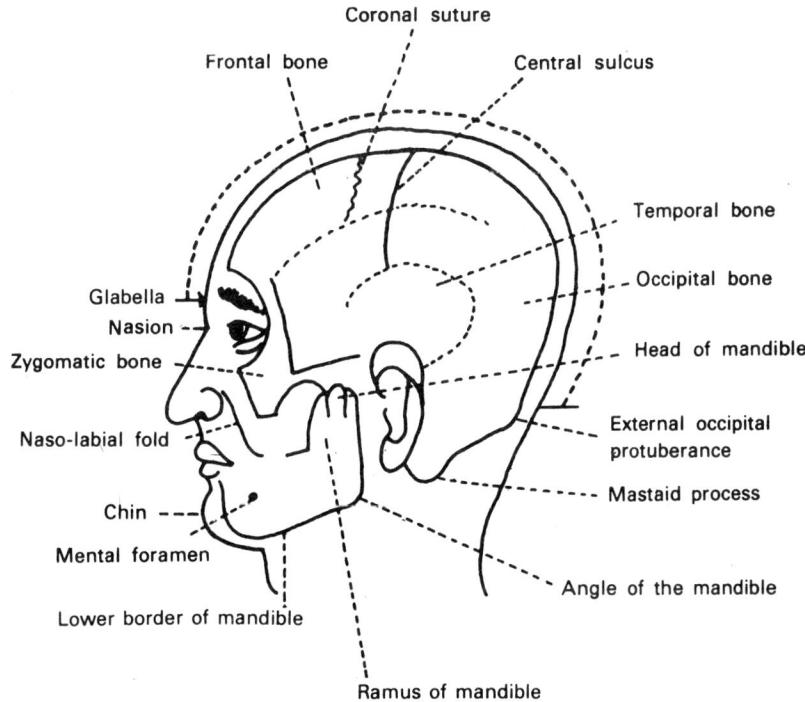

Fig .3.5 Surface land marks of head and face.

Orbits

Place your right index finger on the smooth area between the two eyebrows. This is called glabella. Palpate the thick curved ridges on both the sides of the glabella. These are the supercilliary arches. Deep in the eyebrows supraorbital margins are felt on both the sides. Below the supraorbital margins and bounded by them superiorly are the two cavities of the orbits containing eyeballs. The inferior margin is formed by the zygomatic bone and the maxilla. Palpate the infraorbital foramen a few millimeters below the orbit and a finger's breadth from the side of the nose. The lateral margin of the orbit is formed mainly by the frontal process of the zygomatic bone. The medial margin is mainly by the frontal process of the maxilla.

In the eye, the pupil is an important landmark. The white of the eye is called the sclera and the clear glassy front is the cornea. The coloured part behind the cornea and seen clearly through it is the iris. The black spot in the centre of the iris is a circular aperture called the pupil. The eyelids, provide protection to the eye ball. They join each other at the medial and lateral angles of the eye.

Head

Place your finger on the bony knob felt in the posterior midline where the back of the head joins the nape of the neck. This is called the external occipital protuberance. Pass your finger on the curved ridge extending from the external occipital protuberance towards the mastoid process. This is the superior nuchal line, one on each side. Press the finger tip into the hollow behind the jaw, below the tip of the mastoid process. The bone in the bottom of the hollow is the tip of the transverse process of the atlas vertebra. Put your finger again on the external occipital protuberance and pass it in the midline of the head towards glabella. The highest point is vertex. A line joining the external occipital protuberance and the root of the nose, through vertex, corresponds in direction to the longitudinal fissure of the brain. This line also corresponds in direction to the midline of the frontal bone, sagittal suture between the two parietal bones, and midline of the occipital bone, in that order from before backwards. The suture between the frontal bone and the two parietal bones is called the coronal suture, and the point of junction of the coronal and sagittal sutures is known as the bregma, the site of the foetal anterior fontanelle, which closes during the end of the second year or before it. Suture between the parietal and occipital bones is called lamboid, and at the junction of these sutures posterior fontanelle is located. This fontanelle is closed at or soon after birth. The parietal bone shows an outward bulging at a point rather above its centre, forming the parietal eminence, which is easily seen and palpated on both the sides.

Over the anterolateral aspects of the head two frontal eminences are easily palpated as obvious bulgings (Fig. 3.5).

Brain

The central sulcus (fissure of Rolando): Put your finger tip on a point half an inch behind the centre of an imaginary line drawn across the vertex of the skull from the base of the nose to the external occipital protuberance. Now draw your finger forwards for 3.5 to 4 inches on another imaginary line from this point towards the centre of the zygomatic arch which is felt as a bony ridge between the ear and the eye. This corresponds with the central sulcus. In front of this line is the motor area and posterior to this line is the sensory area. The main centres situated here correspond, from below upwards, to the motor and sensory functions of the face, upper limb and the lower limb of the opposite side of the body.

Face

Put your finger on the root of the nose. This is called nasion. The crease between the angle of the mouth and outer part of the ala of the nose is known as the nasolabial fold. Put your finger on the prominence of the cheek situated on the lower and lateral side of the orbit. This is the zygomatic bone.

Upper Limb

Put your finger on the clavicle and trace it on to the whole of its extent. It ends medially at the sternoclavicular and laterally at the acromioclavicular joints. At this moment palpate the acromion again. It is the flattened piece of the bone about 1 t-sun wide and lies on the top of the shoulder. Identify supra- and infra-clavicular fossas above and below the clavicle. The latter lies below the junction of the lateral and intermediate thirds of the clavicle. Press deep and laterally in the infraclavicular fossa and identify the coracoid process.

Abduct the arm to examine the hollow of the axilla. The two folds (anterior and posterior axillary folds) are brought into view.

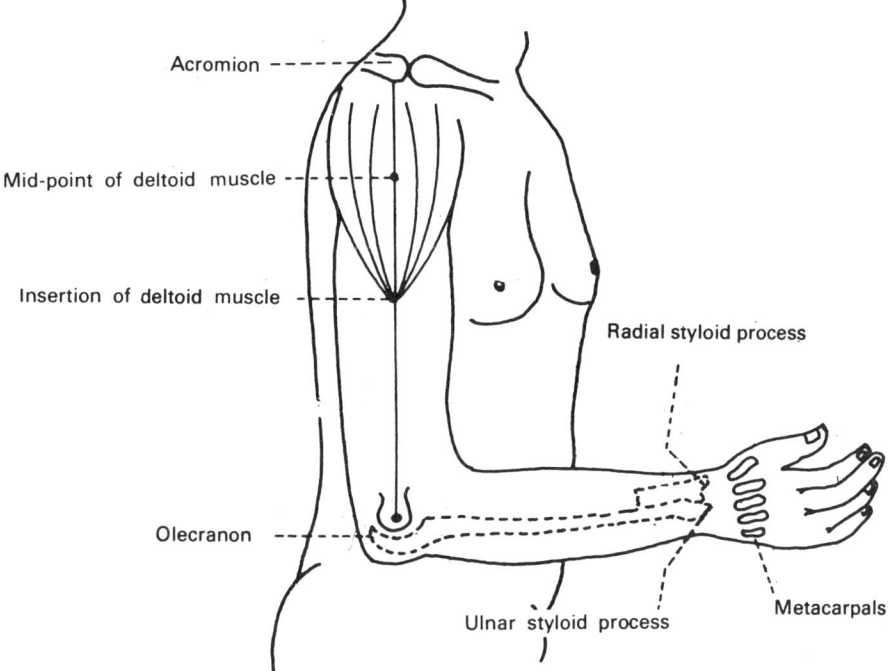

Fig. 3.6 Surface land marks of upper limb.

Palpate the upper end of the humerus under cover of the deltoid muscle, the part of it felt on the outer side of the arm below the acromion is the greater tubercle; the lesser tubercle is palpated on the front. Move your palpating hand on the shaft of the humerus downwards identify the deltoid tuberosity half way down on the lateral aspect of the arm. Near the elbow, the humerus is widened from side to side and two sharp margins the lateral and medial supracondylar ridges are distinctly felt. The projecting ends are the medial and lateral epicondyle of the humerus. Palpate the ulnar nerve behind the medial epicondyle. Between the epicondyles on the front of the elbow, the cubital crease is evident and it is about 9 t-sun from the anterior axillary fold (Fig. 3.6). The biceps brachii muscle is seen as the fleshy bulging on the front of the upper arm. Its tendon can be nicely palpated in front of the flexed elbow as a thick cord. There are two hollows on either side of this

tendon.   Palpate the olecranon process of the ulna on the back of the elbow and then feel
for the posterior border of its shaft which is subcutaneous from end to end.   It terminates
at the styloid process of the ulna, which makes a blunt ridge on the medial side.   The head
of the radius can be palpated below the lateral epicondyle and the shaft can be felt through
the muscles.   Now palpate the lower end of the radius on both sides, back and front, and also
on the lateral side.   Palpate its dorsal tubercle on the back towards the outer side.   Stretch
the thumb out from the palm of your hand and look into the hollow, which is now well seen
on the lateral side of back of the wrist.   This is called the "anatomical snuff-box".   Press
your finger deep in the hollow.   The bone felt in the upper part of its floor is the styloid
process of the radius.   The pisiform bone is felt at the upper end of the hypothenar eminence.
The tendons of the two muscles, the flexor carpi radialis (lateral) end the palmaris longus
(medial), are seen lying side by side in front of the lower third of the forearm and the wrist.
The junction of the forearm and wrist is marked by the skin crease that runs across the front
of the limb at the level of the upper part of the pisiform bone.   The metacarpal bones are
easily felt through the tendons.   The first raw of knuckles is formed by the distal ends (heads)
of the metacarpals while their proximal ends (bases) are felt as the uneven prominence about
1 t-sun below radius and ulna.

The phalanges, metacarpophalangeal and interphalangeal joints, finger tips and nails are
distinct features and need no detailed description (Fig. 3.7).

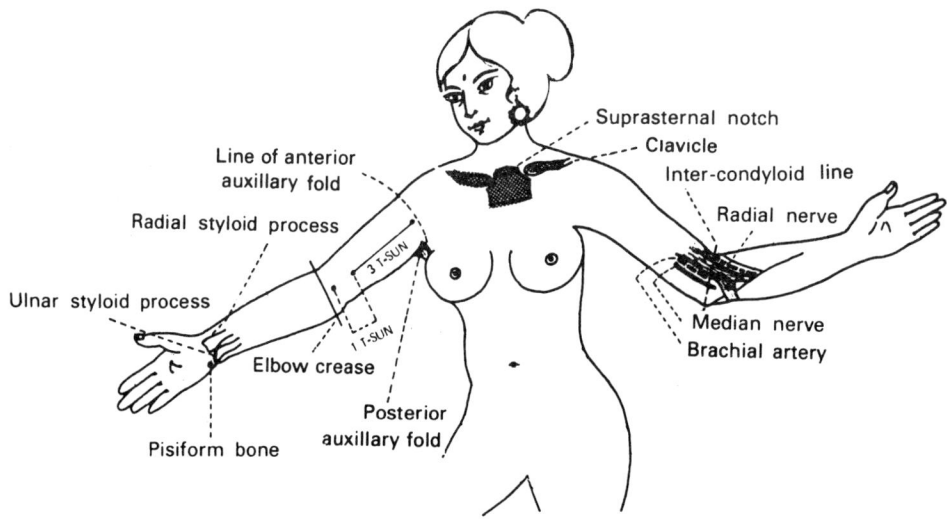

Fig. 3.7 Surface land marks of upper limb.

Back

The spines of the vertebra are felt in the posterior midline furrow.   Start palpating from
the external occipital protuberance downwards in the midline.   The upper most spinous
process to be felt first is that of the second cervical or axis vertebra (the first vertebra or
atlas has no spinous process).   The spinous process of the sixth, seventh cervical and first
thoracic vertebra are usually prominent and palpable.   They are more conspicuous by flexion
of the neck and trunk.   The seventh cervical spine is the upper most of the knobs, in the

posterior midline at the root of the nape of the neck, the seventh cervical vertebra is therefore popularly termed as the vertebra prominence. Palpate the medial border of the scapula and find that the point where the crest of the scapula meets its medial border corresponds with the spinous process of the third thoracic vertebra. The seventh thoracic vertebra is at the level of the lower angle of the scapula. Palpate the sacrum. It has three spines which are readily felt deeply between the buttocks. It reaches almost to the anus and moves slightly under pressure except in the old persons (Fig. 3.8).

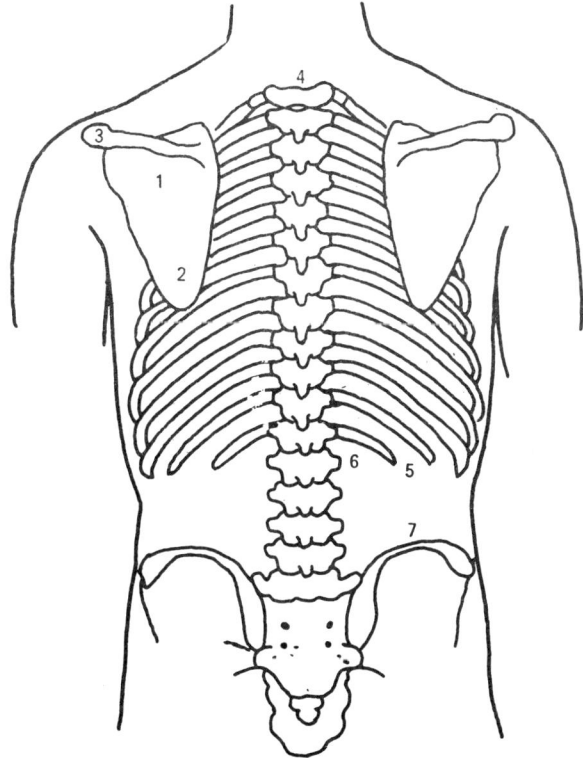

Fig. 3.8 Surface land marks of the back.

1. Scapula
2. Angle of scapula
3. Acromion
4. First thoracic vertebra
5. Twelfth Rib
6. First Lumbar
   Vertebra
7. Iliac crest

Scapula

You have already identified the medial border of the scapula (3 t-sun from midline) and its junction with the crest. Now palpate the crest in its whole length upto the acromion and acromio clavicular junction. Identify the upper and lower angles of the scapula, the former at the level of the second rib and the latter at the level of the seventh rib.

Anterior chest wall

Place the tip of the index finger in the suprasternal notch and trace it downward till it reaches the anterior abdominal wall. Identify from above downwards the sternal angle, body of the sternum and xiphoid process. The sternal angle is felt as a distinct transverse ridge and it marks the union of the manubrium with the body of the sternum. Palpate the cartilages of the second ribs on both sides of the sternal angle. The anterior part of the first rib is about 1 t-sun above the second and covered by the clavicle. The shallow depression at the lower end of the sternum is the epigastric fossa and the bone in the floor is the xiphoid process. Palpate the right and left boundaries of the epigastric fossa formed by the cartilages of the seventh pair of the ribs. The nipple is located usually opposite the space between the fourth and fifth ribs, about 4 t-sun away from the anterior midline. The distance between the two nipples is 8 t-sun and between the two ribs is 1½ t-sun. If the twelfth rib is long enough its tip can be palpated 1 t-sun above the iliac crest (Fig. 3.9).

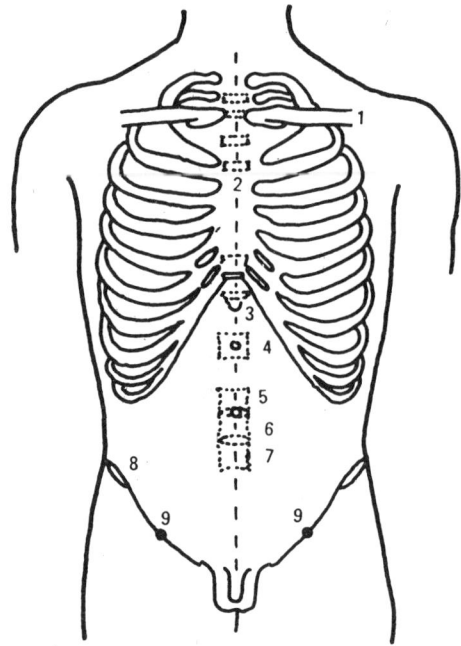

Fig. 3.9 Surface land marks of chest and
abdomen.

1. Clavicle   6. Fourth Lumbar vertebra
2. Sternum   7. Fifth Lumbar vertebra
3. Xiphoid process   8. Anterior superior iliac spine
4. First Lumbar vertebra   9. The mid point of the
5. Third Lumbar vertebra   inguinal ligament

Abdomen

The part of the body between the ribs and the iliac crest is termed as the anterior abdominal wall. Exactly on the midline there is one linear depression extending downwards from the lower end of the sternum towards the pubic region. This is called the linea alba and it marks the position of the median fibrous band. The umbilicus or navel is a well known feature in the midline rather near the pubis than the xiphoid process. The longitudinal prominence on each side of the linea alba is formed by the rectus abdominis muscle. The distance between the umbilicus and xiphisternum is 8 t-sun and between the umbilicus and upper border of the symphysis pubis is 5 t-sun. The symphysis pubis is the bone felt in the lowermost part of the anterior abdominal wall (Fig. 3.9).

Gluteal region

The gluteal region is bounded above by the iliac crest and below by the gluteal fold which marks the junction of the buttock with the posterior aspect of the thigh. The skeleton of the buttock is formed by the ischium bone and its tuberosity (ischial tuberosity) is easily palpated through the bulging of the buttock. The highest point of the iliac crest is at the level of the fourth lumbar spine. Trace the iliac crest in its whole extent. The anterior end of the crest is termed as anterior superior iliac spine and is easily felt. The posterior end is known as the posterior superior iliac spine and it is recognised by a dimple in the skin. It corresponds to the second spine of the sacrum (Fig. 3.10).

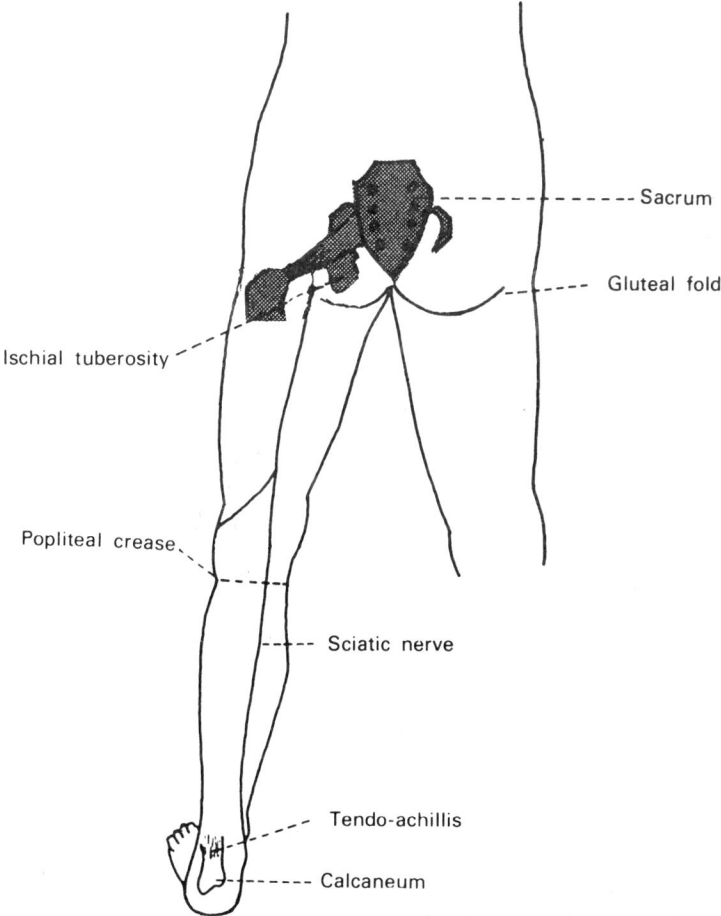

Fig. 3.10 Surface land marks of lower limb.

Lower limb

The bone felt at the lowest part of the abdomen in the anterior midline is symphysis, between the two pubic bones. The upper border of the symphysis when palpated laterally forms a crest, the pubic crest, and ends in a blunt prominence, the pubic tubercle. Palpate an elastic band at the junction of the thigh with abdomen. This is inguinal ligament. It can be traced medially to the pubic tubercle and laterally to the anterior superior iliac spine, which is the anterior end of the iliac crest.

Pulsations of the femoral artery are felt midway between the anterior superior iliac spine and the pubic symphysis. A hand's breadth below the highest point of the iliac crest greater trochanter is felt as a wide prominence, on the upper outer part of the thigh. Front of the thigh is the area between the inguinal ligament and the patella.

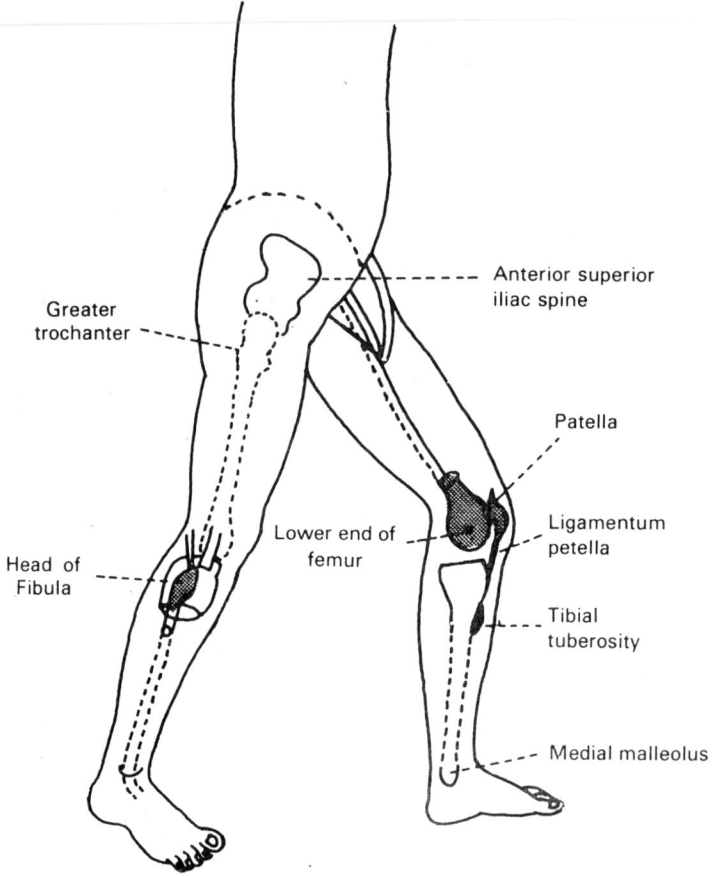

Fig. 3.11 Surface land marks of lower limb.

The distance between the greater trochanter and middle of the patella is 19 t-sun. The ligamentum patellae stretches downwards from the patella and leads the palpating finger to a blunt bony prominence—the tuberosity of the tibia, on the front of the upper end of the tibia. Palpate lateral and medial condyles of the femur and tibia at the side of the knee.

The most prominent points on the sides of the femoral condyles are called the lateral and medial epicondyles of the femur. The fleshy swelling above the medial condyle of the femur is formed by the lower part of a large muscle called the vastus medialis.

The popliteal fossa is located behind the knee, upper part of the tibia and lower part of the femur.

Head of the fibula is palpated below the posterior part of the lateral condyle of the tibia as a well marked bony prominence on the lateral side of the leg, at the same level as the tibial tuberosity. Tendon of biceps femoris is felt as a thick cord on the head of the fibula, specially when the joint is flexed. Lateral popliteal nerve is palpated on the back of the head of the fibula on deep pressure. In the middle of the popliteal fossa, the pulsations of the popliteal artery are felt easily on flexing the knee. The bulk of the calf is formed by the bellies of the gastrocnemius muscles which merge inferiorly into the lower part of the calf. Trace the bellies downwards till they are replaced by a thick strong tendon—the tendo-achillis. Palpate the sides of the ankle joint. The bony prominences felt are the two malleoli—medial and lateral—and they grip the talus between them. The medial malleolus is the downward projection of the lower end of the tibia and the distance between its tip and the medial condyle of the tibia is 13 t-sun.

The lateral melleolus is the lower end of the fibula and is 16 t-sun away from the middle of the patella. The lower part of the shaft of the fibula is subcutaneous and can be nicely felt above the lateral malleolus.

The anterior border of the shaft of the tibia is subcutaneous and readily felt. Medial surface and medial border of the tibia is also felt quite easily from end to end and pulsations of the posterior tibial artery are felt on the medial side of the ankle behind the medial melleolus.

Calcaneous forms the bone of the heel. About 1 t-sun below the medial melleolus a bony resistance felt on the medial side of the heel is sustentaculum tali. Palpate the tuberosity of the navicular bone on the medial aspect of the foot as an obvious prominence. The medial cuneiform and the first metatarsal bones are felt in front of the tuberosity. Midway between the heel and the root of the little toe is a bony projection : the tuberosity of the fifth metatarsal bone. The head of the fifth metatarsal bone is at the root of the little toe. On the dorsum of the foot all metatarsal bones can be felt individually through the tendons. Toes, their phalanges, and joints are the very distinct parts of body and hardly need any description (Fig. 3.11).

4

PHYSIOLOGY OF THE CONTROL OF BODY FUNCTION

Human beings and other complex multicellular organisms have a basic difference from the unicellular organisms from which they have evolved. The unicellular organisms are in contact with the external environment, e.g. sea-water, with which they can exchange nutrients, waste products, oxygen, carbon dioxide, etc. Each cell of a multicellular organism is not in such a direct contact with the external environment. How can these cells perform their basic functions? The answer to this question was given back in the ninteenth century by Claude Bernard who clearly enunciated that each cell is bathed in the extracellular fluid. The extracellular fluid constitutes that immediate environment with which the cells can exchange nutrients, waste products, oxygen, carbon dioxide, etc. This environment is called the internal environment.

For optimum functioning of the individual cells, and consequently of the whole body, the internal environment has to be kept uniform, both physically (e.g. temperature) and chemically (e.g. pH). All the vital mechanisms, however varied they may be, have only one object, that of maintaining the constancy of internal environment. This process is called homeostasis. All the cells in the body act in a coordinated, regulated, and integrated way for the various homeostatic processes. How the coordination and integration of the different cell functions is achieved? It is the purpose of this chapter to discuss these "biological control systems" which serve the function of coordination.

BIOLOGICAL CONTROL SYSTEMS

There are two types of biological control systems:
1. Neural control system—Nervous system
2. Humoral control system—Endocrinal system.

Nervous system

The basic structural and functional unit of the nervous system is neuron (Fig. 4.1). Each neuron is made up of a nerve cell from which various processes, the nerve fibres, arise. One

Dr. P.S. Deshpande, Department of Medicine, Pt. J.N.M. Medical College, Raipur (M.P.), INDIA.

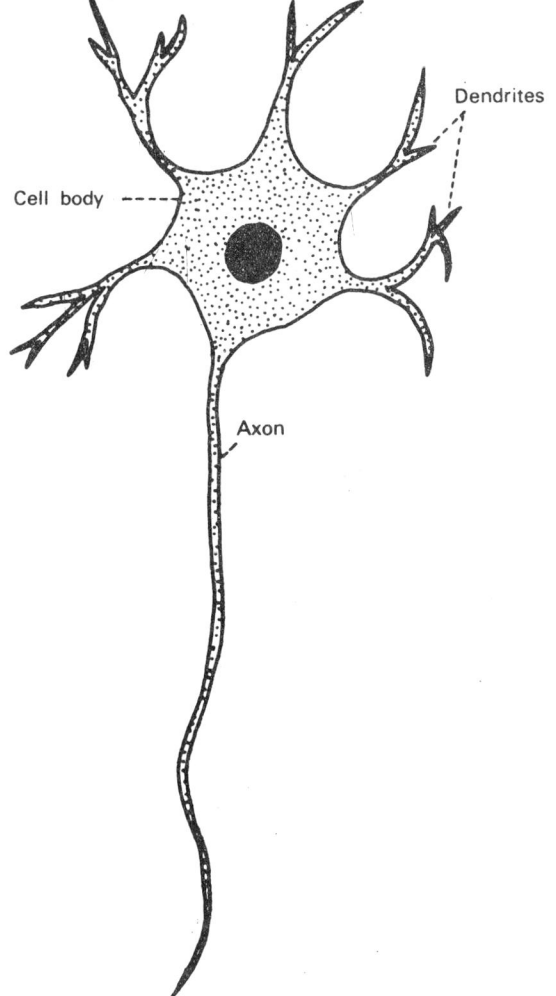

Fig. 4.1 Neuron.

of these is longer than the others and is called axon; others are called dendrons. Dendrons conduct the impulse from periphery to the nerve cell while axon generally carries the impulse away from the nerve cells. In the central nervous system the nerve cells are grouped together in the cortical grey matter of the brain, central grey matter of the spinal cord and the various nuclei; in the peripheral nervous system they are located in the ganglia. The nerve fibres are grouped together to form tracts of the central nervous system and the peripheral nerves.

Propagation of impulse along a nerve fibre is called nerve conduction and is basically an electrical process which involves a progressive change in the transmembrane potential from negative to positive. This change, which is called action potential, is brought about by alternation in the permeability of the cell membrane, allowing an influx of sodium ions. Transmission of impulses from one neuron to another occurs at a synapse—a place where

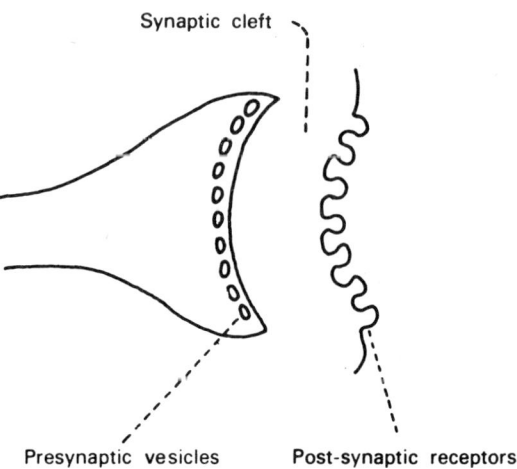

Fig. 4.2 Synapse.

one neuron is in contact with another (Fig. 4.2). The synaptic transmission is mediated through certain chemical substances—the neurotransmitters. These include acetylcholine, norepinephrine, dopamine, serotonine (5-hydroxytryptamine) and GABA (γ-aminobutyric acid). Through a synapse one neuron can exert either exitatory or inhibitory influence on the other neuron.

Parts of nervous system
    A. Central nervous system—brain and spinal cord.
    B. Peripheral nervous system:
        1. Afferent—Sensory nerves.   } Cranial
        2. Efferent : (a) Somatic—motor nerves } spinal
                (b) Autonomic
                    (i) Sympathetic
                    (ii) Parasympathetic   } Visceral nerves

Afferent pathways in the nervous system—Sensory perception with particular reference to pain
    Different types of receptors exist in the skin and some of the deeper structures for each modality of sensation—touch, heat, cold, pain, pressure, etc. Impulses originating due to the stimulation of these receptors travel through the sensory nerve fibres which enter the spinal cord through the posterior roots. The nerve cells of these primary sensory neurons are situated in the posterior root ganglia and the corresponding ganglia of the cranial nerves. In the spinal cord and brainstem the sensations are carried in two pathways. Some fibres of the primary sensory neurons ascend on the same side through tracts of Gall and Burdach situated in the posterior Funiculus (Fig. 4.3). These fibres carry sensations of position, vibration, tactile localisation and tactile discrimination. The tracts of Gall and Burdach end in the nuclei gracilis and cuneatus situated in the lower part of medulla oblongata from where secondary sensory neurons begin, cross to the opposite side and ascends in the brainstem to

reach the thalamus. Thalamus acts as a relay station where all the sensory information is integrated and dispatched through the tertiary neurons to the sensory cortex situated in the parietal lobe.

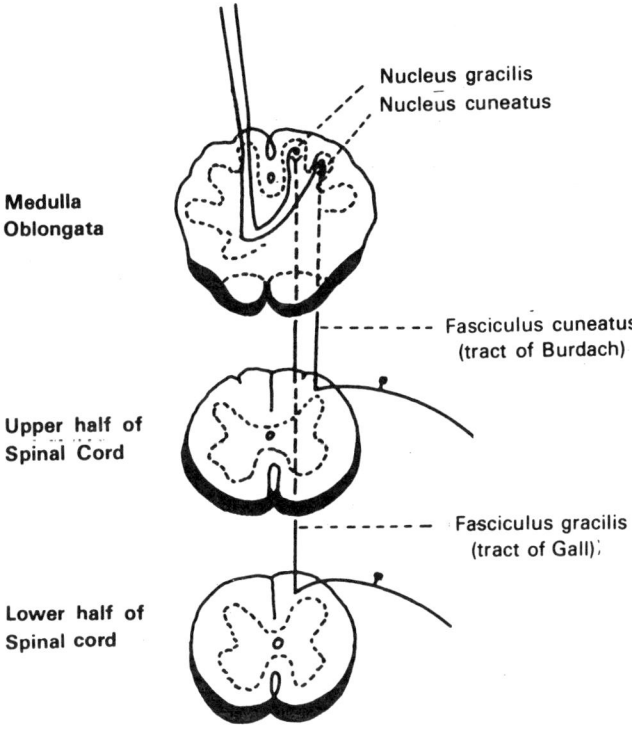

Nucleus gracilis
Nucleus cuneatus

Medulla Oblongata

Fasciculus cuneatus (tract of Burdach)

Upper half of Spinal Cord

Fasciculus gracilis (tract of Gall)

Lower half of Spinal cord

Fig. 4.3   Pathways for senses of position etc.

Crude touch, pain and temperature travel through another pathway from spinal cord to thalamus (Fig. 4.4). The receptors for pain are in the form of free nerve endings. The impulse is carried by two types of nerve fibres—thick and thin. As soon as they enter the spinal cord the thick fibres synapse with large secondary sensory neurons but most of them do so with small neurons of substantia gelatinosa. The axons of these small neurons compose the tract of Lissauer and connect with the large secondary sensory neurons of the same and adjacent segments on which they exert an inhibitory influence. The axons of the secondary sensory neurons cross to the opposite side through anterior commissure and ascends in the form of anterolateral spinothalamic tract through the anterior funiculus of the spinal cord and through the brainstem to end in the posterolateral nucleus of the thalamus. However, some of the ascending fibres leave the tract at the level of brainstem and establish connections with the reticular formation of the brainstem and the hypothalamus. Tertiary neurons transmit the impulse from thalamus to the sensory cortex.

The sensory impulses which enter the brainstem from the cranial nerves also have corresponding pathways upto thalamus.

Perception of pain. Perception of pain is a complex process in the sense that the stimuli which give rise to pain result in a sensory experience plus a reaction to it, the reaction

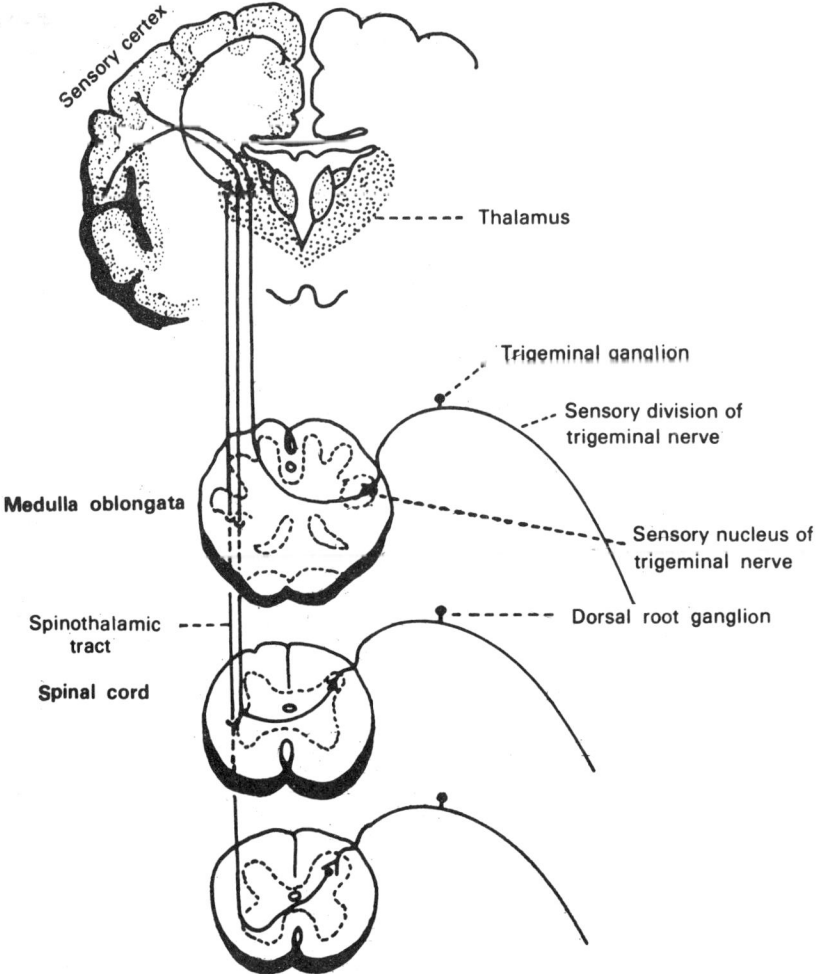

Fig. 4.4 Pain pathways.

including the emotional response (anxiety, fear) and behavioural response (withdrawal). Pain is also associated with a number of physiological changes in the body. The crude perception of the existence of pain is the function of thalamus. Precise information regarding the location, intensity and duration of pain is not received at the thalamic level. This is the function of the sensory cortex. Different areas exist in the sensory cortex representing different parts of the body (Fig. 4.5) which make localisation of pain possible. The intensity coding is dependent upon the frequency of firing by the primary neuron and the number of primary neurons affected. When the intensity of stimulus is more the frequency of firing (rate of generation of action potentials) increases. Moreover, a strong stimulus is capable of stimulating a greater number of neurons—a process called recruitment. The emotional and behavioural reactive component of pain is the function of the frontal lobe which has connections with the sensory cortex and other parts of the brain. If these connections are

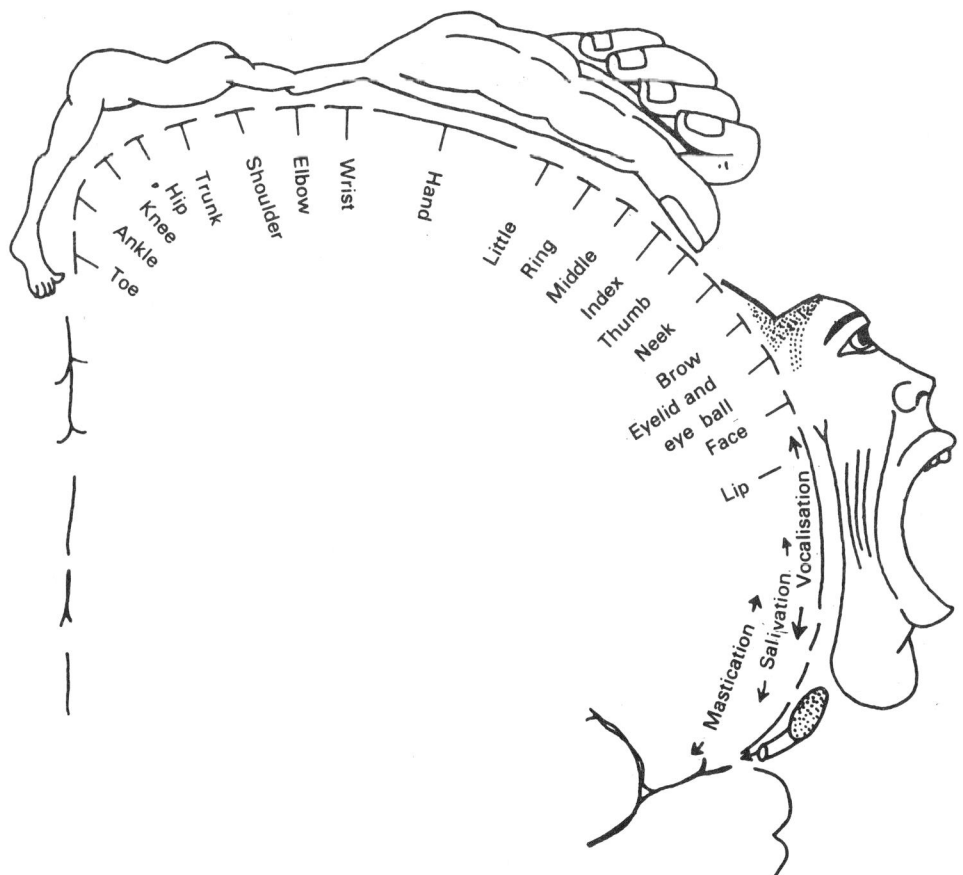

Fig. 4.5 Representation of body in the sensory cortex.

severed, this aspect of pain can be eliminated. The pain would be felt but will no longer be disagreeable. The connections of the "pain fibres" with reticular formation of the brainstem and the hypothalamus are responsible for the behavioural pattern of aggression and defence and for the autonomic and endocrine stress response which causes a number of physiological changes in the body. The physiological changes include greater secretion of epinephrine into the blood stream, faster heart rate, higher blood pressure, increased blood sugar, reduced gastric acid secretion and motility, reduced bloodflow to the viscera and skin, dilatation of pupils, and sweating.

Descending pathways capable of altering the transmission of information in the afferent neurons, spinal pathways or brain centres are known to exist. They are thought to form means by which emotions, past experiences, state of attention, habits and personality of the individual can alter sensitivity to pain in terms of its perception as well as reaction.

Visceral pain—Referred pain. Pain of visceral and deep somatic origin is vaguely localised due to sparce pain sensitive nerve endings in these structures. Visceral pain is not felt precisely in the affected viscus but is projected to that part on the surface of the body which derives its nerve supply from the same spinal segments as does the affected viscus. For example the sensory fibres from the heart terminate in first to fourth thoracic segments of the spinal cord. Pain due to ischaemia of the myocardium is therefore felt in those areas of skin which also send pain sensation to these segments, viz. the mammary region and the inner aspect of the arm. One of the many theoretical explanations of the referred pain is that the visceral sensory fibres are discharging into the same pool of neurons in the spinal cord as the fibres from the skin and an overflow of impulses results in misinterpretation of the true origin of the pain by the sensory cortex.

Root pain—Radicular pain. Irritation of the posterior nerve root is capable of causing pain in the cutaneous distribution of that root. Area of the skin supplied by a particular nerve root is called dermatome. Root pains are strictly localised to the respective dermatomes. In contrast, complete destruction of a nerve root will eliminate all the sensations including pain in the affected dermatome.

Painful stimuli. The stimuli which are capable of producing pain vary for different structures. Skin is sensitive to pricking, cutting, and burning but viscera are not. Pain in the gastrointestinal tract is produced by distention or traction upon the masenteric attachment. Voluntary muscles are sensitive to ischaemia and prolonged contraction. Myocardium is sensitive to ischaemia alone. The solid viscera like liver are sensitive to stretching of the capsule. Arteries are sensitive to vigorous pulsations (migraine).

Somatic efferent pathways—Muscular action

A muscle contracts when it is stimulated by the impulse reaching it through a motor nerve. Each muscle consists of a number of muscle fibres each supplied by an alpha motor neuron situated in the anterior horn cells of the spinal cord and the motor nuclei of the brainstem. The axon of alpha motor neuron ends in contact with a muscle fibre; this place of contact is called neuromuscular junction. Acetylcholine liberated by the axon acts on the motor end plate of the muscle fibre and generates an action potential which causes contraction.

The voluntary muscular contraction is under the control of motor cortex situated in the frontal lobe anterior to the central sulcus and corresponding to the sensory cortex. The representation of the different muscles of the body in motor cortex is similar to the representation of sensations from different parts of the body in sensory cortex. The cells of the motor cortex are called upper motor neurons and the anterior horn cells lower motor neurons. Axons of the upper motor neurons course as the pyramidal (corticospinal) tracts through the internal capsule, brainstem and the spinal cord to synapse with the anterior horn cells (Fig. 4.6). Most of the fibres cross in the medulla oblongata and travel in the lateral funiculus of the spinal cord to innervate the muscles of the opposite half of the body. Some fibres however descend on the same side to provide dual innervation for some important muscles like those of respiration. Though motor cortex can order a muscle to contract the precise extent and duration of the contraction is determined by other connections which the anterior horn cells receive, particularly from the cerebellum. These connections make fine movements possible and prevent overshooting. They also maintain posture and equilibrium. Muscles always maintain a tone which is an involuntary act. This and the involuntary muscle spasms are the functions of local reflex arc. Thus, apart

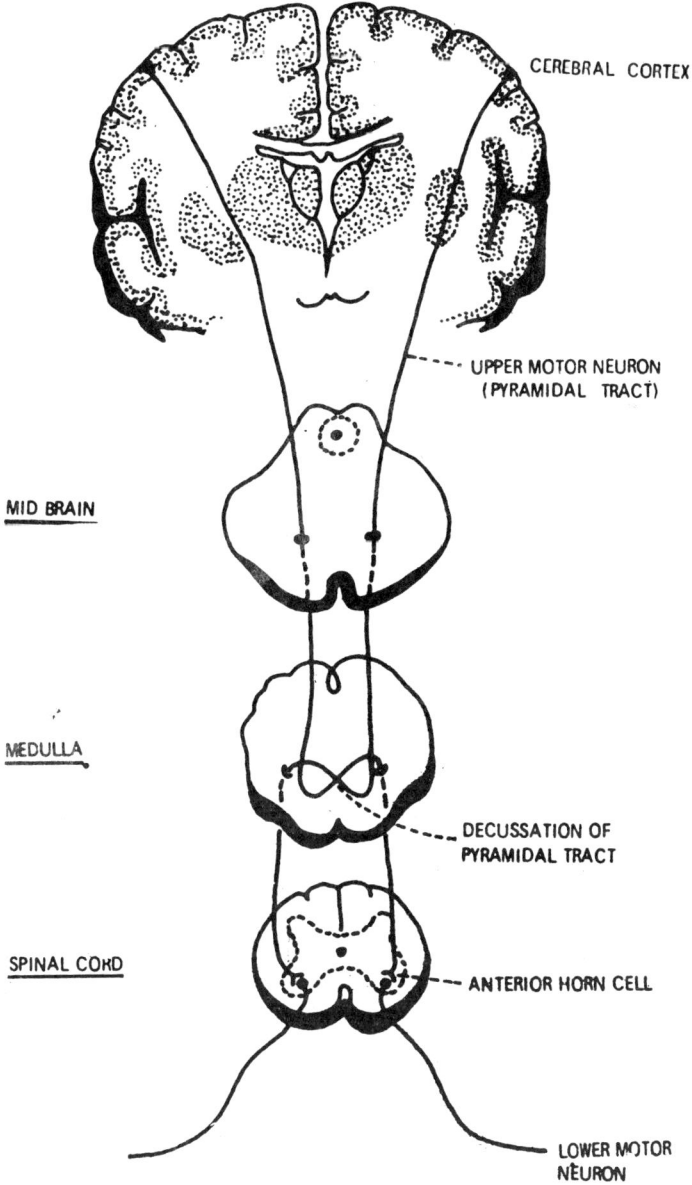

Fig. 4.6 Motor pathway.

from the voluntary pyramidal control the alpha motor neurons are under the local and extrapyramidal control.

Local control of motor neurons. Stretch reflex: Reflex action is defined as that action which occurs subconsciously. It is mediated through a reflex arc which has an afferent (sensory) component which perceives a particular sensation and an efferent (motor) component which orders a muscular action.

There is always an intervening internuncial neuron between these two except in the case of stretch reflex. All these components of the reflex are situated at the local spinal cord level or in the subcortical centres of the brain.

Stretch reflex is the simplest type of reflex (Fig. 4.7). The sensation of stretch is perceived by stretch receptors situated in the muscle spindles lying in between the muscle fibres. Afferent fibres from the muscle spindles enter the spinal cord through the posterior roots and synapse with the anterior horn cells. When a muscle is stretched, the muscle spindles are stimulated, an impulse is generated which stimulates the anterior horn cells and the muscle contracts. At the same time there is relaxation of the antagonist muscle due to inhibitory effect on its anterior horn cells (reciprocal innervation).

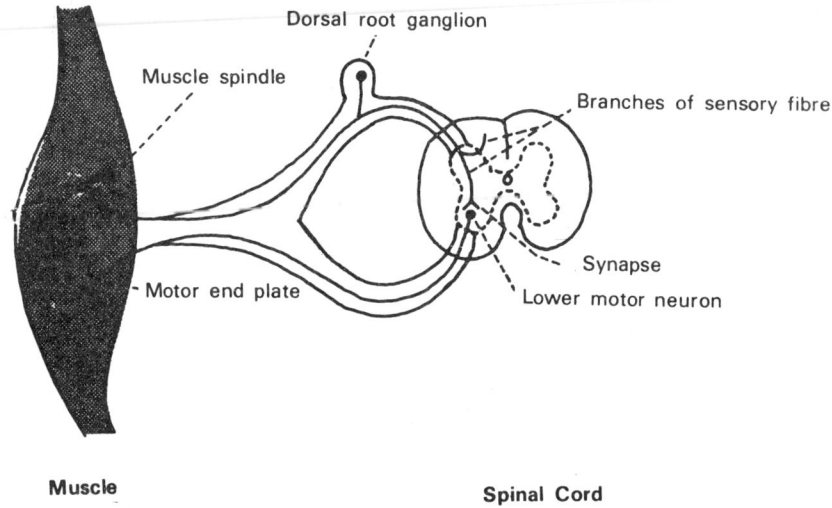

Fig. 4.7 Pathway of stretch reflex.

Gamma motor neurons. These are also situated in the anterior horns. They supply intrafusal muscle fibres of the muscle spindles. Contraction of these fibres increases the sensitivity of the stretch receptors. Thus increase in gamma motor activity would facilitate the stretch reflex and thereby increase the muscle tone (Fig. 4.8). Unlike alpha motor neurons the gamma neurons are under extrapyramidal control.

Tension monitoring system. The receptors which perceive the tension in the muscle when it contracts are Golgi tendon organs. When a muscle contracts they are stimulated. Impulses arising from these receptors exert an inhibitory effect on the anterior horn cells. This reflex prevents overcontraction of the muscle.

Renshaw cells inhibition. This is another mechanism by which excessive muscular contraction is prevented. When an alpha motor neuron is stimulated and sends an impulse to the muscle fibre it also sends an impulse through a collateral to the Renshaw cell situated in the vicinity of the anterior horn cell (Fig. 4.9). Renshaw cells have an inhibitory influence on the motor neurons. This mechanism allows a muscular contraction to be self-limited.

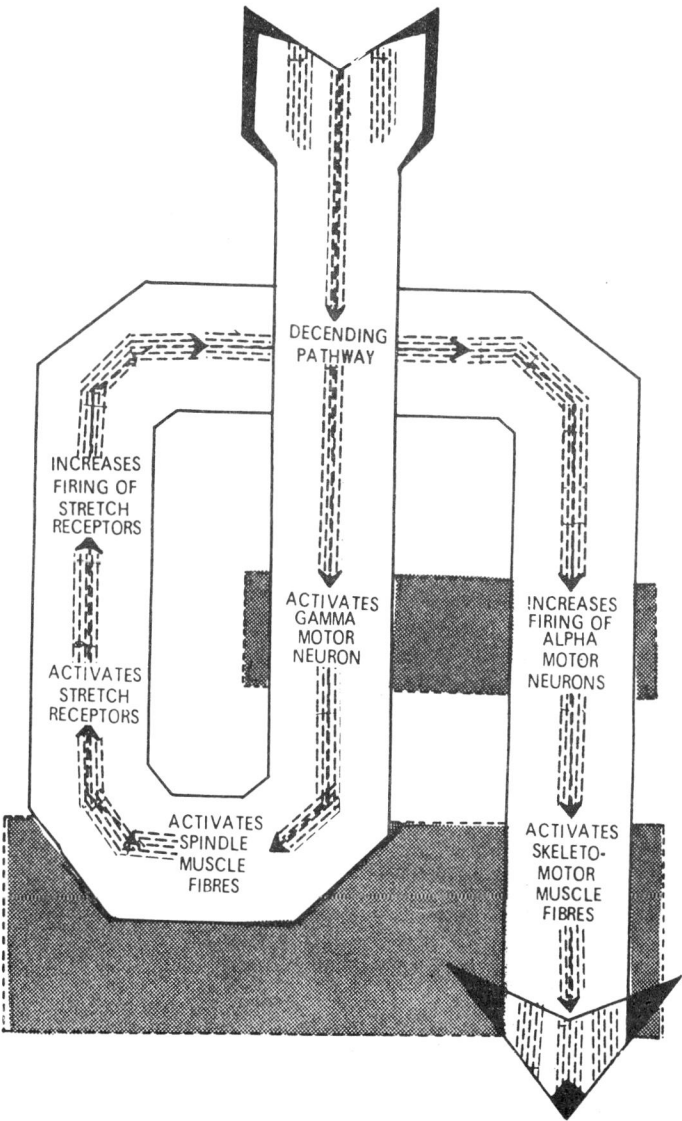

Fig. 4.8 Gamma loop.

Extrapyramidal control of motor neurons through descending pathways. Vestibular nuclei, brainstem, reticular formation, cerebellum and the basal ganglia exert their influence on the anterior horn cells through various pathways. These neuronal centres have an important influence on the coordination of muscular activity.

Muscular spasm. This is a reflex muscular activity which is often seen in association with the painful arthritic conditions. Basically a protective phenomenon, it is self-perpetuating because long-standing muscular contraction itself stimulates the pain receptors in the muscle. Consequently a vicious circle of pain-spasm-pain is produced.

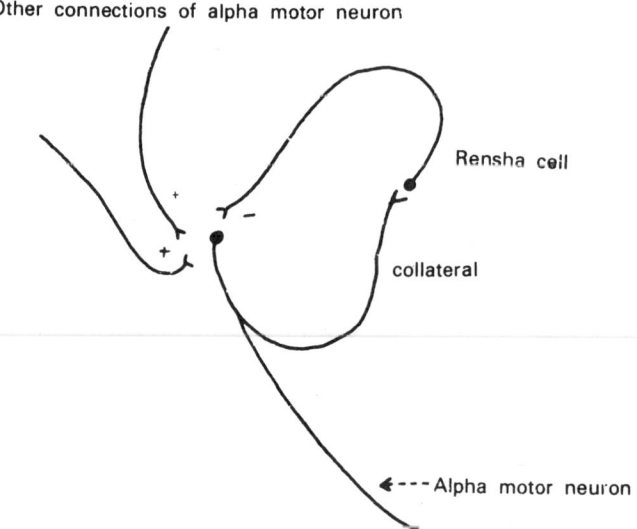

Other connections of alpha motor neuron

Rensha cell

collateral

Alpha motor neuron

Fig. 4.9   Renshaw cell.

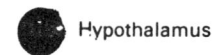

Hypothalamus

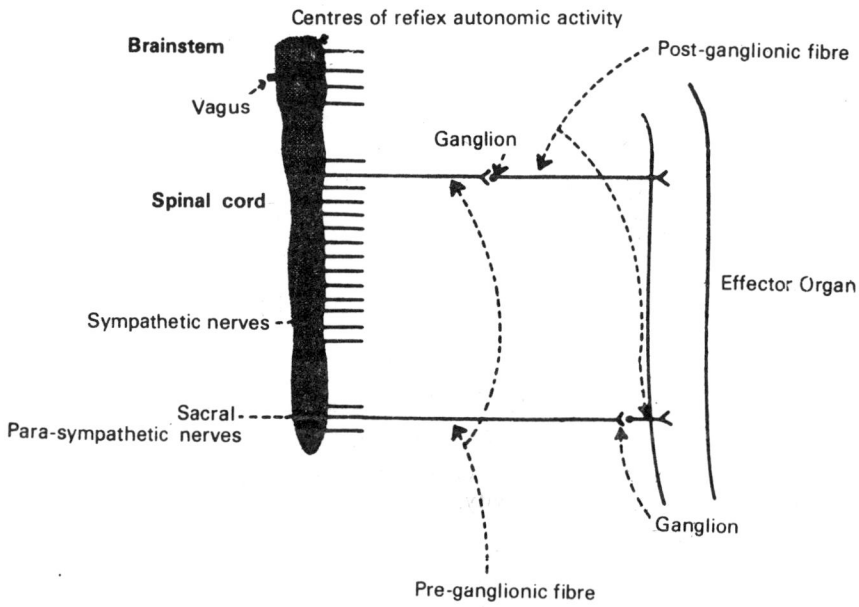

Centres of reflex autonomic activity

Brainstem

Post-ganglionic fibre

Vagus

Ganglion

Spinal cord

Effector Organ

Sympathetic nerves

Sacral
Para-sympathetic nerves

Ganglion

Pre-ganglionic fibre

Fig. 4.10   Autonomic nervous system.

Autonomic nervous system

Unlike somatic nervous system this is not under the voluntary control. The highest cerebral centre for the control of autonomic activity is hypothalamus. Some centres also exist in the reticular formation of brainstem which regulate such reflex autonomic activities as respiration, heart rate, blood pressure, etc. The peripheral division of the autonomic nervous system consists of two parts—sympathetic and parasympathetic. Sympathetic division emerges from the thoracolumber part of the spinal cord and parasympathetic from the brainstem (vagus) and the sacral spinal cord. All the autonomic nerves have ganglia where preganglionic fibres synapse with postganglionic (Fig. 4.10). The neurotransmitter at all the ganglia and at the postganglionic nerve endings of the parasympathetic system is acetylcholine, and that at the postganglionic nerve endings of the sympathetic system is norepinephrine.

All the glands, smooth muscles of the viscera, blood vessels and myocardium are innervated by both the divisions of autonomic nervous system. The actions of sympathetic and parasympathetic systems on these structures are usually opposite to each other and are shown in Table 4.1.

Table 4.1: Effect of sympathetic and parasympathetic stimulation on various organs

Organ	Sympathetic	Parasympathetic
Heart rate	Increase	Decrease
Coronary arteries	Dilation	Constriction
Blood vessels to the muscles	Dilation	Constriction
Other blood vessels	Constriction	Dilation
Bronchi	Dilation	Constriction
Pupils	Dilation	Constriction
Gastro-intestinal tract		
Motility	Decrease	Increase
Secretion	Increase	Decrease
Bladder		
Detrusor	Inhibition	Contraction
Sphincter	Constriction	Inhibition
Uterus		
Pregnant	Contraction	—
Non-pregnant	Inhibition	——
Sweat glands	Secretion	—
Adrenal medulla	Secretion	—
Liver	Glycogenolysis	——

Looking to its functions it follows that the autonomic nervous system has an extremely widespread and important role in the homeostatic control of internal environment. Sympathetic system helps the body to cope with the challanges from the outside environment and the parasympathetic system seems to be more responsible for internal house keeping such as digestion, defecation and urination. The sympathetic system is utilised in conditions of stress or strong emotions while the parasympathetic system is most active during recovery or rest.

Hormones

The hormonal system or endocrine system constitutes the second great communications system of the body, the hormones serving as blood borne messengers which regulate cell function. Hormone is a chemical substance synthesised by a specific organ or tissue and secreted into the blood, which carries it to other sites in the body, where its actions are exerted. Hormones are secreted by endocrine (ductless) glands. They control many important physiological functions such as reproduction, organic metabolism and inorganic metabolism. Inspite of the ubiquitous distribution in the body through the blood, hormone acts specifically on its target organ. Table 4.2 gives various endocrine glands, their hormones, control of their secretions and their actions.

Control of hormone secretion by feed-back mechanism

The secretion of hormone is controlled by the effect which it produces on its target organ. ACTH secreted by anterior pituitary stimulates the adrenal cortex to produce cortisol. When the cortisol level in the blood rises, it suppresses the anterior pituitary and ACTH production is reduced. Parathormone produced by the parathyroid glands increases serum calcium which in turn suppresses the parathyroid activity.

Hypothalamic control of hormone secretion

Hypothalamus is the supreme control organ of the humoral system. Hypothalamus is to the endocrine glands like what brain is to the nervous system. All the major endocrine glands except the parathyroid glands, the pancreas and adrenal medulla, are under direct or indirect control of hypothalamus. Tne posterior pituitary receives neural impulses from hypothalamus while the anterior pituitary is governed by the hypothalamus by means of chemical substances travelling through the blood stream by way of the hypothala mico-hypophyseal portal system. Scuh chemical substances are TSH releasing factor, ACTH releasing factor, etc.

Local hormones

Local hormones are produced locally anywhere in the body in response to injury, for example, histamine, serotonine and kinins. Their basic function is local vasodilation so that the area receives an increased blood flow.

Interrelation between neural and humoral control systems

These two systems do not work in an isolated way. Their coordinated action is achieved through hypothalamus. Hypothalamus receives neural connections from different parts of the brain. It also receives chemical signals regarding various metabolic parameters through the chemoreceptors. It sends neural impulses to reticular formation of the brainstem through which the autonomic activity is controlled. How it controls the humoral system has already been discussed.

Response of the body to stress and trauma

Such response is local and general. The local response consists of liberation of histamine from the mast cells, production of serotonine, and activation of kinins. The general response

Table 4.2 : Hormones

Endocrine gland	Hormone	Secretion controlled by	Main functions
Anterior pituitary	Growth Hormone (GH)	GH releasing factor	Growth
	Thyroid stimulating hormone (TSH)	TSH releasing factor and thyroxine	Stimulates thyroid secretion
	Adrenocorticotropnic hormone (ACTH)	ACTH releasing factor and cortisol	Stimulates adrenal cortical secretion
	Follicle stimulating hormone (FSH)	FSH releasing factor and sex hormones	Growth of ovarian follicle and estrogen secretion, spermatogenesis
	Leutinising hormone (LH)	LH releasing factor and sex hormones	Stimulates progesterone/ testosterone secretion
	Prolactin	Prolactin inhibiting factor	Development of breast and milk secretion
Thyroid	Thyroxine and triodothyronine	TSH	Increases tissue metabolism
	Calcitonin	Plasma calcium level	Calcium metabolism
Adrenal cortex	Cortisol	ACTH	Organic metabolism, protection against stress
	Aldosterone	Angiotensin II and plasma potassium level	Inorganic metabolism
	Sex hormones	—	—
Ovary	Estrogen and progesterone	FSH and LH	Normal functioning of female sex organs
Testis	Testosterons	LH	Spermatogenesis, secondary sexual characteristics
Posterior pituitary	ADH	Neural impulses from hypothalamus	Increases resorption of water by renal tubules
	Oxytocin	-do-	Contraction of pregnant uterus
Parathyroid	Parathoromone	Plasma calcium level	Calcium metabolism
Pancreas	Insulin and glucogan	Blood sugar level	Maintenance of normal blood sugar
Adrenal medulla	Epinephrine and norepinephrine	Sympathetic neurons	Similar to sympathetic stimulation
Kidneys	Renin and angiotensin	Ischaemia	Stimulate aldosterone secretion
	Erythopoietin	Hyposeia	Erythorpoiesis
Gastro-intestinal tract	Gastrin, secretin, glucagen, CCK-PZ	—.	Local actions
Local hormones	{ Histamine, serotonine Bradykinin, kalleicrein	—	Local defence

occurs due to the neural impulses received by hypothalamus.   Due to increased production of ACTH releasing factor by the hypothalamus the anterior pituitary secretes more ACTH, consequently the adrenal cortex produces more cortisol. Cortisol, the stress hormone, stimulates protein catabolism, favours gluconeogenesis, and potentiates the action of nore-pinephrine.   Under stress, hypothalamus also triggers the sympathetic activity which has the following effects:

1.   Increased glycogenolysis.
2.   Increased breakdown of adipose tissue triglyceride.
3.   Increased alertness.
4.   Increased muscle contractility and decreased fatigue.
5.   Increased cardiac output.
6.   Increased ventilation.
7.   Increased coagulability of blood.

The other hormones which are definitely released during stress are aldosterone, ADH and growth hormone. It is likely that the secretion of almost every hormone is altered; for example that of prolactin, thyroxine and glucagon is increased, while that of pituitary gonadotrophin sex hormones and insulin is decreased.

5

THE LIVING BODY AND ELECTRICITY

There is a multiplicity of relations between the living body and electricity. For the last 10 years many theses [1–20] related to this theme have been reported in the journals of the Kyoto Pain Control Institute. A general classification has been made of the relations between the living body and electricity:

1. Electrical method for treatment and examination.
2. Relations between the living body and electricity under electric stimulation from the outside.
3. Electrical properties of the internal environment of the living body.
4. Electricity which originates in the living body.
5. The electromagnetic factor as the mechanism of the treatment effects.

It can be assumed that there are many other facets to the relationship between the living body and electricity. The object of this chapter is to write as definitely as possible about electrical treatment, electrical properties of the internal environment of the living body, and electricity which originates in the living body, adding a basic explanation about electricity.

ELECTRIC TREATMENT

How electricity flows in the living body

In most cases, both "low frequency treatment" which was originally used for rehabilitation or home treatment, and "electro-acupuncture treatment", which has been highlighted recently, have employed the method of placing two terminals (plate terminal and needle terminal) on the body, and making electricity flow between these two terminals.

In the case of negative electric potential charge, only one terminal is placed on the body, and with a vinyl sheet between the body and bed, the bed which is against the back can indirectly be the other terminal [3, 4, 9, 10, 12, 13].

Now, as Fig. 5.1 shows when the two terminals are placed and the electro-stimulation carried out, most of the electricity will, in simple terms, flow along the shortest way as shown

Takeshi Sawa, Department of Anaesthesiology, Faculty of Medicine, Tokyo Medical and Dental University, Tokyo (Japan).

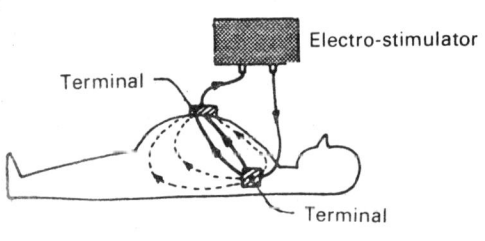

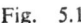

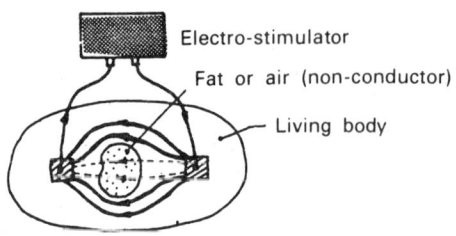

Fig. 5.1   Fig. 5.2

by the solid line (—◄—)   between the two terminals.   This means that the amount of electric

current which flows along the roundabout way, as shown by the dotted line (--◄---), is small.

But this assumption is made on consideration that electricity can flow equally in any part
of the living body.   However, in clearer terms, the flow path of electricity does not depend
on the distance, but instead it can be said that it "choses the easiest path to flow on".   For
example, as shown in Fig. 5.2, if there is something like fat or air which is difficult for
electricity to flow through (a non-conductor) between the terminals, not much electricity will
flow that way.   Even if it is farther, it choses the easy way to flow.   This phenomenon is
just like water running.   A river blocked by a mountain runs around its bottom.

The parts in the living body through which electricity flows easily are the ones which have
a high concentration of ions* in an aqueous solution like blood and body fluids.   Therefore,
the electricity flows freely through parts which contain many blood vessels.   On the other
hand, parts like adipose tissue or lungs (with air) do not conduct electricity so freely.   Since
the structure on the living body is not homogenous, if we examine each part, its complicated
conduction path would probably be discernible.   But on the whole, as shown in Fig. 5.1,
electricity flows along a fairly short way between the two terminals.

If the electricity which is sent to the body from the electro-stimulator and returns to it
again after passing through the body is considered as water, the cycle can be like Fig. 5.3.   If
we compare Figs. 5.1 and 5.3, the electro-stimulator is equivalent to the pump, the electric
wire to the hose, the terminals to the funnels and the living body to the cloth bag full of
cotton through which the water flows.

Nerves are connected like long electric wires between each part of the body and the spinal
cord or brain.   Therefore, it is easy to think that the electricity sent into the body from the
outside runs along these nerves to the spinal cord and brain.   But actually this is not so.   As

shown in Fig. 5.4, the current   (⌐ᴧᴧ⌐)   sent from the outside into the living body enters

from the terminal on one side and flows along the easiest path of flow to reach the other
terminal.   Then from there it just returns again to the electro-stimulator.

If this current size from the outside reaches a certain value called threshold), a special

type of electricity (called impulses or action potential)   (⌐◄─)   in Fig. 5.4 is

evoked in the nerves. This evoked impulse   (◄─)   ,which is transmitted along the

* An ion is an atom or a molecule which has a positive or a negative charge.   Molecules placed in water are
dissolved by it, and become ions.   This phenomena of creation of electrified atoms and molecules is called
ionisation.   Water has this ionisation capability.   Before positive and negative charges are neutralised and
they dot not display any electrical characteristics.   Ions and electrons are particles carrying electrical charge.

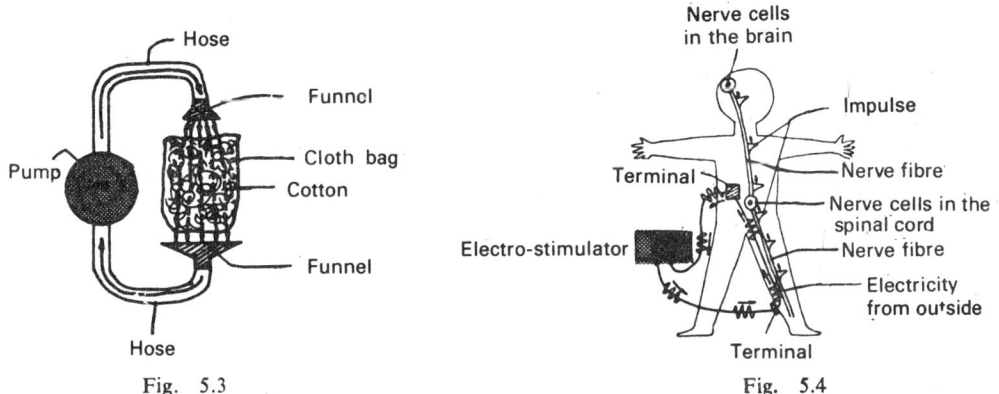

Fig. 5.3   Fig. 5.4

nerve fibre from the point of generation, reaches the nerve cells (⊙) in the spinal cord, and from there is transmitted to the nerve cells (⊙) in the brain. Conversely, the electricity which is transmitted from the nerve cells in the brain and in the spinal cord to the organs and muscles in each part of the body also flows along the nerve fibres in the form of an impulse.

The living body can also store electricity

As mentioned above, the living body has the property of not only permitting electricity to flow through it, but also of storing it. In Fig. 5.3 the property of the living body which permits electricity to flow through it was represented by the cloth bag full of cotton. However, if we try to represent the property of storing electricity, it will be like a rubber bag (Fig. 5.5). Rubber bag does not let the water in but it can stretch elastically and thus increase its storage capacity a good deal. The living body has a part like this which can store electricity. The way that the rubber bag stores water is that it is stretched by the water thrust into it. So more water can be stored. Since this rubber bag has elasticity, if water is no longer thrust into it from the outside, the rubber bag presses the water back out to the pump.

The part which stores electricity in the living body also has the property similar to this rubber bag. The difference is that in the case of the rubber bag, the molecules in the material expand or press back elastically, but in the case of electricity, are the electric particles. When electricity is thrust into the living body from the outside, the positive and negative electric particles which exist in the electrical storage part of the living body are separated. As shown in Fig. 5.6(a), before electricity is introduced from the outside, the positive and negative particles which exist in the electrical storage part of the living body are in a disorganised chaotic state, repulsing and attracting each other. When electricity is sent from outside by the electro-stimulator, negative electric particles are forced to gather around the positive terminal and positive electric particles are forced to gather around the negative one [Fig. 5.6(b)]. These separated electric particles are former atomic nuclei or electrons in the atoms or molecules which compose the living body. Or they are ions which exist inside and outside of the cell membranes. In this way, electricity is stored.

The detached negative and positive electric particles electrically attracting each other try to return to their former chaotic condition, just like the molecules of the stretched

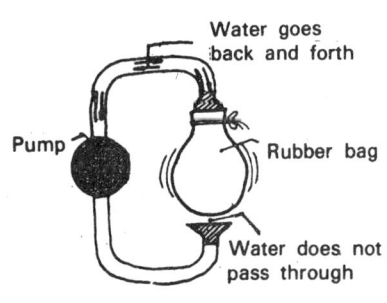

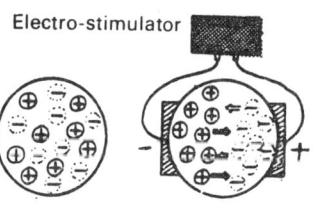

(a) Condition before   (b) Condition of
    electricity is   attraction
    introduced   and repulsion

Fig. 5.5   Fig. 5.6

rubber trying to contract to their former positions. There is much more electric energy in the separated state than in the disorganised chaotic state. Therefore, if the electro-stimulator stops sending electricity, the electricity which has been stored as in the condition shown in Fig. 5.6(b), pushes the current back to the electro-stimulator using this energy. This is like the rubber bag, where if the water being sent from pump was stopped, the water in the rubber bag would be sent back to the pump.

That which allows the electricity to be stored and sends it back is a "non-conductor". In the living body, as mentioned before, fat or air and cell membranes, do not transmit electricity but can store or release it. Again using the example of the water pump and rubber bag, the conducting part and the storing part of electricity in the living body can be explained as in Fig. 5.7. While the water is being sent by the pump, water flows through the part which allows it to, and at the same time a certain amount of water is kept in the part which allows water to remain. Once the pump stops sending the water, the water flow in the part which allows water to go through would stop also, but water in the part which allows it to remain would be pushed back in the direction of the pump. Therefore, after the pump is stopped, water would flow back for a short time.

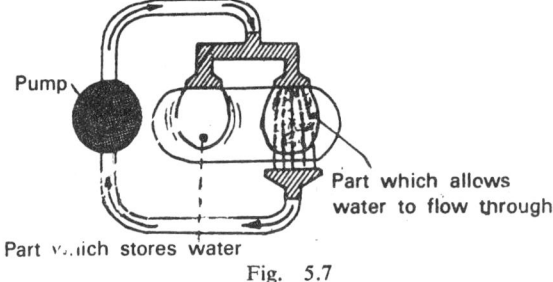

Fig. 5.7

In the case of electricity, the part which conducts electricity is called "conductingpart" and is symbolised by ─⋀⋀─ and the part which stores electricity is called "electrostatic capacity part", symbolised by ─| |─. So if we show the electrical character of the living body with these symbols, it would be like in Fig. 5.8. The electrical character of the living body shown in Fig. 5.8 is called the "electric equivalent circuit" of the living body.

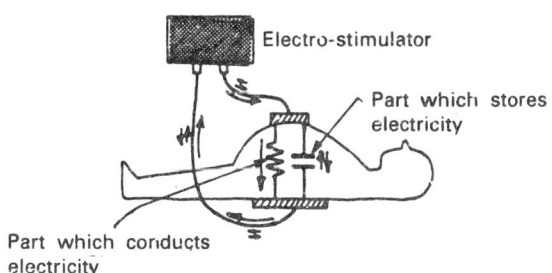

Fig. 5.8

Now, as shown in Fig. 5.9, when electricity is thrust into the living body by the electro-stimulator which generates negative rectangular waves, the negative current flows during the stimulation period. And after the electricity is off, we can see that the current is sent back towards the electro-stimulator from the opposite positive direction from the living body.

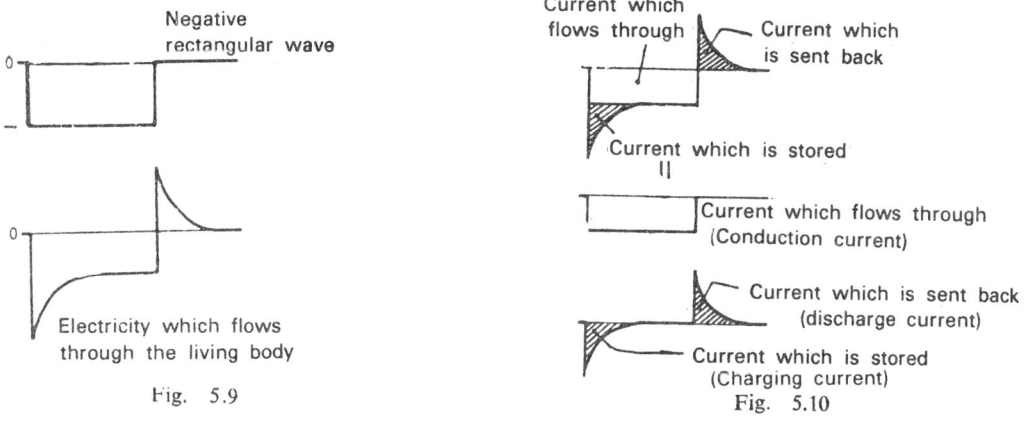

Fig. 5.9   Fig. 5.10

As mentioned above, the current during the stimulating period is a mixture of "conduction current" which flows through the conducting part in the living body and "charging current" which is stored in the electrostatic capacity part. This is analytically shown in Fig. 5.10. The conduction current, which flows through the conducting part, has the same type of negative rectangular wave as the one sent from the electro-stimulator. And the charging current which was stored in the electrostatic capacity part is the type of current which reaches its maximum at the beginning of stimulation and then falls off after that.

The current which is sent back towards the electro-stimulator from the living body just after the stimulation is called "discharge current". We can see that it is just like the charging current except that it flows in the opposite direction. Since this current, which is the one stored in the living body, is sent back completely, it has exactly the same size and form.

The power of the electric stimulation is proportional to the density of the current

This treatment is performed by placing a pair of terminals on the surface of the body in order to send electricity through it. As shown in Fig. 5.11, if one of the plate terminals is bigger than the other, the amount of electricity which flows from the smaller terminal into the body and out through the bigger terminal will not change, but the voltage will. The electric density in the body tends to be generally higher around the smaller terminal and lower around the other. Since the power of the electric stimulation is proportional to the density, the part of the body around the smaller terminal, which gives off a high electric density, receives a bigger electric stimulation. Thus, that part can feel the electric stimulation more acutely than that near the bigger terminal; also, its muscular movement becomes more active. The smaller plate terminal, which contains, in general, a higher electric density and stronger stimulation, is called the "treatment terminal" or "negative terminal". Therefore, we must place this treatment terminal on the affected part or on a meridian point and then make our diagnosis and give subsequent treatment. On the other hand, the bigger plate terminal receives a lower electric density and has a weaker ability for stimulation; it is called a "positive terminal" (earth terminal or opposite pole) and is the "returning gate" for the electricity which is flowing back. Treatment using extremely small terminals is called "needle treatment" and is used for electro-acupuncture. In this case, as shown in Fig. 5.12, the electric density for the part of the body at the needle becomes very high compared to that around a plate; the body feels the stimulation mostly just around the needle. When using the needle the plate terminal becomes the earth side.

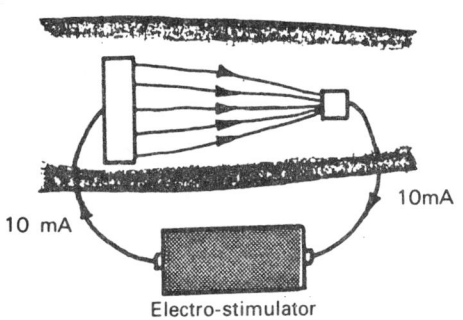

Fig. 5.11 Sending electricity, one terminal is smaller than the other.

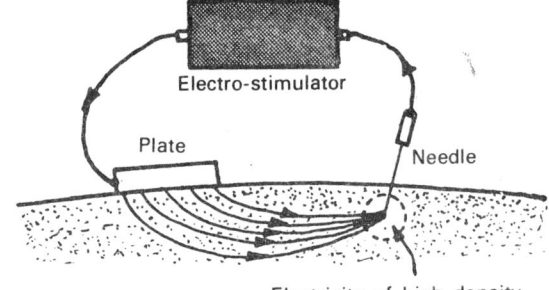

Fig. 5.12 Needle terminal *vs.* Plate terminal.

Negative electricity gives better stimulation using less electricity

When using the same size plate terminals or two needle terminals (Fig. 5.13), in general it can be said that it is the negative terminal which causes a quicker reaction than the positive terminal, although sometimes the reaction is influenced by the sensitivity of the nerves around that terminal. This is because the living body is more sensitive to negative than to positive electricity.

It was observed that less current was needed by the human body in order to be able to feel the electricity by means of a negative terminal than that of a positive one. The result was that half to one-third less quantity of electricity was needed. One of the reasons is due to the characteristics of the nerves in the living body; another reason is because the nerves around a negative terminal cause the action potential (or impulse) to begin with less electricity (Fig. 5.4) which is transmitted to the brain as a stimulation, or is transmitted to a related muscle causing contraction. Therefore, unless there is some special reason to do otherwise,

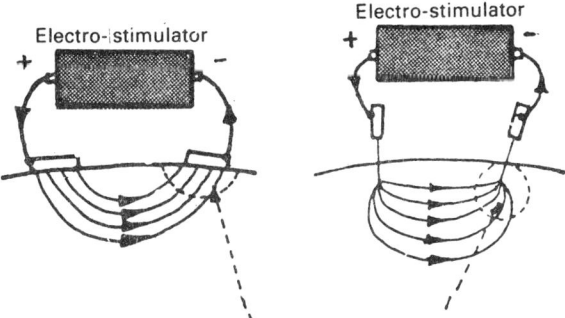

These parts sense the stimulation quicker

Fig. 5.13 The part at the negative terminal can sense
the stimulation quicker than the part at the
positive terminal.

we should perform our treatment connecting the treatment terminal to the negative terminal,
thereby saving some electricity.

What are voltage and current

Voltage

Voltage is the action which pushes out or pulls in (moves) the electrons. Let us review
some simple basic electric theory. When the voltage of a dry battery is 1.6 volts (Fig. 5.14),
this action which pushes electrons out of the negative terminal and pulls electrons in through
the positive terminal is indicated in voltage units, as 1.6.

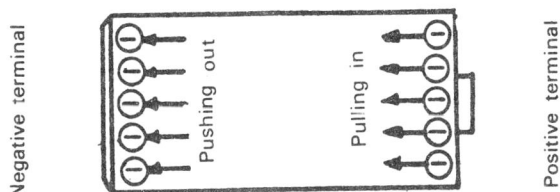

Fig. 5.14 The positive terminal of a dry baterry tries to
pull electrons in and the negative terminal
tries to push electrons out. The strength of
this pulling and pushing action is voltage.

The 100 volt wall outlet is based on this same fact—one of the terminals pushes electrons
out and the other in, and the power of this action is indicated as 100 volts. Therefore,
when an electric apparatus is pluged in, electrons move in and out (electricity flows) through
the fittings producing energy. Since the electricity used in our homes is the alternative type,
it switches the direction of its flow between the two terminals frequently. This switching
frequency is 50 times per minute (50 hertz) in the Tokyo area of Japan and 60 times per
minute (60 hertz) in the Kansai area. Because voltage refers to the power of the action
which pulls in and pushes out electricity, voltage always exists even without electricity.
That is why even from a dry battery or a home wall outlet, having no apparatus connected
we can nevertheless get voltage.

The voltage of lightning is from 10 million to one hundred million volts. The giant cloud in a hot summer sky is formed by an ascending current of air which, by moving quickly past and rubbing against water droplets or ice grains in the cloud, cause friction. The lower part of the cloud which is closer to the earth gathers many negatively charged electrons while the upper part, because of the lack of electrons which went to the lower part, becomes positively charged. In this bottom part of the cloud these electrons thrust against each other, pushing others away, because similar electrons repel each other (Fig. 5.15a). This mass of negative electrons forms a huge electric field which then naturally tries to attract the positive electricity around it, since opposites attract. Under this influence, in the earth below our giant cloud a positive electric mass is formed. The mass of negative electricity in the cloud and that of the positive electricity in the earth pull towards each other. This power strength is from 10 to 100 million volts.

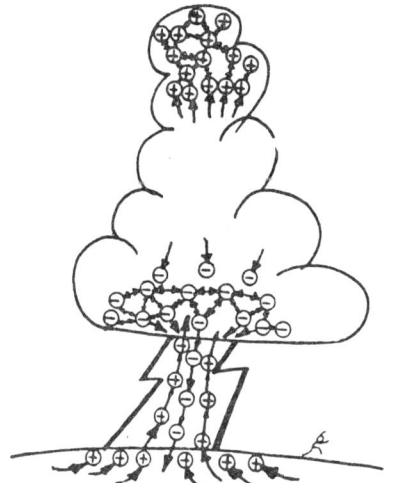

Fig. 5.15(a) Electrons push each other in the giant cloud, and these pushed ones reach the earth. Also the positive ions go up to the cloud and cause the falling of a thunderbolt.

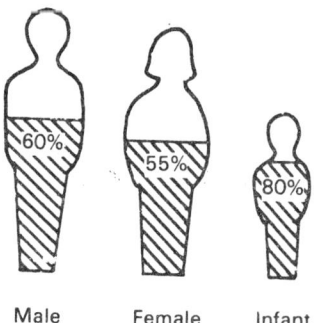

Male   Female   Infant

Fig. 5.15(b) The proportions of water (% of weight).

As mentioned before, usually air is a non-conductor. But when the expelling power in the thunder cloud becomes too strong, even air cannot keep from getting involved any more and lets the electrons race through to "kiss" the soil. Once a road between the cloud and the earth has been cleared, it becomes easy for electrons to go through. Also, the positive electricity in the earth rushes up to reach the giant cloud along this road; there then happens the sudden electric neutralisation and the electrons in the cloud disappear. This phenomenon is called the fall of a thunderbolt and the road is seen as a flash of lightning. In the case of electric acupuncture treatment, the negative terminal which is put on the surface of the body thrusts with electrons, or negative ions, the positive ions out from the body. On the other hand, the positive terminal pulls the electrons or negative ions out of the body thrusting positive ions in. But the quantity of these moving electrons or ions is not such that can influence the quantity of ions already in the whole body—but it is just enough to stimulate the nerves so that they sense the electric flow, causing muscles to move.

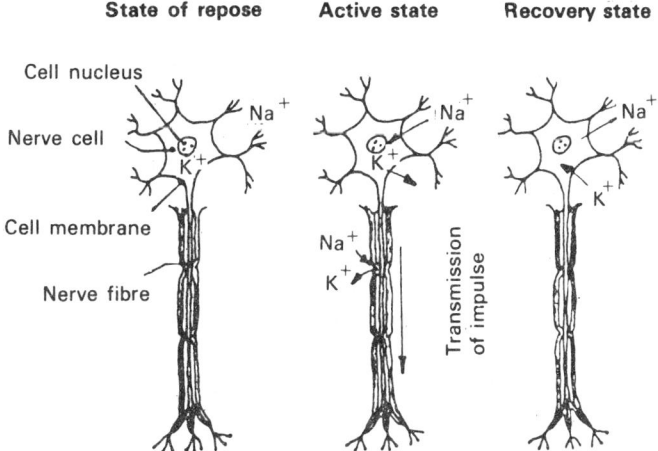

Fig. 5.16   The distribution of ions outside and inside the cell
and its movement through the states of repose,
active and recovery.

Electric current

Electric current means the quantity of electricity, of electrons or ions which flow.   Usually it is measured by how many electrons and ions flow during 1 minute.   The electricity which flows in and out of the body in the case of the "electric treatment" is very small, ranging 1/1000 to 20/1000 amperes (1-20 mA).   The electricity which a 20 W fluorescent tube requires is 0.2 amperes (200 mA).

That which affects the living body is not the size of the voltage but the quantity of current or electricity (electric volume or amperage).   If 1 mA (1/1000 A) flows into the heart directly, it will stop the heart's beating.   Electricity flowing in a body causes heat.   Since the number of electric vibrations (frequency) of the electricity used in electric treatment is only 5-100 times per second, it works mostly for stimulating nerves and the low heat therapy caused can be ignored.   In case the frequency increases to more than a million times a second, the electricity will induce a great amount of heat which can be used for "heat therapy".   The reason why the increase in frequency produces heat is because the electrons and ions in the body are being shaken violently, the same number of times as the frequency, which is more than a million times per second.   By that action a kind of friction begins that results in the production of heat.

ELECTRICITY AS AN ELEMENT OF THE INNER ENVIRONMENT OF A LIVING BODY

Acidity and Alkalinity

Sometimes it is said that because human bodies are naturally maintained in an alkalined condition, alkalinic food is better than acidic food.   This acidity and alkalinity of the body is due to the electrical nature of the blood and the body fluids, which are charged by ions and their proportions.   Electricity exists in the body not only in the form of electric current or voltage, but also in the form of electrically charged particles, a countless number of ions which play an all important role in our bodies.

Acidic and alkalinic food

As first, I want to talk about the acidity and alkalinity of food. There is no doubt that the blood and the body fluids around the cells are kept on the weak alkaline side. However, this does not mean that taking too much acidic food will decrease the alkalinity of the blood and body fluids suddenly, while increasing their acidity. Calling some foods acidic (or alkaline, for that matter) means that they contain some elements which are able to produce acid (or alkali) when they are taken into the body. This has nothing to do with the inherent acidity (or alkalinity) of the foods themselves. The food taken into the body is broken down and digested by various digestive enzymes, then delivered to the organs in the form of elements and molecules to be absorbed into the body.

For instance, sour tangerine juice is surely considered to be an acid, but we cannot say that the tangerine itself is an acidic food. Once it is taken into the body, the acidity of the juice does not remain but in fact is digested and resolved into several forms of non-sour substances, elements and molecules. Among these resolved elements, there are "metal elements" which help the body produce alkaline substances. Therefore, sour umeboshi (pickled plums) and tangerines belong to the alkaline food category. As mentioned above, since acidic and alkalinic foods do not affect the acidity or alkalinity of the body directly, we should not concern ourselves about whether one is acidic or alkalinic, but just eat a proper balance of various kinds of food.

The balance between cells in the whole body

The most important thing about the acidity and alkalinity of the body is the presence of these two in the blood. This theory of the "equilibrium between acid and base" plays an important role in the field of medicine. As was mentioned earlier, the blood is slightly alkaline. The reason is that the body cells produce acid continuously, as long as they are living so to neutralise somewhat this acid, the blood is made to be alkaline. Like this human bodies are made quite well to be naturally balanced.

Well, it is a rule of nature that only well-balanced animals can survive. All animals and plants which we see in our daily lives, including man, regardless of their sizes are composed of a collection of countless tiny cells. Taking man as an example, the skin can be thought of as a sort of "sack" filled with an aqueous solution (blood and body fluids) where elements similar to those in sea water are found and where an astronomical number of living cells soak themselves.

But these cells are not self-existent, like amoebae in some kind of pond, but are rather gregarious. For these cells to function together as one unified living body, there are various mechanisms working to make connections between them. The transferring media, "blood", circulates throughout the body touching every cell; also, they have constant contact with each other via their information media, the "nerves", "hormones" and "minerals" which are carried in the blood help the whole body to be balanced.

Inside the body, when some local disorder occurs, the whole protective mechanism works itself up to settle the situation as quickly as possible, and this mechanism is well used by oriental medicine, the treatment method for various kinds of pain and disease which involves inserting one thin needle into the body or sometimes includes giving finger massage.

The way of managing the acid produced in the body, and its elimination

The blood acts as a transmitting media for carrying nutrition, hormones and oxygen to each cell as well as carrying exhaust products from them to the kidneys and lungs in order to eliminate waste matter from the system. It also carries wastes to the liver for disposing or resynthesising. The blood goes around each cell and functions to balance "the inner environment" of the body keeping these cells alive.

The reason why living cells produce acid continuously will be delt with as follows: Cells produce energy by oxidising the nutritive substances with the oxygen carried from the lungs, both of which are carried by the blood to the cells. The cells synthesise protein (a process called assimilation) which is a necessary substance making up the cells: or they resolve old exhausted substances and discharge them (a process called catabolism). The nutritive substances, after being oxidised and turned in to energy, will be exhausted and (finally) resolved into water and "carbonic acid gas". This carbonic acid gas (cag) melts into the water and becomes "carbonic acid". Therefore, as along as cells live this acid is discharged from them into the blood endlessly.

When a shortage of oxygen happens, in order to keep the cells alive, a stronger acid called lactic acid will be released into the blood. That is why the blood usually leans to the alkaline side. That which keeps the blood a little on the alkaline side is sodium bicarbonate ($NaHCO_3$) synthesised in kidney. This is what you take when you have heart-burn, or use sometimes when you are baking. The blood contains much sodium and this neutralises the acid produced by each cell, protecting the blood from becoming acidic.

This neutralised acid is carried to the lungs and taken into the alveoli again as aeroform carbonic acid gas (cag), after which it is eliminated into the air through our breathing. As the quantity of cag decreases, naturally carbonic acid which is made by the gas in the blood and body fluids decrease too. The quantity of eliminated cag from the body into the air daily is up to about 300 litre in aerial volume, and 600 g in weight.

The relationship between hydrogen, hydroxide ions, acid and alkaline

Both the blood and the body fluids are aqueous solutions. Water is an electrically united substance composed of "hydrogen ions" (H^+) and "hydroxide ions" (OH^-). In water at normal temperatures, besides the united form (H_2O), are also disassociated forms of H^+ ions and OH^- ions. The quantity of these ions is usually equally balanced. The aqueous solution which contains equal amounts of hydrogen ions and hydroxide ions is called a "neutral" solution. The solution containing hydrogen ions and less hydroxide ions than this neutral solution is called "acidic", and the opposite case is called alkalinic.

Water itself is a neutral solution containing the same amount of H^+ and OH^-. But in the body, the cag eliminated from the cells and melting into the water, where it is turned into carbonic acid, increases the amount of hydrogen ion H^+ in the blood, which then tends to be slightly acidic. But as mentioned above, blood contains sodium bicarbonate and its ion (bicarbonate ion HCO_3^-) which unites with H^+ and neutralised the blood to protect it from becoming too acidic.

The hydrogen ion H^+ and hydroxide ion OH^- existing in neutral water are only in slight quantities, each number of ions in 1 litre of water at normal temperatures is about $1/10,000,000$ mol (mol is the unit used to count ions or molecules; $10,000,000$ is described as 10^7).

As described earlier, when the amount of hydrogen ion H^+ increases, hydroxide ion OH^- decreases; this means that their multiplied number remains the same as long as the temperature remains the same. When hydrogen ion H^+ increases its number 1000 times more than that of neutral water, then hydroxide ion OH^- will be $1/1000$. That product stays always the same. Blood in its usual condition keeps H^+ a little less than OH^-. The amount of H^+ is 1/2.5 that of neutral water, while that of OH^- is 2.5 times more. Their product $[(1/2.5) \times 2.5 = 1)]$ is always the same as neutral water. Describing them in terms of mol, the amount of H^- in 1 litre of normal blood would be $(4/10^8)$ mol and OH^- $(2.5/10^7)$ mol; their product is $(1/10^{14})$, since $(4/10^8) \times (2.5/10^7) = 10/(10^8 \times 10^7) = 1/10^{14}$ mol/l. A normal water solution contains $1/10^7$ mol/l of H^+ and $1/10^7$ mol/l of OH^- their product is also $1/10^{14}$. Therefore, we can say that the product of H^+ and OH^- in any solution, either alkalinic like blood or neutral like water, always stays at $1/10^{14}$ mol at normal temperatures.

pH as a measuring unit for acidity and alkalinity

Now we know that in ordinary water at normal temperatures, the density of both H^+ and OH^- is $1/10^7$ mol per 1 litre. As it is not convenient to write figures such as $1/10^7$ each time, it was decided to describe them simply as 7, the power to these members. The density of ions (especially the density of H^+) is indicated in terms of the value of pH. pH is the shortened form for "power of hydrogen ion". Since the density of H^+ in plain water is $1/10^7$, we say "the pH of pure water is 7". Also, the density of H^+ in normal blood is $4/10^8$ which is $1/10^{7.4}$ and so is put: "the normal value of pH in the blood is 7.4". Remembering that the pH of weak alkalinic blood is 7.4 and that of water is 7, it can be said that when the pH value exceeds 7, then it leans towards alkalinity.

When we put alkalinic substances like sodium hydroxide into water, the amount of H^+ will decrease while that of OH^- increases and ends up at the point of pH 14. 14 is the "power number" of product of H^+ and OH^- $(1/10^{14})$ in a solution.

On the other hand, when we put hydrochloric acid into water to increase the density of hydrogen ions, the pH will be less than 7 and will reach pH 0. So now we understand that pH 7 means neutrality, pH 0 to pH 7 shows an acidity and pH 7 to pH 14 shows an alkalinity. The fact that the pH of blood is 7.4 means that it is slightly alkalinic; as mentioned earlier, this is caused by sodium bicarbonate produced in the kidney getting into the blood.

In a normal state, the pH of blood is kept around 7.4 (7.3-7.5); but as cells in the body generate carbonic acid gas which turns into carbonic acid, the cells become slightly acidic. In those cases (*1*) in which there is some trouble with the lungs, and the function of eliminating carbonic acid out into the air via breathing is reduced (the cag staying in the blood); (*2*) when the acid called "ketone body" caused by diabetes stays in the blood; or (*3*) when trouble in the kidnies resulted in the production of smaller quantities of sodium bicarbonate, the amount of acid in the blood should be increased so that the pH goes down close to 7 and the blood loses its alkalinity.

In most cases, urine is slightly acidic. Although the quantity of hydrogen ion H^+ caused by cag, which is discharged into the blood from the cells, is reduced by the bicarb ion HCO_3, all of it cannot be neutralised completely. So, the rest of the acid is excreted through the kidnies into our urine. Also, a part of the acid will be needed for synthesising sodium bicarbonate $NaHCO_3$. Therefore, the density of H^+ in urine increases and pH goes down. However, the amount of acid and alkaline in urine depends on their presence in the blood. Table 5.1 shows the acidity and alkalinity for blood, cells and urine.

Table 5.1 : The normal value of acid and alkaline in blood, cells and urine

Blood	Cells	Urine
Slightly alkalinic	Slightly acidic	Usually slightly acidic but sometimes alkalinic
pH 7.3-7.5	C. 7.0	4.6-7.8

Geriatric respiratory diseases and the acidity of the blood
(*the importance of abdominal respiration*)

The above title seems to be strange, but to breathe in and out correctly is the most important way to protect the blood from being too acidic.

Recently, the average life span of humans has become longer; but more and varied kinds of geriatric diseases are beginning to be noticed. The pain and paralysis which can be objects of acupuncture and moxibustion treatment in Oriental medicine are the main constituents of geriatric diseases. Also, chronic respiratory diseases are counted as being some of the principal geriatric diseases too, and because of the recent increase in air pollution, respiratory diseases are also increasing in number.

As mentioned before, where the cag generated in the body is eliminated, out of the body through respiration. For cag to be well eliminated, the lungs should function normally; the quantity of air in one's breathing (called "tidal volume") should be large and the number of breaths per minute should be normal. In a typical adult's case, the tidal volume is around 500 ml and the number of breaths in one minute is about 15 (times). We are doing this rhythmically, unconsciously, through the reflective actions of the automatic nerves. When breathing in, our diaphragm and chest muscles contract and the space in the chest expands so that which is inside (our lungs) becomes bigger, too.

The fresh air (mixed gaseous body of 20% oxygen and 80% nitrogen) flows into the expanded space of the lungs. When breathing out, by merely relaxing the diaphragm and chest muscles, the lungs through their own elasticity naturally contract, pushing the air out (just like a blown-up balloon, when it shrinks). Therefore, when you breathe out there is no need to use any muscles, but just relax. However, when people get older, sometimes the elasticity of their lungs becomes weak, or many of the small ramified air roads, the bronchial tubes, becomes smaller making it difficult for the air to go through. When these situations advance morbidly, chronic geriatric obstructive respiratory diseases occur.

Pulmonary emphysema and pulmonary fibrosis are the principal diseases. A discription of these would be—the bronchial tubes become smaller, lungs have no elasticity, just like an already stretched out balloon, and people even have difficulty in breathing in and out. In these conditions, not only when breathing in but also when breathing out, one must make an effort by using more muscles; the breathing begins to get shallower and one breathes quickly using his shoulders. This kind of shallow and quick breathing does not allow enough air in and out through the lungs; one must make a great effort and soon gets tired. This causes the elimination of cag to become slower, its density in the blood increasing extremely high. If we leave this situation alone, theoretically the pH of the blood will get lower than 7 and become terribly acidic (called hyperoxemia).

But the human body is quite well organised, such that in this case, the production of sodium bicarbonate in our kidney increases; even though the cag in the blood is high, the H+ is neutralised, thereby protecting the blood, keeping its pH down (it stays around pH 7.1-7.3). But once the chronic obstructive respiratory diseased person catches a cold, he will then develop dyspnoea; the carbonic acid in the blood will get too high suddenly; sometimes he may fall into a coma.

Therefore, these patients should be careful not to catch a cold, trying to develop their physical strength as well as properly exercising in order to make a "slow and deep abdominal respiration" instead of a quick and shallow shoulder breathing in their daily life.

In the case of pulmonary emphysema, the bronchial tubes are thinner than normal so one must breath slowly to get the air into the depths of the lungs. Though not sufficiently, nevertheless to some degree or other, by slow abdominal respiration one can protect his blood from carbonic gas, keeping the proper balance of ions in the body and protecting the blood from becoming too much acidic. Like this, "breathing in and out well" plays an important role in arranging the electrical environment of the living body, by making a good balance of our ions.

Returning to food as in the beginning, we should not concern ourselves about whether "this is acidic or that is alkalinic"; eating a proper balance of various kinds of food is the most important thing for keeping the best inner environment of our living body.

When you become ill, even if it is with a chronic disease, you should follow the correct ways of living, trying to keep a good balance in your body.

The function of body fluids and ions

It may seem that acidity and alkalinity is a matter of chemistry, having no connection with electricity but in fact a chemical nature occurs via the electrical nature of the outer nuclear electrons and the nucleus of atoms and molecules. In this connection we will also explain the electrical phenomenon of ions more directly so that you can understand the connections between the living body and electricity more deeply.

When it comes to discussing the nutritive balance of food, always it is suggested that we should take the following three kinds of elements in an adequate balance:
1. Carbohydrates as a source of calories (energy).
2. Protein and minerals which produce the elements of the body.
3. Minerals, which arrange the body environment, and vitamins as the lubricant. Plus taking necessary amount of water.

Among these, minerals in category 3 have an important electrical function. These ions exist inside and around all the cells and in the blood in solution. Let us look at the water and ions in the body and their functions from now.

The quantity of water in a body

The human body does not seem to contain so much water because it never comes out when we push against the flesh. However, as shown in Fig. 5.15b, it contains much more water than we imagine. In an adult man 60% of the body weight is water and in an adult woman 55% on the average. This means a man who weighs 70 kg carries 42 kg of water and a woman of 50 kg carries 28 kg of water. Bodies of infants contain even more water: 80% of the body weight. So, a 5 kg baby contains 4 kg water. An adult on the average, discharges 2000 to 2500 ml of water from the body in a day (1000-1500 ml in urine, 900 ml in breath and sweat and 100 ml in stool). So we must take the same amount of water in a day by drinking or other ways in order to keep the balance.

When you peal a tangerine and open it up, you can see the beautiful orange coloured granular cells packed to the full. We can say that human body also is a collection of small cells; each cell is filled with a water solution (aqueous). In this water solution there exist various kinds of substances or tiny organs either in dissoluted form or undissoluted form. The water solution inside the cells is called intracellular fluid and the whole solution outside the cells is called extracellular fluid which is divided into two groups. One is the "blood" which flows inside blood vessels, and the other is intercellular fluid which circulates between the cells. Intracellular fluid is kept in a tremendous number of cells and accounts for three-fourths of the water solution in a body. The other one-fourth is extracellular fluid; both blood and intercellular fluid.

Ions which are dissolved in the water solution

As mentioned above, the human body contains a large quantity of water, both inside and around the cells and there also exists many kinds of ions, "the electrified atoms and molecules". Cells are wrapped by a thin membrane called "the cell wall". There is a big difference in the constitution of the ions inside and outside of the cells which are partitioned with the cell membrane. When positive ions are dissolved inside and solutions of the cells K^+ (kalium) and Mg^{++} (magnesium) form the majority, and when negative ions are resolved HPO_4^- (phoperic acid ion) and protein make up the majority. On the other hand, outside the cells, among intercellular fluid and the blood, Na^+ (natrium) is largely contained in the form of positive ions and many Cl^- (chlorine) HCO_3^- (bicarbonate) ions are contained as negative ions.

The cells themselves are living units soaked in intercellular fluid, to which nutrition and oxygen are supplied for them to take in. Also waste matter from the cells is discharged into intercellular fluid to be eliminated out of the body through the blood, or to be resynthesised. The components of ions in intercellular fluid and blood (both belong to extracellular fluid) are very similar to that of sea water. Life originally came into existance in the sea and the first unicellular animal or plant (something like an amoeba) lived in an environment of sea water. These animals came out of sea with sea water wrapped by a skin soaking cells in it, like present human beings, animals and plants. Of course, the animals and plants still living in water are the same. The reason why the blood tastes as salty as sea water is that the components are almost the same in both cases, most of them contain Na^+ and Cl^- (basic NaCl).

The exchange of ions across the cell wall and the transmissive action of the nerves

As was explained in Fig. 5.4, when electricity flows into the body from an electro-stimulator, an impulse (or action potential) is evoked in the nerve cells, which is transmitted to the spinal cord and brain, causing a sensation or perception. Even though the electricity is not sent by the device, since there are many special nerve cells (receptors) which can sense pain, heat, light, sound, taste, and so on, existing on the surface of body, eyes, ears, tongue and other parts. When each receptor gets various kinds of stimulation, the electric impulse (action potential) is evoked and transmitted to the sensory nerves, reaching the brain through the spinal cord which causes a sensation or perception. On the other hand, from the brain and spinal cord, impulses are transmitted retrogressively through another kind of nerve (called motor nerve) to each part of the body's muscles so that arms, legs, eyes and every organ works well. These impulses (action potential) of the nerves are generated through the instantaneous action of the ions moving between the inside and outside of the nerve cells; the nerve fibres then transmit this action. As shown in Fig. 5.16, when a nerve is not active (a state of repose) there are many kalium ions (K^+) distributed inside it and the nerve fibre. Many natrium ions (Na^+) are distributed outside the cells. This is the same as above mentioned pattern for cells in general when various kinds of stimulations (for example, pain, heat, light, sound or taste) are given to the nerves from outside the body, the nerves react to them, the character of walls of nerve cells change, and instantaneously numerous natrium ions rush into the nerve cells. In the meantime, kalium ions are going out. At this very moment it loses its electrical balance and the voltage (impulse, action potential) rises instantly, which is transmittted in a wave-form to the spinal cord through the nerve fibres, then the brain where it courses various perceptions (like pain, heat, etc.). Like this, then by being given some kind of stimulation, the character of walls of nerve cells change with outer and inner ions exchanging places. Thus arises the action potential. We call this phenomenon the "excitement" of a nerve. After one excitement is finished, natrium comes back in its position. The movement of the ions in this restorative stage is caused by the nerve cells having spent their natural energy in taking in and pushing out these ions by force. This action is called "active transport". Thus the nerve cells generate electricity by the movement of ions between nerve fibres; this movement" is what's transmitted.

Now let us look more closely at the process of how nerve transmission takes place when your finger touches a hot pot. By reflex, you pull your finger away from it instantly. In the first place the moment your finger touches the hot pot, the heat is transmitted to the heat receptor nerves on the skin of the finger. These nerve cells get excited and generate their impulses, which are conveyed to the nerve cells on the dorsal of the spinal cord through "sensory nerve" fibres. Some part of this impulse is also transferred to the nerve cells on the frontal side of the spinal cord (this is called the transmission of nerves by "reflection"). This impulse is transmitted again to the muscles of hand and finger through motor nerve fibres, contracting these muscles in order to pull the finger back. Since this process is performed by the electrical transmission of impulses, the whole action is carried out very speedily. Therefore, the very moment we touch the hot pot, we pull our finger back to avoid being burnt. This whole quick action is not performed voluntarily but is due to the unconscious reaction of impulses reaching the spinal cord and coming back. That is how we can pull our finger back "reflectively". At the same time, the other part of the electric impulse which has been transmitted to the nerve cells on the dorsal of spinal cord from the tip of the finger is transmitted to the sensory nerves and goes up to the brain, then we get the perception of "heat". This perception is memorised in our mind so that we become careful before touching a hot pot again. We can say that reflection is an unconscious protective function and perception is a learning function for future use. Electricity in the living body is involved directly with these functions.

Transmission properties of nerves and electro-stimulating treatment
The muscles which we can move any time by our own will are controlled by motor nerves and they are called voluntary muscles. As these voluntary muscles are used mainly for moving various parts of our frame, they are also called skeletal muscles. When the brain nerve or spinal cord nerves are incapacitated because of cerebral apoplexy or whiplash

injury, the motor nerves which are linked with those nerves lose their function, with the result that the connected muscles do not move or get convulsive attack and are "paralysed". Nerves in our body usually generate impulses by the excitement of their own cells; these impulses are transmitted to the muscles and then the muscles contract.

Besides voluntary muscles, there is another kind of muscle in our body which cannot be cotrolled by our own will. These are called involuntary muscles. Most of them belong to the category termed "smooth muscles." These muscles are controlled mainly by the "autonomic nerves" and activate the inside organs' functions. These autonomic nerve cells exist in the diencephalon, the mesencephalon, the medulla oblongata and the spinal cord, from where inpulses are sent endlessly in order to beat the heart, to breath and let the endocrine, stomach and intestines work.

There are various causes for paralysis—the nerve cells lose their functions and cannot generate impulses, or the transmission channel is broken and stops sending the impulses, or the muscles themselves have some trouble moving, and so on In the former two cases, since the muscles themselves are capable of movement, we can send low frequency electric waves into the body, which mechanism is similar to that of the impulses racing through the nerves, getting them excited enough to generate the impulses needed to move the muscles. This is the treatment method for paralysis using a low frequency electro-stimulator for rehabilitation in hospitals or at home. It is said that this treatment is performed by applying the electro-physiology of the nerves and muscles directly.

The relationship between acupuncture treatment and nerves

On the other hand, the treatment by electro-stimultor which recently is often used seems to have much effect because of a more complicated mechanism. In the case of simple acupuncture treatment, it has been using the method whereby stimulation is given to the meridian points by the use of twirling technique and pecking technique. Basically, the electro-stimulator has the same principle of twirling technique and pecking technique. That is, as shown in Fig. 5.4, the nerves around the insertion point of the needle are stimulated by the electricity, get excited, and cause an impulse., Twirling technique and pecking technique have the same mechanism. Because of the mechanical stimulation, the nerves get excited and generate impulses. It is true that patients feel the electro-stimulation or the vibrations from the needle. But it cannot be thought that impulses generated from the nerves can be transmitted to the diseased parts directly and relieve the pain or sometimes heal, say, shoulder stiffness. All twirling technique and pecking technique and the electro-stimultor seems to have the following treatment mechanism—at first, the nerve gets excited because of the stimulation given to the meridian points, which activates the "central nerves" of the brain or spiral cord and then stimulates the other nerves, hormones or enzymes. Sometimes this treatment gives a psychological influence to the patient, causing a reaction in the whole body and getting the abnormal part back to normal. Of course, by choosing certain merdian points, it is possible to get a certain effect at the diseased part. However, it may not be due only to the direct connection between the meridian point and the diseased point; it is considered that a polyhedral reaction takes place in the central nerves of the brain and, as a result, there appears some effect at the diseased part. Also there is another reasonable theory that there may exist many routes from the sensory nerves to the autonomic nerves, so when sensory nerves feel the stimulation from the needle, it causes various reactions in the whole body through these routes. Therefore, the treatment by electro-stimulator, acupuncture using twirling technique and pecking technique, moxibustion and finger massage surely involves the sensations from the peripheral nerves or the perception by the cerebrum in the first stage; but the importance should be put on the overall sequential reactions caused by the stimulation. It may take a long period of time to elucidate the mechanism of this reaction after medical science advances further. So instead of discussing about it too much, we should make efforts to improve the methods of treatment or clinical studies applying a short of phenomenalism. Therefore, simply insisting on the validity of the nerve theory or the hormone theory, or trying to explain with knowledge gained from Occidental Medicine, or explaining anything only referring to the meridian points should be rather refrained from. But, we should record our experiences steadily, keep them in order, study the past theories and go on step by step towards the future objectively.

References

1. Yoshio Manaka et al., A study on electrical characteristic of the skin, especially in relation to meridians and meridian points. *Kyoto Pain Control Institute Journal, (JKPCI)*, **3** (1), 1970.

2. Kunzo Nagayama et al., The theory on the effectiveness of acupuncture: The theory of electric energy and magnetism of the living body. *JKPCI*, **3** (4), 1970.

3. Keisuke Komagate et al., A study on clinical results of the combined use of negative potential and magnetism (negative pole), *JKPCI*, **4** (1), 1971.

4. Dumitrescu, I.F. et al., The "Fenestration Occlusion" phenomenon. *JKPCI*, **4** (2), 1971.

5. Keisuke Komagate et al., A study on the prevention of burns caused by galvanization in a low frequency and on sensory and motor system. *JKPCI*, **4** (3), 1971.

6. Keisuke Komagate et al., A study on clinical results of the combined use of negative potential and magnetism (negative pole)—an additional report. *JKPCI*, **4** (1), 1971.

7. Masamichi Himoto et al., Metal magnetic grain therapy and intracutaneous needle therapy. *JKPCI*, **4** (3), 1971.

8. Calude Pinet, Introduction a L'Etude bioelectroque des points Chinois, *JKPCI*, **4** (3) 1971.

9. Kunzo Nagayama et al., A study of ion needle (I). Ion (negative potential) electrostatic needle-like therapeutic terminal. *JKPCI*, **5** (2); 1972.

10. Masamichi Himoto et al., A stuty of ion needle (V). Influence of acupuncture, moxibustion static electricity (negative potential) and local stimulation. *JKPCI*, **6** (3), 1973.

11. Masamichi Himoto et. al., A study of the ion needle (VI). Reanimation of incipient wilted cut plant by ion needle stimulation. *JKPCI*, **6** (4), 1973.

12. Kunzo Nagayama et al., A study of the ion needle (VII). Experimental results of ion needle treatment. *JKPCI*, **7** (1), 1974.

13 Kunzo Nagayama et al., A study of the clinical effectiveness of the combined treatment using a negative potential charge and a dry hot pack. *JKPCI*, **7** (2), 1974.

14. Takeshi Sawa et al., A study of the waveforms of an acupuncture electrical stimulator. *JKPCI*, (7) 3, 1974.

15. Kunzo Nagayama et al., Needleless and drugless energy control therapy. *JKPCI*, **7** (4), 1974.

16. Tancomi Yoshida et al., A study of electro-acupuncture treatment (II) : Pulse duration. *JKPCI*, **8** (1), 1975.

17. Takeshi Sawa et al., A study on polar effect of galvanization. *JKPCI*, **8** (2), 1975.

18. Kunzo Nagayama et al., Application of plate vs. Plate low frequency electro-stimulation for classical acupuncture modality needle setting therapy. *JKPCI*, **9** (4), 1976.

19. Takeshi Nakazono et al., Prototype manufacture of a skin electrical fluctuation indicator. *JKPCI*, **10** (2), 1977.

20. Takeshi Nakazono et al., The monitor of Tokki (RK-7198), *JKPCI*, **10** (2), 1977.

6

ELECTRIC STIMULATOR USED
FOR ACUPUNCTURE

VARIOUS KINDS OF THERAPY BY USING ELECTRICITY

The electric current or electromagnetic waves have been used for treating various diseases for a long time. Many kinds of electricity have been used and the difference in their effects are mainly caused by the difference in the frequency as shown in Table 6.1.

Table 6.1 : Various kinds of therapies by using electricity

Therapy	Electricity	Frequency	Main effect
Static (ionic) therapy	Static charge	—	—
Direct current therapy	Direct current (DC)	0 Hz**	Electric stimulation
Low frequency therapy	Pulse or alternate current (AC)	1-1000 Hz	Electric stimulation
Microwave therapy	AC electric field	100 MHz**	Heating effect
Ultrashort microwave therapy	Electromagnetic	2450 MHz	Heating effect
Ultrared rays ultra-violet rays, radiation	Light X-rays γ-rays		Heating effect Chemical effect Others

*NOTE : Hz (Hertz) is a common unit of electric current frequency used these days in place of CPS (cycles per second) which was used in the past. Hz stands for the number of waves or pulses of electricity per second and MHz (megaHertz) stands for one million Hz.

Takeshi Sawa, Department of Anaesthesiology, Tokyo Medical and Dental University, Tokyo, Japan.

Here the electric stimulator used for acupuncture is explained. The sort of electricity used for acupuncture is so-called "low-frequency electric current". This is almost same as the low-frequency electric current which has been used for the "low-frequency therapy" in orthopedy, In the traditional low frequency therapy, a pair of plate electrodes are put on the surface of the body and electric current is flown into the body through these electrodes. Differing from this, in the acupuncture therapy electric current frequency used for the acupuncture therapy is from one up to some hundred hertz (so called "low-frequency").

BASIC DESCRIPTION OF THE ELECTRIC STIMULATOR

The electric stimulator used for acupuncture can be divided into two types. One is the "bipolar wave" generator (Fig. 6.1a) which is used for needle-to-needle stimulation. In the needle-to-needle stimulation a pair of needle electrodes are used and both needle electrodes can cause stimulation. The other is the "mono-polar wave" generator (Fig. 6.1b) which is used for needle-to-plate stimulation. In this case needle electrode alone is effective for stimulation and this is similar to the traditional low frequency therapy. In the needle-to-plate stimulation, needle must be connected to the negative terminal of the stimulator output and plate is connected to the positive terminal. If the needle is connected to the positive terminal by mistake it corrodes during stimulation and breaks in the body.

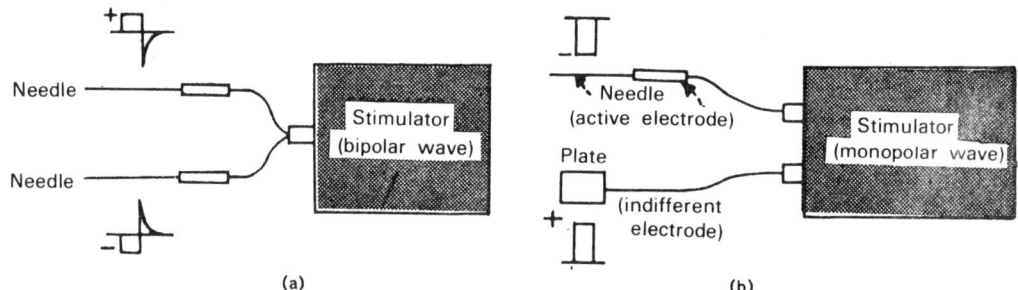

Fig. 6.1 Two kinds of stimulators (wave forms) used in acupuncture treatment.

The electrode which is effective to stimulation (in this case it is the needle) is called "active" electrode, and another electrode which is ineffective to stimulation is called "indifferent" or "ground" electrode.

As stated above, although the electric stimulator used for acupuncture can be divided into two types, both basically have almost same composition and function except the difference of electrode (whether needle or plate) and wave form (whether bipolar or monopolar). The basic composition of stimulator is shown in Fig. 6.2. The stimulator is operated by two power sources; one is battery (DC) powered machine and the other is AC powered machine (sometimes two-way machine is available). The common components which are equipped in all kinds of stimulators are: (1) output terminals, (2) output adjuster, (3) frequency adjuster, (4) power switch, and (5) stimulation indicator (sound or light or both). Some stimulators are equipped with (6) output indicating meter, (7) timer, (8) battery checker, (9) power source indicator, and (10) selector switch for continuous or intermittent, but they are not always equipped (see Fig. 6.2).

GENERAL CARE ON USE

(1) The output leads should be kept in good order after use and electrodes (particularly

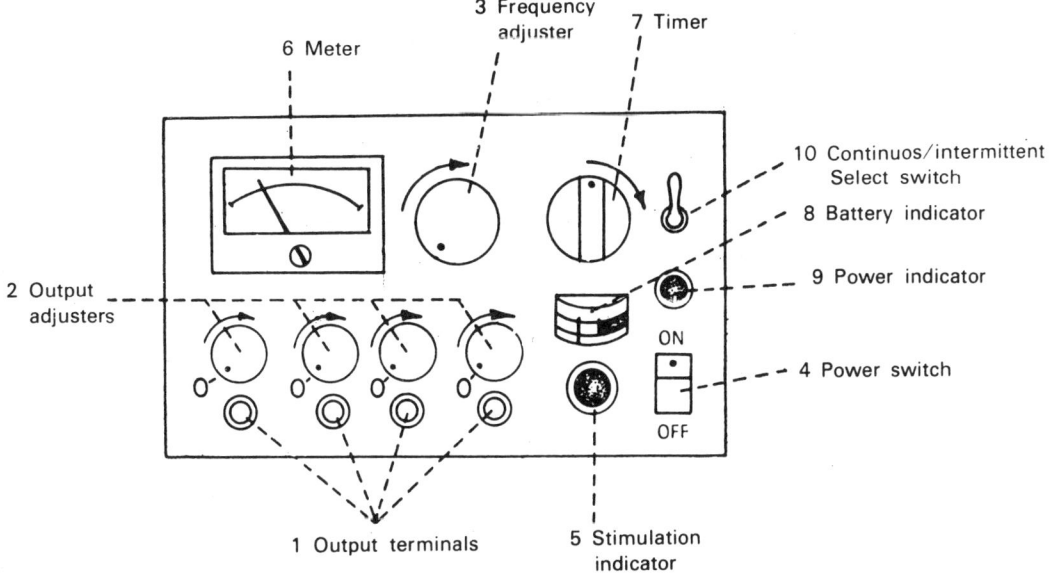

Fig. 6.2   Basic composition of stimulator used for acupuncture.

wet type) should be cleaned. As the soldering of the pinch clips at the tips of the output leads and the thin copper wires in the output leads are easily broken, the output leads should be handled carefully and should avoid kinking.   The spare output leads should be prepared.

(2) Before stimulation is applied to a patient, make sure that all output adjusters are returned to their zero position (usually fully counter-clockwise).   Some stimulators provide a safety device such that stimulation cannot be applied unless all output adjusters are returned to zero position.

(3)   Power switch should be turned off before power cable is disconnected.

(4) The voltage of battery should always be checked and batteries should be taken off when stimulator is not to be used for several months.

EASILY PRACTICABLE TROUBLE SHOOTING

(1) When the stimulator does not work, your operating procedure should be checked again according to the operating manual before thinking that the machine has trouble. Particularly, as stated above, in the machine which has a safety device, check first whether all output adjusters are returned to zero. For the purpose of checking it is important that the operating manual should be kept near the machine so that it could be located easily.

(2) In the case of the AC powered machine, damage to the power cable in plug or at any location near the machine or a loose screw in the plug must be inspected first.

(3) In the case of the DC-powered machine, checking by battery checker alone is not sufficient.   Open the cover of battery case and make sure whether the contact of battery is loose or the electrolyte spills out of battery.

(4) If the banana tip of the output lead is loose, press it against the desk and make its spring action stronger (Fig. 6.3).

(5) We can check the stimulation voltage on the output terminal by tester (voltage—resistance tester).   The AC-range lower than 50 volts is recommended for use and each tester

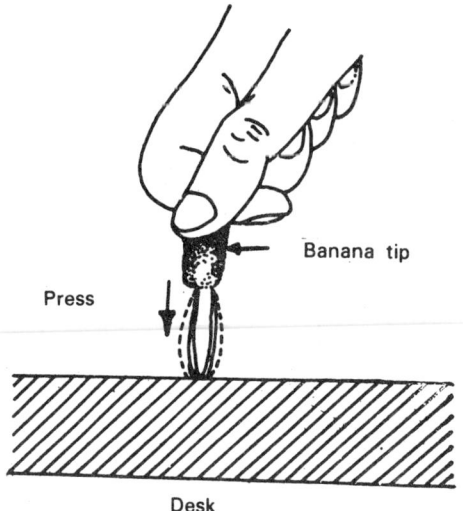

Fig.6.3   Press the banana tip against desk and make its spring action stronger.

leads are connected to needle-needle or needle-plate electrodes. This method is only for checking. If exact output voltage measurement is needed, a synchroscope cathode-ray oscilloscope) should be used.

BASIC KNOWLEDGE CONCERNING ELECTRIC STIMULATION FOR ACUPUNCTURE

How much voltage or current is adequate for treatment

According to the results that we measured in the out-patients of our university hospital by applying negative square wave of pulse width more than 1 msec, the range of adequate peak voltage was 2 to 25 volts and that of adequate peak current was 0.5 to 4 mA per needle. Such a wide variation in voltage or current is due to personal difference and/or the difference in sensitivity of the part where the needle is inserted.

How does the sensible current differ by the difference in pulse width

We measured the change in adequate peak current due to the difference in pulse width of negative square wave in the out-patients. The peak current necessary to get adequate stimulation increased largely as the pulse width became less than 1 msec. Figure 6.4 shows the relative change in peak current when the peak current at the pulse width of 5 m sec. is regarded as a unity (1.0). This relationship is quite similar to the response curve of nerve or muscle to electric stimulation (intensity—duration curve). Such a relationship could not be seen in voltage.

How quick does the electrolytic corrosion of needle occur by positive current flow

The test was done for No. 5 stainless steel needle (diameter 0.25 mm) by flowing positive square wave current of 1 msec pulse width. With the peak current of 20 mA (mean value of 1 mA) and 50 Hz, needles corroded within 9.2 ± 3.5 (SD) hours in saline solution and 44 minutes in rabbit flesh. With the peak current of 10 mA (mean value of 1 mA) and 100 Hz needles corroded within 3.2 ± 0.9 hours in saline solution and 47 min in rabbit. As

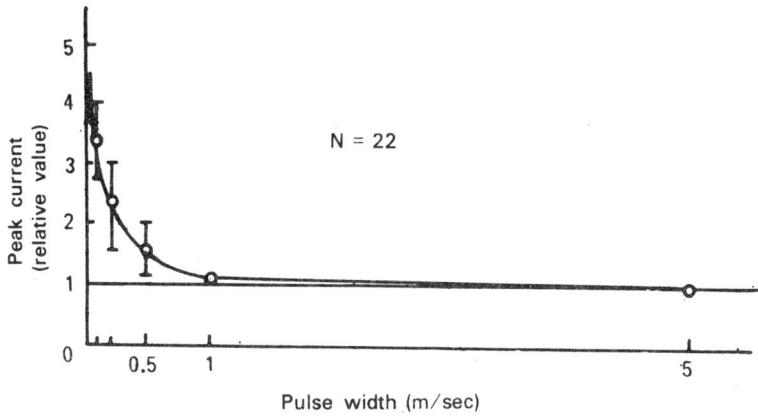

Fig. 6.4 Relationship between pulse width and peak current.

seen above, when needle is inserted in living body and positive current is flown it corrodes within one hour. This result suggests us that the application of positive square wave current to the needle electrode should be avoided strictly.

The polarity effect of electric stimulation

Positive and negative square wave current (50 Hz pulse width 0.1-5 msec) was applied alternatively to the same needle of the same patient and the amount of current and voltage necessary to get adquate stimulation was determined. As a result, the same strength of stimulation was obtained by less negative current which was 37% of positive one and by less negative voltage which was 38% of positive one. This shows that the negative current is more effective than the positive one for electric stimulation but this does not necessarily mean that negative current is more effective in treatment. It has not been made sure which polarity is more effective in treatment. However, negative current is recommended because it never causes electrolytic corrosion of needle and also it can make adequate stimulation by lower amounts of current.

The comparison of negative and positive phase of bipolar wave

Bipolar wave has negative and positive phase as a pair and is used frequently in acupuncture treatment. We wondered which phase is effective to stimulation. To clarify this, six types of waves (Fig. 6.5) were applied to the same needle of the same patient and their effects were compared.

The 1st half-wave and the 2nd half-wave were made by rectifying the whole wave. As a result, negative waves (1N and 2N in Fig. 6.5) could give enough stimulation by less current and voltage (less than half of 1P and 2P). This indicates, that negative phase alone is effective to stimulation in a pair of bipolar waves and the positive phase of bipolar wave does not play its role as electric stimulation (Fig. 6.6).

What should be used as the index of the strength of stimulation

Figure 6.7 shows the no load voltage waves (top row), the voltage waves under loading (middle) and the current waves under loading (bottom).

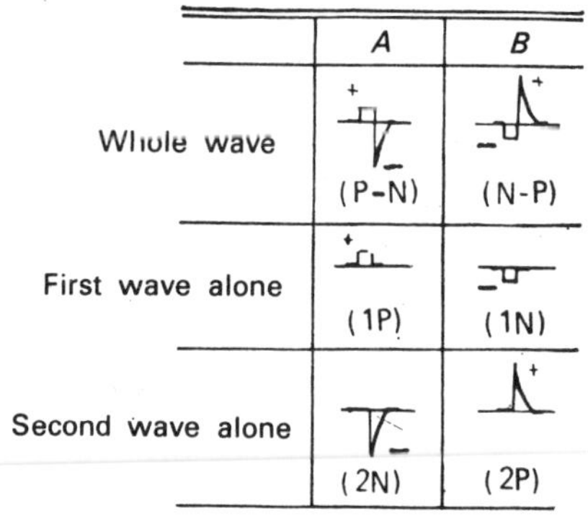

	A	B
Whole wave	(P-N)	(N-P)
First wave alone	(1P)	(1N)
Second wave alone	(2N)	(2P)

Fig. 6.5   Six types of waves.

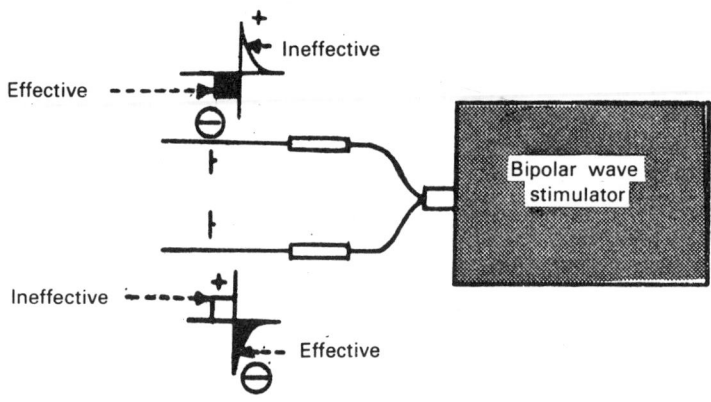

Fig. 6.6   In a bipolar wave, negative phase alone is effective for stimulation.

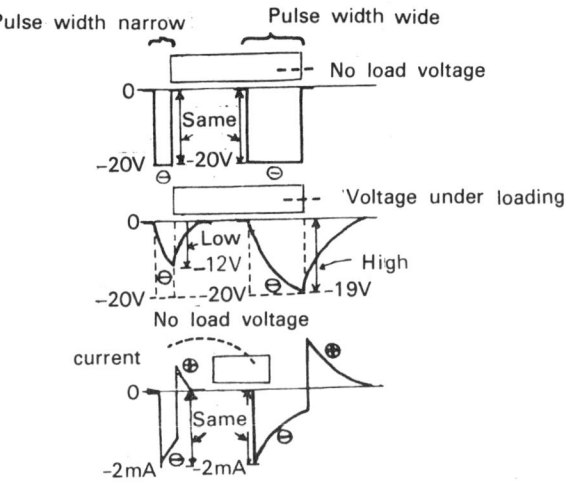

Fig. 6.7   Voltage and current waves distort by flowing the current to patient (under loading.

Here, no load means that stimulator is not connected to patient and loading means that stimulator is connected to patient and current is flown into the patient's body. As shown in Fig. 6.7, no load voltage (top) and current (bottom) do not change by the change in pulse width but voltage under loading (middle) varies as the pulse width change. This means that either no load voltage and current can be used as the index of the strength of stimulation but voltage under loading cannot be used. As no load voltage and peak current correspond to the setting position of output adjusting dial, the setting position of output adjusting dial can be used as the easiest index of strength of stimulation for clinical purpose.

7
STIMULATION IN ACUPUNCTURE.

In the beginning of acupuncture it was found that Stimulation of a few specific areas on the human body was capable of maintaining the equilibrium of the energy flow in the human body. In the stone age stimulation was carried out with sharp pieces of stone, bone and bamboo. This was called as "bians". With the advancement of knowledge different types of metal needles like gold, silver and brass came to be utilised for the stimulation of acupuncture points. In the modern age many new methods of treatment have been introduced in this field of acupuncture for stimulation of acupuncture points.

TYPES OF STIMULATION IN ACUPUNCTURE

According to the traditional Chinese concept, the acupuncture points are located on the body surface following the meridian system. When they are stimulated by different methods, they are capable of bringing the equilibrium in the disturbed energy or Qi. By adopting different methods of stimulation this energy can be tonified or sedated.

According to the modern concept, the acupuncture points are low electrical resistance spots scattered all over the body; when there is disease of an organ the electrical resistance falls down in it. When these points are stimulated, they can bring about the cure by maintaining the energy equilibrium. Chart 7.1 broadly classifies the different methods of stimulation, both the ancient system and the modern methods adopted by the practitioners of acupuncture.

Ancient system of stimulation

1. Heat stimulation
In the olden days it was a practice to heat acupuncture points and the following methods were used for it.
   Direct heat. This was being done by putting a hot coin or by scarring the acupuncture point with red hot iron or by putting direct fire on the Ah-shi points.
   This technique involved crude methods. In modern society this technique is not being used as this is painful and permanent scar formation also takes place.

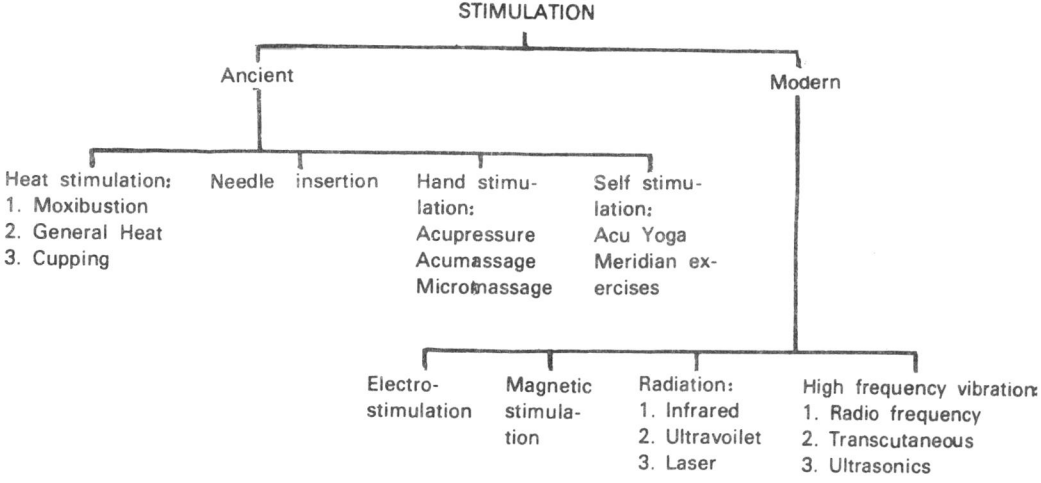

STIMULATION

Ancient   Modern

Heat stimulation:	Needle insertion	Hand stimu-	Self stimu-
1. Moxibustion		lation:	lation:
2. General Heat		Acupressure	Acu Yoga
3. Cupping		Acumassage	Meridian ex-
		Micromassage	ercises

| Electro-stimulation | Magnetic stimula-tion | Radiation: 1. Infrared 2. Ultravoilet 3. Laser | High frequency vibration: 1. Radio frequency 2. Transcutaneous 3. Ultrasonics |

Chart 7.1

Moxibustion. Moxibustion therapy involves treating the disease by heating a point by burning moxa wool to produce the heat on the certain points of the human body. The details of the moxa therapy are explained in Chapter 11.

Cupping therapy. Cupping was known as the "horn method" in ancient times. This means the treatment of the diseases through local congestion or blood stasis by using a small jar or cup in which a vaccum is created by burning a piece of cotton soaked with alcohol kept inside the jar or cup (Fig. 7.1) so that the oxygen inside is consumed and the vacuum is created. Now a days the cup is attached by suction to the skin surface over the selected points.

2. By insertion of a needle

Acupuncture points can be stimulated by inserting the needle in different ways to get the desired effect. Two kinds of desired effects were achieved by different methods:

a. Tonification (*bu*) or by inforcing energy, and

b. Dispersion (*xie*) or by reducing or sedating energy.

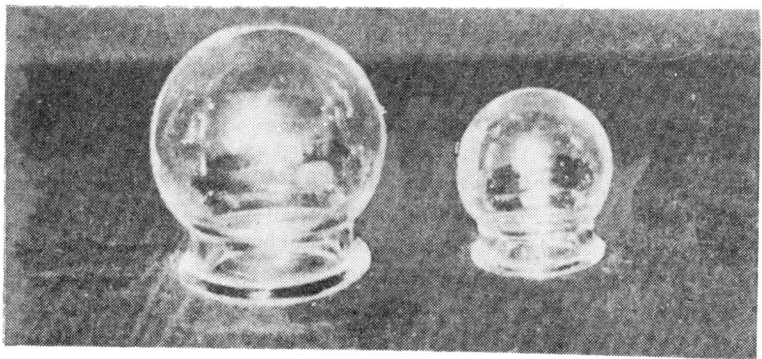

Fig. 7.1 Apparatus for cupping therapy

The different types of needle insertions are explained below.

A. *Superficial needling.* Superficial needling of about ½ t-sun and less than that or subcutaneous needling in the body will tonify the energy or will increase the energy. It is used in chronic cases, in polio paralysis, hemiplegia, paraplegia, etc.

B. *Deep Needling.* Putting a deep needle at the point will sedate the energy and hence it is used in acute cases with painful conditions.

C. *Along the direction of energy flow.* Every meridian has a particular direction of flow of energy. When from a particular point if we pass a needle along the direction of flow of energy, it will tonifiy the energy or will increase the energy.

D. *Against the direction of energy flow.* If the needle is inserted against the direction of energy flow, it will sedate the energy.

E. *If we put the needle during inspiration it will tonify the energy, if we put the needle during expiration that will sedate the energy.*

F. *Slow or fast needling.* Putting the needle rapidly and removing it slowly will cause the tonification of energy and putting the needle slowly and removing it rapidly will cause the sedation of energy.

So the effect of tonification and sedation or dispersion can be achieved as follows:

Tonification	*Sedation*
1. Using a gold needle.	1. Using a silver needle.
2. Inserting a needle during inspiration.	2. Inserting a needle during expiration.
3. Putting the needle along the direction of energy flow.	3. Putting a needle against the direction of energy flow.
4. Rotating anticlock-wise.	4. Rotating clock-wise.
5. With little force, superficially mild stimulation.	5. With forcefully deep and strong stimulation.
6. Retain the needle for long time.	6. Retain the needle for short period.
7. Remove needle slowly.	7. Remove needle rapidly.
8. After removal of needle close the point with fingertip.	8. Leaving the point open after removal of needle or bleeding.

Now we will see the different types of needle hand stimulation.

Tapping. On the head of the needle with a finger tip very slow tapping can be done about 20 to 30 times in a minute. This is mild stimulation.

Up and down movement. Needle is held between the thumb and the index finger and slow up and down movements are carried out without taking out the needle from the skin at that point in the range of 1 cm and 5 to 20 times a minute. This is mild stimulation.

Rotating. The needle is held between the thumb and the index finger and is rotated by the fingers either clock-wise or anticlock-wise about 15 to 20 times a minute.

Flicking. The needle is held between the thumb and the index finger and up and down movement is carried out with needle moving in the range of 2 cm and at a very fast rate about 50 to 60 times per minute. This is strong stimulation.

Vibration. The needle is held between the thumb and the index finger and given the vibration sideways and up and down movement about 30 to 40 minutes. This is again a strong stimulation.

Snapping. The needle is held between the thumb and the index finger and then with very fast rotatory movements by the fingers up and down movements are carried out about 40 to 60 times a minute. This is very strong stimulation. Rotatory or pin rolling movement is carried out simultaneously with up and down movement.

Heat stimulation to the needle. After the needle is inserted at the point moxa is applied to the head of the needle and ignited or alternatively the needle head is given a direct heat with a fire to the inserted needle for ½ to 1 minute. This gives both the effects at a time where tonification as well as sedation or dispersion of energy is desired.

3. Hand stimulation

There are different ways to stimulate acupuncture points with the use of hand. Putting pressure over an acupuncture point is called acupressure and massaging the point or giving a peculiar type of vibration during massage is called as micromassage or acumassage.

Acupressure. Light pressure at the point will tonify the energy while the hard pressure at the point will disperse or sedate the energy. Hard pressure is applied for some time and immediately released after one or two minutes and again the pressure is applied. This method is very good to give fast relief in pain. Slow increase of pressure at particular points and slow release of pressure will give better results in some nervine conditions and psychosomatic diseases.

Acumassage. By massaging at the point we can either tonify the energy or sedate the energy.

Massage is of different types: *1. Tui* massage with palm and fingers, *2. Na* with the heel of palm deep massage is carried out, and *3. Ning* catching or pinching the body points in the hand and giving massage.

With *Tui* we can tonify the energy while with *Na* we sedate the energy and with *Ning* we can reduce the pain very fast by releasing the spasm of muscles.

Micromassage. If biceps muscle is tightly contracted then a few vibrations can be produced in the fingers. While creating these vibrations slow massage is given or hand massage is given with putting full force to vibrate whole body of the acupuncturist and this will give a micromassage.

With light micromassage we can tonify the energy while with deep micromassage we can sedate the energy.

There are many other methods of stimulating the acupuncture points with hand, and one of these is called *shietsu*, a Japanese system of giving pressure and massage at the acupuncture points.

With light type of massage circulation of blood is improved and with deep type of massage and pressure spasm of the muscle is reduced as well as due to the increase in muscle tone and release of endorphine pain is reduced.

Self stimulation

Acu Yoga. With self-exercises or typical types of yogic positions the pressure is located at the particular points and that is called Acu Yoga. These yogic exercises were practised well in olden days by saints in India. Now also many people practise it by themselves to maintain their health. Many different positions are described to get different types of curative effects.

Meridian exercises. Different meridian exercises are advised to the patients to maintain their body energy aquilibrium. These exercises resemble yogic positions with slight difference in it. These are the peculiar positions so that these slight difference in it. These are the peculiar positions so that these strech the meridians to stimulate total meridians with combination of self-massage at perticular points with hand. These can be very conveniently practised by a patient and are an additive factor to get better and quicker results.

Meridian exercises are the different ancient ways of stimulation which do not need any costly instruments and were practised for very long period giving very good results. But with the modern equipment being available other methods of treatment have come to be used in practice.

MODERN METHODS OF STIMULATION

Electrostimulation

After inserting the needle and to stimulate with the hand, it was rather clumsy and even disturbing when used for acupuncture anaesthesia. Electrostimulator was divised in 1966 in China to give electrical stimulation to these needles with different types of stimulation like: (*1*) Adjustable impulses, (*2*) dense and disperse impulses, (*3*) discontinuous type of impulses, (*4*) ripple type impulses, and (*5*) saw tooth type impulses (Fig. 7.2).

In the same instrument there is a point detector also, as it is proved that acupuncture points are the low electrical resistance points.

In most cases both 'low frequency electrical stimulation', which was used for rehabilitation or home treatment, and electroacupuncture treatment, which has been highlighted recently, are employed using the method of placing two terminals (plate terminal and needle terminal) on the body and making electricity flow between these two terminals.

The power of the electric stimulation is proportional to the density of the current; hence the part of the body around the smaller terminal that gives off a high electric density receives the bigger electric stimulation. The smaller plate terminal which transmits a higher electric density and stronger stimulation is called the "treatment terminal" or "negative terminal". The treatment therefore should be placed on the affected part or on a meridian point which is diseased or is showing a very low electrical resistance.

Negative electricity gives better stimulation using less electricity and therefore unless there is some special reason, the affected part should be treated by the treatment terminal (the negative terminal).

The treatment by electrostimulator, which is being used commonly, seems to have much effect because of a more complicated mechanism. In the case of simple acupuncture treatment, the practioners have been using the method whereby stimulation is given to the meridian points by the use of twirling and pecking technique. Basically, the electrostimulator works on the same principle of twirling and pecking technique, that is, the nerves around the insertion point of the needle are stimulated by the electricity, get excited and cause an implse, whereas the mechanical stimulation excites the nerve in hand stimulation.

The advantage of electrostimulator over the hand stimulation lies in the fact that it has the stimulating capacity around the acupuncture point within a field of 5 mm around the point in all lirections.

Electrical stimulation apparatus

The Electro-Acupuncture, model Apee-Stim AFI 8103 is a push button multipurpose acupuncture therapy apparatus which transmits five kinds of pulsating currents of different frequencies and intensities through the acupuncture needles to the human body for therapeutic

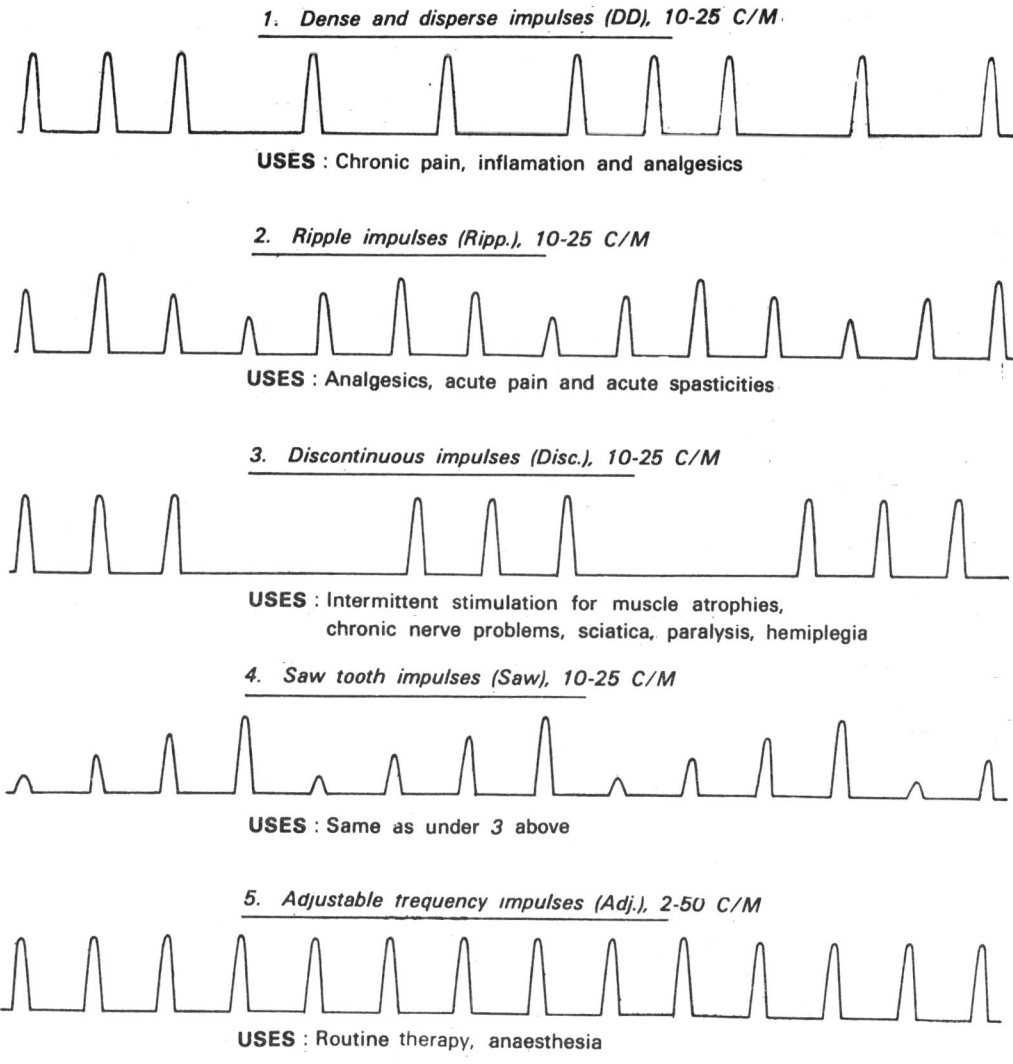

1. *Dense and disperse impulses (DD), 10-25 C/M*

USES : Chronic pain, inflamation and analgesics

2. *Ripple impulses (Ripp.), 10-25 C/M*

USES : Analgesics, acute pain and acute spasticities

3. *Discontinuous impulses (Disc.), 10-25 C/M*

USES : Intermittent stimulation for muscle atrophies, chronic nerve problems, sciatica, paralysis, hemiplegia

4. *Saw tooth impulses (Saw), 10-25 C/M*

USES : Same as under 3 above

5. *Adjustable frequency impulses (Adj.), 2-50 C/M*

USES : Routine therapy, anaesthesia

Fig. 7.2 Wave patterns in electrostimulation

purposes or anaesthesia (Fig. 7.3). This apparatus is used in the treatment of various diseases in clinical operation for an acupuncture anaesthesia. It is also suitable for use in order to promote the efficiency of acupuncture treatment or acupuncture therapy.

The specific character of the stimulator is if in any disorder only *yin* or *yang* current is required it can also be adjusted by using the switches located above the output knobs.

Acuscope
Acuscope is the instrument which is used for measuring the electical resistance of skin. It is designed to detect the specific point where electrical resistance of skin is below normal. This gives an indication of the acupuncture point. If electrical resistance drops down further, the

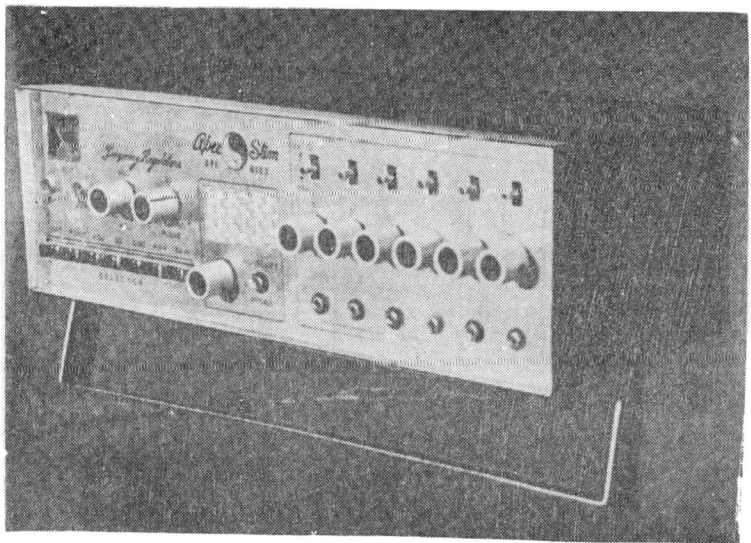

Fig. 7.3 A typical electrostimulator

abnormally lowered electrical resistance indicates the diseased point. In acuscope (Fig. 7.4) sound is the indication for measuring electrical resistance. If the frequency of sound is low it shows that electrical resistance it low, but if the frequency of sound is high, it shows that the electrical resistance is further dropped down and hence it is the diseased point. If acuscope does not produce any sound, it means that the skin is normal or it is the normal acupuncture point.

Magnetic stimulation

With the help of magnets the energy can be stimulated in a meridian. If we want to tonify a point, put the south pole of one magnet over the diseased point and the north pole seeing the direction of energy flow in that meridian proximal to it. So to tonify we have to stimulate along the direction of energy from the north pole to the south pole. For immunity improving we can use the north pole on the diseased place or immunity improving point.

For the upper half of the body we can use the north pole at the left palm and south pole at the right palm, and in the same way we can use for lower half body disorders north pole at left sole south pole at right sole.

There are a few newer instruments called as magnetrones which create magnetic field all around the body and can be controlled by electric field so that the energy can be chanalised as desired.

Stimulation by rays

A simple infrared lamp or ultraviolet lamp can be used to stimulate the acupuncture points. Infrared light usually causes reliving of pain and ultraviolet rays have the immunity-improving and tonification effects.

There are a few instruments which are manufactured by using modern techniques to give the infrared rays and ultraviolet rays in a narrow beam which can be used to stimulate the acupuncture points to get the desired effect.

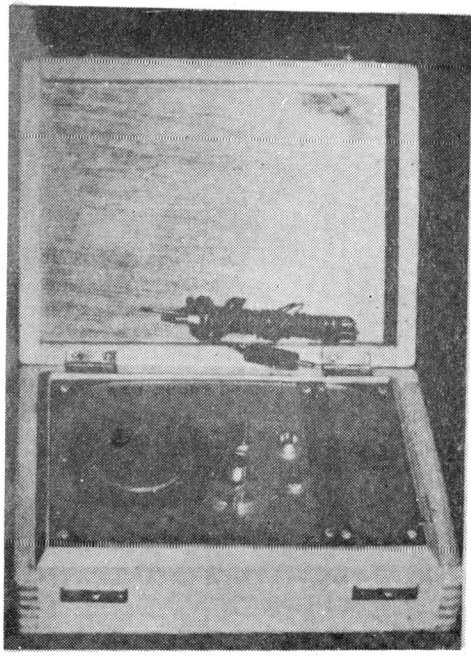

Fig. 7.4 Acuscope

Instead of inserting the filliform needles, these rays can be used safely without the painful pricking of the needles, especially in the case of very old people, small children and the extremely sensitive patients.

With the introduction of the laser technology, laser acupuncture machines have been introduced to help the acupuncturists in modernising their methods of treatment (Figs. 7.5 & 7.6).

High frequency vibrations

Radio frequency acupuncture. When the radio-frequency sound wave is converted to produce vibrations and used for the acupuncture points stimulation that is called as "radio frequency acupuncture."

The frequency of electroacupuncture is about 1 to 1000 Hz per second while in radio-frequency it is from 1000 Hz to 10,000 Hz per second. With these ranges of stimulation we can create even acupuncture anaesthesia.

Transcutaneous acupuncture. Since 1970, the Army General Hospital in Canton, China, has used cutaneous electrodes instead of needles, in several hundred surgical operations; with a reported 98 per cent success rate. Skin electrodes, applied over the chosen acupuncture points, have also been used in conjunction with electrical stimulation in acupuncture therapy, especially in paediatrics, for obvious reasons. The method consists of a small metal plate affixed to the particular acupuncture point and stimulated electrically in a fashion similar to the conventional electroacupuncture using transcutaneous acupuncture needles (Fig. 7.7). It has certain

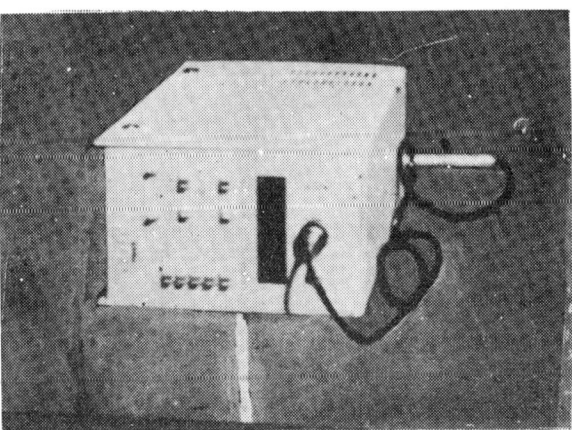

Fig. 7.5 Laser equipment

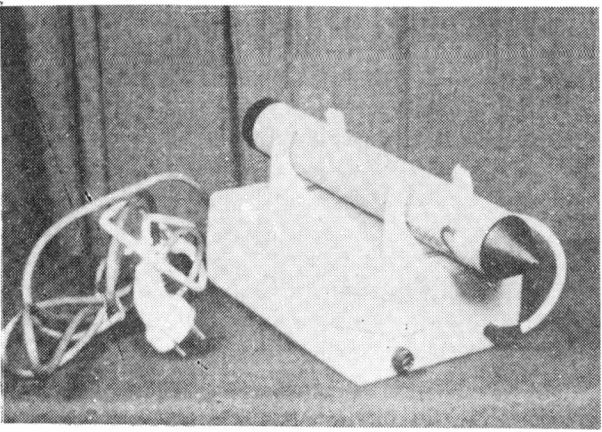

Fig. 7.6 Laser stimulator

advantages, the most obvious of which is the absence of skin puncture and its possible consequences like pain and infection, etc. Many cases, however, do not respond to this type of stimulation for long periods and also chronic cases do not show better results with this type of stimulation, especially the patients of polio and paralysis, who do not show the similar results as obtained from using the routine acupuncture.

It has been suggested that cutaneous stimulation is more acceptable for most patients, especially children, old aged patients and very sensitive patients. This method, therefore, should be used in preference to the others for children as well as for patients anxious and frightemed at the anticipation of pain by needles.

Recently developed and advanced machine is very small, handy and can stimulate with case at the point desired instead of putting the cutaneous plates. The intensity and frequency also can be adjusted as desired and hence can be used for the minor anaesthesia purposes i.e. for dental extraction, etc.

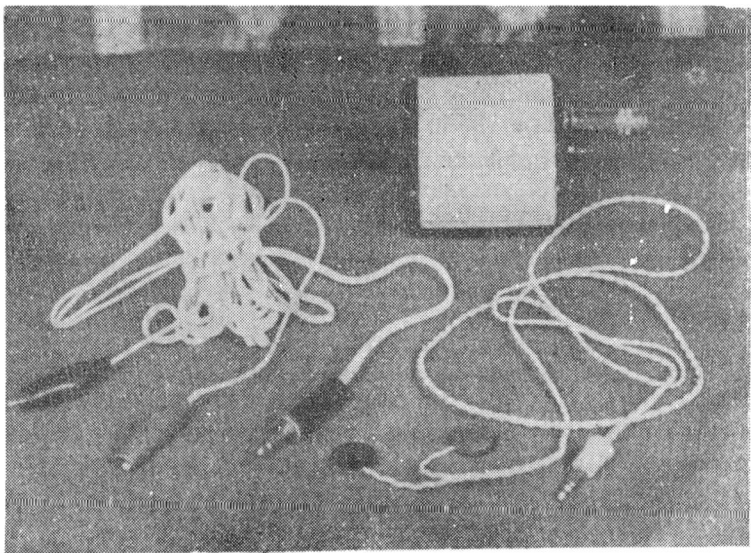

Fig. 7.7 Transcutaneous stimulator

There are many recently developed instruments like ultrasound and radio frequency stimulator which transmit transcutaneous stimulations. The bipolar biphasic electrical impulse by the stimulator created when transmited through the nerves gives the desired effect. Hence an accurate knowledge of the dermatones is necessary for transcutaneous stimulation with acupuncture points.

Ultrasonic Stimulation. In 1946 Horvath reported that malignant tumours respond favourably to the application of ultrasonics but later on it was found to be wrong. However, Horvath's claim stimulated the development of ultrasonic therapy and its ecritical evaluation. Many scientists and hospitals are involved in evaluating the effects of ultrasonics. At first only two components of the effect of ultrasonic waves were regarded as biologically significant, the thermal and the machanical action respectively. Afterwards it was realised that physio chemical and highly specific neurotrophic effects contributed to the biological actions of ultrasonics. It was well known that in the effect of thermal action simple conceptions did not account for the effects and that the heat librated by the ultrasonic waves was of critical importance at the interfaces where these are penerated by the wave bundle. As to the neurotrophic effects, their recognition is mostly due to the studies by Stublfauth and Tschannen. These scientists have proved that the effect of ultrasnonics is largely indirect one evoked through relfex arches or head's zones. Physiochemical factors have been studied by Homy Kie Witsch. His studies, as well as the observations of Denier, Henker and Butehtala, provide a theoritical background to the empirical fact that even relatively small amounts of ultrasonic energy may have pronounced clinical effects.

Investigations carried out since 1946 have also shown that it is very difficult to choose appropriate dosage of ultrasonics and that may create some clinical difficulties than expected. First, it is generally acknowledged that the patient by reporting subjective pain determines the permissible limit of dosage and similarly reports subjective skin sensations if the contact between sound head and the skin is impaired. However, determination of dosage is still of importance in many critical investigations and where comparative analysis of results is intended. The conclusion has been reached that the simple dosage indicators are inadequate for estimating the amount of energy actually applied and that the following data are required for an accurate description of dosage.

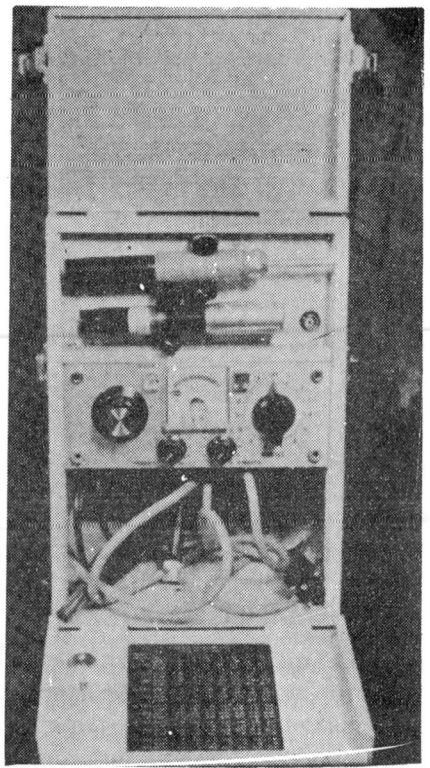

1. Wattage per unit area of skin (per square centimeter)
2. Area of the sound head surface emitting the waves
3. Frequency
4. Modulated or unmodulated waves
5. Precise indication of usage of continuous or impulse waves
6. Nature of contact medium
7. Type of application (massage type of fixed application)

Fig. 7.8 Ultrasonic stimulator

"Using such data with estimating different results, it is concluded that an out put of 3 watts per square centimeter has to be demanded, although, a fixed sound head requires only a fraction of this intensity. In theory, it might be possible therefore to work with lower intensities than 3 watts per square centimeter but the fixed sound head is not always applicable and modern instruments have a total output of 25 to 40 watts, thus providing for an adequate area of emission. Higher intensities have not proved to be of any value in clinical practice. Extended investigations have also shown that the frequency of the waves has little effect upon the clinical result provided that it lies somewhere between 300 and 1500 kc with the frequencies usually employed are 800 to 1200 kc or a half value of 3.5 to 4.5 centimeters is assured and this enables us to reach any of the targets provided the approach is not impeded by intervening interfaces such as that are produced by air spaces, periosteum, etc.

The choice between the modulated and the unmodulated waveform has been decided in favour of the former. As to the alternative between impulse and continuous waveforms, no general decision can be made, but it is said that the impulse therapy is not invested with any specific advantages.

It is also belived that the risk of excessive dosage is possible with the use of impulse waves similarly no therapeutic advantage has been observed from the use of devises which produce a convergence of the wave bundle. Figure 7.8 shows a typical ultrosonic stimulator currently being used by the acupuncturists.

8

METHODS OF DIAGNOSIS

We will consider the diagnostic methods under three headings : (1) Modern diagnostic methods, (2) the traditional Chinese diagnostic methods, and (3) methods which should be adopted by practitioners of the acupuncture in the modern times.

MODERN DIAGNOSTIC METHODS

History taking

The patient is interrogated for the complaints, duration of illness, occupation, social status, environment in which he lives, past illness and the family history.

Clinical examinations

(a) General examination is done as follows:
Pulse, temperature, nails, pupils, conjunctiva, neck veins, glands, visible pulsations throat, etc. are examined and findings are recorded systematically.

(b) Systemic examination:
Digestive, respiratory, cardiovascular, musculoskeletal nervous and genito-urinary systems are examined by four standard methods : Inspection, palpation, percussion and auscultation.

(c) Special clinical tests:
Certain clinical tests are carried out to rule out specific diseases.

(d) Local examination of the part affected is carefully done.

(e) Special examinations are performed as follows:

PR	Rectal examination by finger
Proctoscopy	Rectal examination with proctoscope
PV	Vaginal examination by fingers
PS	Vaginal examination with speculum

Investigations

Investigations are done for the confirmation of the diagnosis provisionally made by clinical examination.

83

(i) Simple laboratory tests, e.g., urine, blood, stool and sputum examination.

(ii) Advanced investigations, e.g., X-ray, scanning, screening, ECG, EEG, electromyogram, serum levels of electrolytes, sugar, cholesterol, urea, VDRL, Widal, antigen-antibody tests, etc.

(iii) Surgical exploration, biopsy and histopathology.

(iv) Autopsy. If the patient dies, the body may be subjected to an autopsy to know the real cause of illness leading to death. In such cases autopsy constitutes the final diagnosis, enriches the clinical experience of the clinicians and provides an opportunity of correlating the signs and symptoms with the pathological findings.

THE TRADITIONAL CHINESE DIAGNOSTIC METHODS

The clinicians in the the past were devoid of the knowledge of laboratory investigations, histopathology and exploratory surgery. Autopsy was not possible due to social and religious reasons. The diagnostic methods advocated by the traditional Chinese clinicians are described below.

1. *Inspection.* The first step in diagnosis used to be, without putting question to the patient, inspecting the patient in various ways as in the modern times.

2. *Auscultation.* Ancient clinicians did not have the benefit of the stethoscope and used their ears for the purpose. However, a modern acupuncturist has the added advantage of the use of stethoscope.

3. *Smelling.* Some diseases can be diagnosed just by smelling, e.g. ketoacidisos and coma, can be detected by the typical smell of breath.

4. *History taking No. 1.* This comprises the history obtained from the patient himself.

5. *Percussion.* The body is percussed at various places as is done in the systemic examination of modern medicine.

6. *Palpation.* This is the most important step in the diagnosis.
   (a) Palpation of whole body.
   (b) Palpation of Ah-shi points of particular diseased area.
   (c) Pulse diagnosis: This has been described in details in a separate chapter.

7. *Special tests.* These consist of naked eye examination of excreta, e.g. urine, stool, sputum, vomitus, semen, etc. They may be done at the pathological laboratory if patient can afford.

8. *Special examination.* These consist of examination of eyes, tongue, lips, skin, hair, nails, formation of bones, etc. This is similar to general examination of the modern medicine.

9. *Examination of the ear.* According to the ear acupuncture chart, sometimes there is change in the colour of a particular area of the ear or a reddish nodular lesion appears on specific area which indicates disease of that particular organ.

10. *History of dreams.* Traditional Chinese acupuncturists used to believe that dreams indicate present or future disease. It is, however, a specialist job and may therefore be treated as optional.

11. *History No. 2.* The disease and pre-illness health of the patient is enquired after from the relatives or close friends, e.g. wife, husband, children and neighbours.

METHODS WHICH SHOULD BE ADOPTED BY PRACTITIONERS OF THE ACUPUNCTURE IN THE MODERN TIMES

It is strongly recommended that the history be taken in all the ways—detailed history as in modern medicine, history No. 1 and history No. 2. Clinical examination as described in modern diagnostic methods should also be made. If needed, help of special examination and modern investigations should also be taken. In certain difficult cases histopathologic investigation is also helpful.

Smelling is also helpful but not in all the cases. A thorough palpation of all the alarm points and Ah-shi points is essential.

Every acupuncture specialist must have a good practice of pulse diagnosis and it must be done in every case. Ear must be examined as already described. Additional help can be obtained from an instrument called point detector (acupuncturoscope).

9
PULSE DIAGNOSIS

Traditional Chinese pulses described in the Nei Jing are entirely different from the pulse described in modern medical science. For the Western trained physician the pulse is one and its rate, rhythm, tension, volume, etc. indicate a condition to which some name is given, e.g., bradycardia, tachycardia, thyroid toxicity, cardiac arrhythmia, jaundice, enteric fever, etc. The pulse for an acupuncturist is the outward expression of the flow and rhythm of 'Chi' and its imbalance inside the body either within or between the meridians. Its knowledge and perfection is the basic requirement in the making of an acupuncturist because it not only suggests the diagnosis but also the time and manner of treatment. Much of the prescription depends upon the diagnosis.

Pulse diagnosis is a very sensitive matter—it is both an art and a science. An acupuncturist has to learn the art of listening and appreciating the music of pulses on the wrists of the patient through his own finger tips. The real skill requires on the part of the clinician, a constant effort to palpate the pulses religiously with great patience, receptive mind, and apt touch of his finger on the wrists of the patient, a great concentration, and above all a very keen desire to know his patient from within. Pulses never lie. They tell in great detail the past, present and future of the patient's body and illness, provided one knows how to listen them. Their music is the music of life. The Chinese believe that every illness reflects in the pulses before it causes obvious symptoms.

TRADITIONAL PULSE POSITIONS

Traditionally there are twelve pulse positions, each related to one meridian and a viscera. Six pulses are positioned on the right wrist and six pulses on the left wrist. Out of the six on each side three are superficial (Fu) and other three are deep (Chen). The location is on the front of the wrist, where the radial pulse is felt by the trained physician. The radial pulse is divided into three sections—the one close to the hand is called the t-sun or inch (first position); the middle one is called the Chih or bar (second position) and the remaining one is the kuan or cubit (third position). On these sections pulses are both superficial and deep. The superficial ones are Yang and felt by light touch while deep ones are Yin and appreciated by pressure. The superficial pulses on the left side are small intestine, gall bladder and urinary bladder; and on the right side, large intestine, stomach and triple warmer on the cun, guan and chih positions. On the same positions, the deep pulses are heart, liver and kidney on the left side and lung, spleen and pericardium on the right side (Figs. 9.1, 9.2, 9.3).

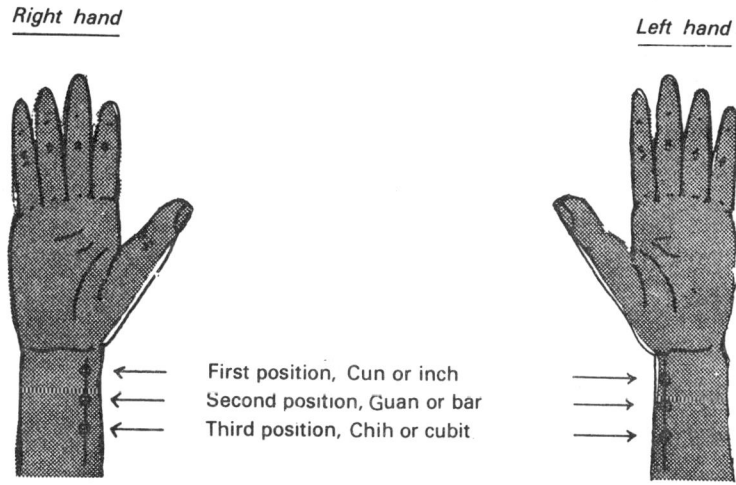

Fig. 9.1   Traditional pulse positions.

METHODS OF PULSE DIAGNOSIS

1. The physician should take his own pulse as the standard before taking the patient's pulses. This also indicates that the physician must be in good health.
2. The physician must be relaxed, calm and receptive.
3. There should be complete silence during pulse diagnosis.
4. The best time for pulse diagnosis is between 5 AM and 1 PM.
5. Position of the patient—
   (a) The patient must be asked to rest for at least ten minutes quietly before the pulse diagnosis for calming down any emotional upset or physical exertion.
   (b) The patient should be comfortably recumbent and the physician should face the patient while taking the pulse. A small pad or cushion should be kept under the back of the patient's arms and wrists, so that his hands are slightly dorsiflexed. This makes the palpation of the pulse easier.
6. If the patient is male, the left wrist pulse is taken first; if the patient is female, the right wrist pulse is taken first.
7. While taking the pulses the practitioner should place the finger tips of his index middle and ring fingers on the first, second and third positions of the radial artery of one hand and then the other hand of the patient's left wrist. Pulses are taken by the practitioner's right hand and the right wrist pulses by his left hand.
8. The practitioner should first keep the finger tips gently and read the pulses in the three different positions. Then he should press deep till the pulses disappear. The pressure should then be released gradually till the pulses just start reappearing again. This should be done in all the three positions, using the pressure with only one finger at a time.

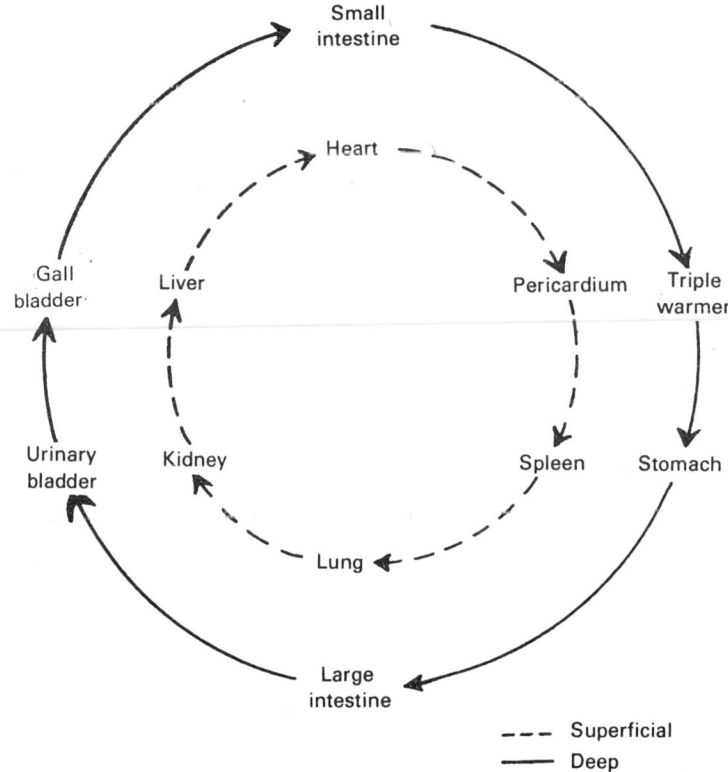

Fig. 9.2 Pulse circulation.

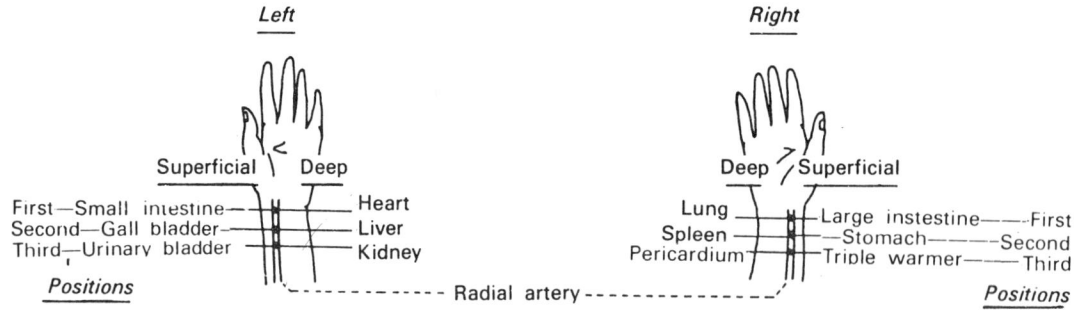

Fig. 9.3 Indication position of 12 pulses.

9. During the pulse diagnosis, every time, the practitioner must concentrate and imagine the organ, meridian and flow of the 'Chi'. He should silently tell himself about the pulses. While palpating the urinary bladder pulse he can just say—I am listening to urinary bladder pulse and it is telling me about the flow of the 'Chi'.

10. In case of weak pulse Yangchi (TW-4) can be stimulated. This will increase the strength of the pulse.

11. After finishing with the taking of the pulses, the practitioner must record his findings in systemetic way on a chart and start making various correlations and interpretations.

NORMAL PULSE

A normal pulse is rhythmic, smooth, free flowing, calm, elastic and compressible but with a certain amount of tension.

The pulses on the left wrist are normally stronger than those on the right wrist (husband-wife law).

Normal pulse—respiration ratio is 4 : 1 (four pulse beats for one full respiration).

Seasonal variations

In spring it is slow, slippery and gentle. In summer it is stronger but fades away quietly. In autumn it beats lightly and wanes quickly. In winter it is deep and urgent.

What to record in pulse diagnosis

1. Rate : Count the pulse beat and respiration per minute. Calculate pulse—respiration ratio.
2. Strength
3. Rhythm
4. Volume
5. Character
6. Regular, irregular or intermittent.
7. Influence of age, sex, constitution, background, temperament, weather, time of the day, season of the year.

The basic qualities of a pulse

There are twenty-eight commonly used pulse qualities. Because of minor differences and impracticability of differentiating, they are classified into the following groups.

1. Floating—Superficial feeling, like a piece of wood floating on water
2. Deep (Ch'en)—Deep feeling like a stone thrown into the river
3. Rapid (Hsu)—Beats six or more times in one respiratory cycle
4. Slow (Ch'ih)—Beats three or four times in one respiratory cycle
5. Sippery—Feels like stone rolling along the bottom of a smooth kettle
6. Hollow—Feels like an onion stalk
7. Hard—Tense like the surface of a drum.

Other qualities of the pulses are as follows:

Sinking, fragmentary, buoyant, bounding, continuous, empty, long, full, short, small, tense, overflowing, thready, wiry, taut, slender, running, tremulous, scattering, intermittent and irregular.

The most important characteristics of the pulses

Rate and strength of the pulse are the most important characteristics, the rest are secondary in the meridian diagnosis. The secondary characteristics help in progress and prognosis.

Number system of pulse readings

This system is a comfortable way of recording the state of the pulses in their respective positions.

On the Yin or deficient side

......3—2—1—0

0—Patient is as good as dead

3—Deficiency sufficient to warrant action

On the Yang side

......5—6—7—8

8—Patient is in the extremes

Fatal pulses

Classically there are 27 fatal pulses, e.g. in the case of enteric fever a thready small and soft pulse is a fatal pulse and suggests a poor prognosis.

The characteristics of a good diagnostician

1. He should be in perfect health himself.
2. He must possess a very good concentrating capacity.
3. He should be able to detect the illness long before the symptoms manifest.

What a traditional Chinese diagnostician does

1. He keeps his own pulses healthy and uses them as standard.
2. He studies the pulses for 10 minutes to 3 hours.
3. He tries to differentiate in each of the twelve pulses, upto twenty-seven different qualities.
4. He judges more than three hundred distinct characteristics in a patient's pulse.

Readings and Interpretations

1. The state of Yin and Yang
   (a) The Yin and Yang imbalance is to be recorded. Left is the character of Yang, right is the character of Yin.
   (b) Wheather Yin or Yang has moved out of proportion—if all the pulses are too strong, hard or full, too much Chi is present in one organ or another.
   (c) If the superficial pulses are too stong, hard or full, too much Yang is present.
   (d) If the deep pulses are light, hesitant or wavering, too much Yin is present.
   (e) Relative strengths of pulses. If t-sun is stronger than Kuan, Yin is over-powered by Yang. The opposite means that Yin has become too powerful.

2. The meridian affected and the exact nature of any illness in the body
   A wiry pulse at large intestine tells that large intestine meridian is imbalanced and the patient has intestinal parasites. An elevated, hard pulse in the same spot indicates constipation. Rapid pulse indicates chronic physiological imbalance and a wiry pulse is found in spasm, pain and nervousness. Deficiency states are indicated by a hollow pulse on greater pressure.
   Biliary and renal stones are suggested by the hard, round and incompressible pulses. Blow up pulse in stomach position indicates aerogastria while the same type in heart position is suggestive of cardiac hypertrophy.

3. *The state of the related meridian*

The first position on the right wrist yields the pulses of the lung (deep) and large intestine (superficial). These two organs are paired. Lung is deep. It is an internal pulse and corresponds with a Yin organ.

4. *Strengths on the two sides*

Comparison of the strength of the pulses on the two sides can be of great help in the diagnosis. For example, in the case of a pregnant woman, rapid pulses on right wrist means she has a female fetus and rapid pulses on left wrist means she has a male fetus.

5. *Seasonal variations*

Pulses that do not behave as they should according to season indicate illness.

6. Whether the treatment is effective or not.

10

METHODS OF ACUPUNCTURE

ACUPUNCTURE NEEDLES

Needles made of stone, bone and bamboo were used in the past to stimulate acupuncture points on the body for getting desired response. In the course of evolution primitive needles were replaced by those of metals. Ultimately stainless steel was found to be quite effective and economical, and it is now the most commonly used material for the manufacturing of the needles. Originally nine different types of needles were used but at present only three to four types of needles are in common use.

VARIOUS TYPES OF NEEDLES AND THEIR USAGE

1. Common needle (filliform needle)

This type of needle has five parts as shown in Fig. 10.1. These needles are available in all the lengths ranging from 0.5 t-sun to 8.0 t-sun sizes and they are selected according to the site and desired depth of insertion.

Diameter. The needles are available in different diameters. Since the thick needles produce more pain, while thin needles are less painful, the thickness of the needles should be selected according to the site of needling.

The methods of selecting the needles for acupuncture. The following way of the selection of the needles for different places is advised.

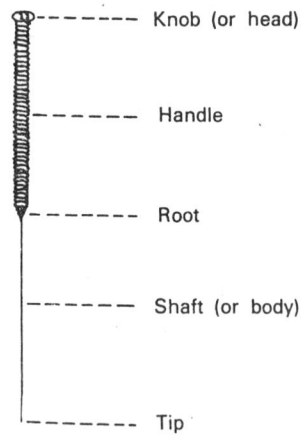

— Knob (or head)

— Handle

— Root

— Shaft (or body)

— Tip

Fig. 10.1 Showing parts of needle.

The size and depth should depend on the location of the point and the type of the point which is being stimulated.

Body area	Needle size in mm	Length
1. Scalp	28, 30	1.5 to 2 t-sun
2. Periorbital	32, 34	0.5 to 1 t-sun
3. Face	30, 32	0.5 to 1 t-sun
4. Ear	30, 32	0.5 t-sun or less
5. Chest	30	0.5 t-sun or less
6. Abdomen	30	0.5 to 1 t-sun
7. Upper extremity	30	1 to 2 t-sun
8. Buttock	28, 30	3 to 5 t-sun
9. Lower extremity	28, 30	2 to 3 t-sun
10. Hand and foot	30	0.5 to 1-tsun

2. Triangular needle (sanlingchen)

This is also known as prismatic needle. It has three cutting edges (triple cutting edge). It is generally used during acute emergencies like high fever, coma, shock, convulsions, etc.

The technique. These needles are used for bleeding from Jing-well points. The needle is held between the thumb and the index finger and a superficial rotation is made until bleeding occurs. After a few drops of blood ooze out from the point, the spot is pressed to stop any further bleeding.

3. Seven star needles (Plum-Blossom needle)

Seven small needles are arranged like a star over a hammer. This is used to prick the skin surface to produce very superficial puncture by light touch until the area becomes red (Fig. 10.2).

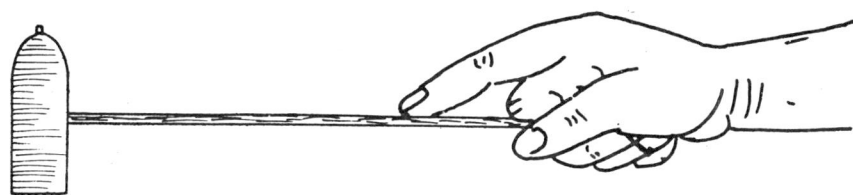

Fig 10.2 Holding a seven star dermal needle.

Indications. All skin diseases like eczema, psoriasis, dermatitis, leucoderma, alopacia, etc.

4. Press needle

It is round in shape and has a small thorn connected with a round base (Fig. 10.3). The length of the tip is about 1 mm. This needle is commonly used when a continuous stimulation is required on ear points in the conditions like bronchial asthma and addictions.

Technique. The needle should be fixed on the ear point and covered with adhesive leucoplast to prevent it from falling.

Duration. The needle can be kept for 3 to 5 days and the patient is advised to massage over it 3 to 4 times a day.

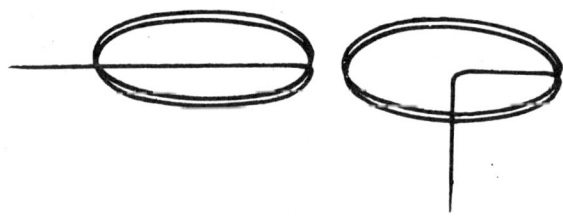

Fig. 10.3 Showing round body press needle.

5.   Hidden subdermal needles

These needles are of small size, 0.3 to 0.5 t-sun in length.   They can also be kept in place for 3 to 5 days and covered with sticking plaster.

Indications.   Asthma, headache, hepatitis, myopia, etc.

Sterilisation of the needles

The needles are kept immersed in 70% alcohol for a period of 24 hours.

Boiling in water should be avoided as it may destory the sharpness of the tips of the needles.

TECHNIQUE OF ACUPUNCTURE

Hold the needle between the thumb and index finger.   Bring the tip of the needle near the acupuncture point and use it rapidly for piercing the skin.   After crossing the skin the needle can be passed further with a firm rotation and pressure over it and if the needle has gone more deep it can be withdrawn.   After inserting the needle it should be manipulated by hand until Te-chi is achieved.

Te-chi (taking of vital energy)

When the tip of the needle is inserted to the correct depth at the acupuncture point a sensation of pain, sourness, numbness, heaviness, fullness and distension may be experienced by the patient. This is the proper response sought.   There should be no pain if the procedure is done properly except for certain points on the hand, foot, face and ear points.

Different areas on the body have different Te-chi, i.e.

Scalp and face	Only numbness
Fingers and toes	Slight pain
Chest and abdomen	Localised numbness
Extremities	All the sensations of Te-chi

Direction of the needle (Figs. 10.4 and 10.5)

Straight or perpendicular	90°
Used for extremities	
Slanting or oblique	30-60°
where there is not very thick	
muscle such as on the chest and head	10-20°
Horizontal	

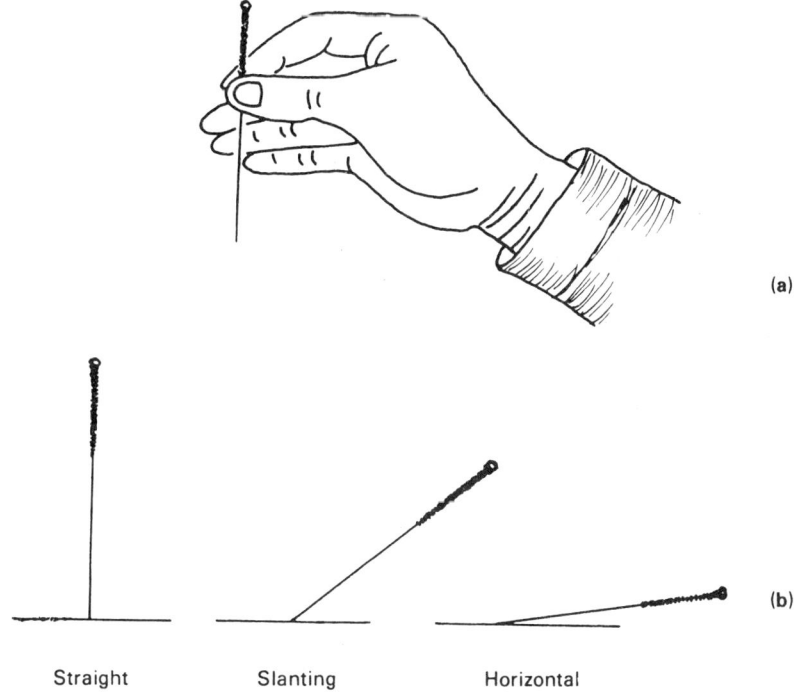

Fig. 10.4   (a)—Holding the needle; (b)—Showing direction of needle insertion.

Straight   Slanting   Horizontal

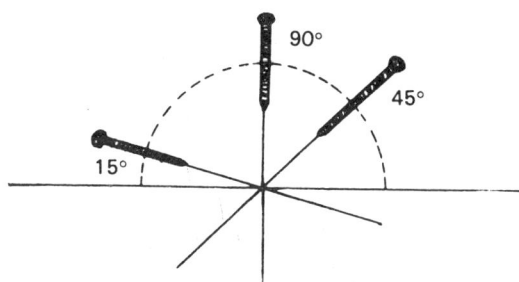

Fig. 10.5   Angles of needle insertion.

Point to point (PP)

Means the needle from one point penetrates through the tissue to another point, e.g. Yingling Quan (Sp-9) to Yangling Quan (GB-34) in lower limb paralysis.

NOTE: Oblique and horizontal directions are usually used for face, skull and chest area. The straight direction of the needle may cause visceral puncture.

Type of stimulation

After the achievement of Te-chi the needle is stimulated by the following methods (Fig. 10.6):

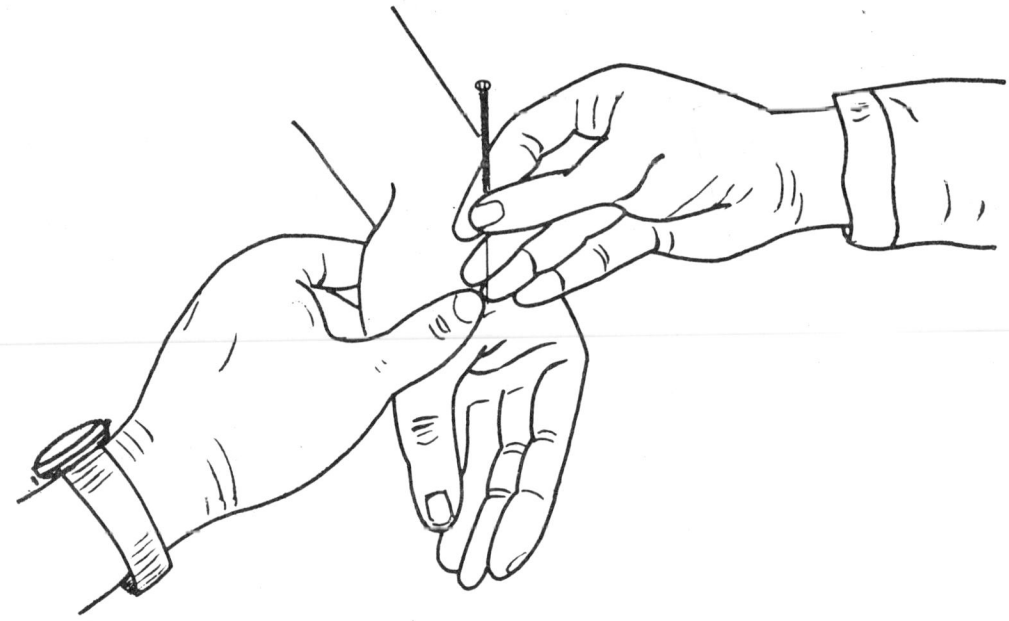

Fig. 10.6 Showing method of needle insertion.

1. Up and down movement: Within 1 cm.
2. Rotation: To and fro rotation of the needle between the thumb and index finger. Rotation should be equidistant to prevent needle dystocia.
3. Flicking: Produced by the thumb and index finger. Usually 20 flicks per period of stimulation. This procedure causes strong stimulation.
4. Vibration: 1 to 2 mm rapid up and down movements done with the fist for 1 to 2 minutes.
5. Snapping: Produced by the snapping of the middle finger on the needle gently.

Manipulation of needle (Fig. 10.7)

It is affected in three ways:
1. *Common method.* After insertion the needle is rotated 240 times back and forth with a steady force.
2. *Supplement method.* The needle is strongly inserted and gently lifted up. This is also called 'Po' method in China.
3. *Deflecting method.* The needle is inserted gently but lifted strongly. This is also called 'Hsiehs' method in China.

Degree of stimulation

1. *Strong stimulation.* Up and down, snapping, flicking for acute cases and younger patients.
2. *Medium stimulation.* Up and down, snapping, flicking similarly as above except that it is gently or slowly applied.
3. *Weak stimulation.* Slow rotation, slow flicking used for older patients and chronic cases. It is also used for sedation and insomnia.

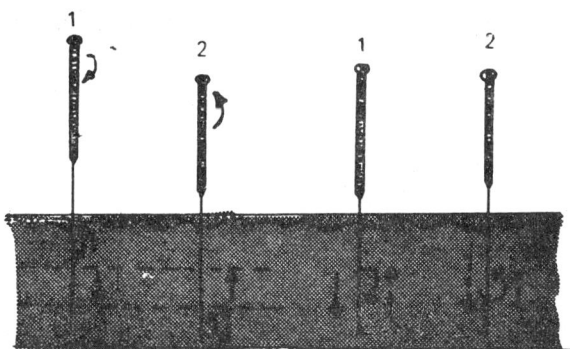

Fig. 10.7 Showing manupulation of needle.

Duration of stimulation

1. *Short*. Needle insertion until Te-chi is accomplished, then use all the types of stimulation techniques for about 20 seconds and remove the needle. Used for general problems such as toothache, headache, etc.

2. *Intermediate*. Following Te-chi rotate needles for several seconds, stop for 2—3 minutes then repeat the rotation. Total time for this course is 10—20 minutes according to the response desired. Used for chronic conditions such as sciatica, migrane, arthritis, etc.

3. *Continuous*. Following Te-chi, continuous twisting of needle for 1 to 2 hours or until patient has relief from his symptoms. This is used for renal colic, acute headache, etc.

NOTE : Generally for acute cases such as early appendicitis the course is 1-3 treatments per day until symptoms subside, in chronic cases 1 treatment per day for 10 days. Following each 10-days period give rest to the patient for 5-7 days before resuming next course. This is done to prevent insensitiveness and point tolerance.

POINT INJECTION THERAPY AND EMBEDDING THERAPY

Point injection therapy

It is observed that the acupuncture points when injected with aqua or drugs remain stimulated for a long time. This forms the basis of the point injection therapy. When Te-chi is achieved and drug is injected, it produces a local inflamation and the acupuncture point is kept stimulated for a longer period.

Embedding therapy (cat-gut therapy)

A piece of cat-gut is tied on the point, it serves the same purpose of prolonged point stimulation. Such a technique is known as embedding therapy.

11

MOXIBUSTION

The dry powder of the leaf of *Artemisia vulgaris* is known as 'moxa' and when used for acupuncture therapy, the method is termed as 'moxibustion'. Moxibustion was introduced in the field of acupuncture during 1102 to 1106 A.D. It serves a purpose similar to that of acupuncture; normalising the flow of 'Qi' in Yin and Yang. That the application of heat over a painful area in the body is capable of relieving pain is a well known fact and the results are much better when the centre of the painful area is selected for heating. The same principle forms the basis of moxibustion. It is suggested that as the heat forms the basis of moxibustion it is Yang in nature (Dr. Nakayam of Japan). It is known to increase the number of red blood corpuscles and the percentage of haemoglobin in the blood.

PREPARATION OF THE MOXA WOOL AND ITS USE

The leaves of *Artemisia vulgaris* are dried in the sunlight and powdered after the soil and sand are removed. The powder thus prepared appears as a yellowish, white soft textured wool like substance and is known as moxa wool.

Moxa wool can be coarse and fine in quality depending upon its texture. Fine textured moxa wool is used in direct moxibustion while in indirect moxibustion coarse textured moxa wool is used. For prolonged moxibustion old moxa wool is the best material.

Storage

Storage of moxawool should be done only in the dry containers, otherwise it loses its properties. It should be prevented from becoming mouldy and every year it should be exposed to sunlight for the times sufficient enough to keep it dry.

The moxa podwer is used in acupuncture in the following ways:

1. Moxa cone : Moxa podwer as such is being used by making "moxacones" and burnt over the acupuncture and Ah-shi points (Fig. 11.1).
2. Moxa roll : Moxa powder is compressed into a cigar like structure known as "moxa roll" and burnt. It is then kept 2 to 4 cm away from the selected point till the point becomes pink (Fig. 11.2).

*Dr. K. L. Tiwari, Department of Botany, Govt. College of Science, Raipur (M.P.), India.

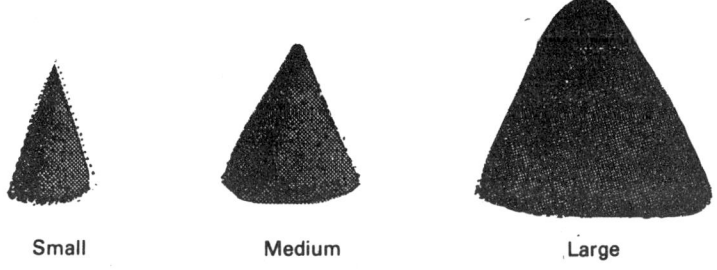

Small   Medium   Large

Fig. 11.1   Moxa cone.

Preparation of Moxa roll

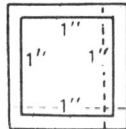

6 Shi t-sun (Chinese inch) × 0.5 Shi t-sun

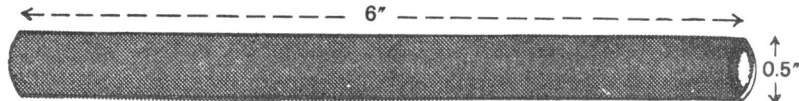

Fig. 11.2   Showing moxa-roll.

3.   Drugs : Recently a few drugs have also been made in the Peoples' Republic of China in the form of capsules, oral and nasal spray.

DIFFERENT METHODS OF MOXIBUSTION

Moxibustion therapy on the basis of treatment is divided into two categories:
1.   Direct moxibustion.
2.   Indirect moxibustion.

1.   Direct moxibustion

In this method the moxa wool is kept over the selected point on the body and burnt. Direct moxibustion is of two types—

(i)   Scarring moxibustion

Moxa wool is kept directly over the acupuncture point of the body and ignited until the skin is burnt. As the term "scarring" indicates, the burning leads to the scarring of the skin and the scar persists.

(ii) Non-scarring moxibustion

In this method moxa wool is kept over the selected point on the body and ignited. But burning of skin is prevented by removing the moxa wool when skin becomes very hot.

Direct moxibustion is capable of producing many other beneficial effects, particularly those of the histotoxins which are the humoral substances produced by the burning skin. They activate the functions of the reticuloendothelial system, which in turn increases the body resistance. It is known to possess anti-allergic properties also.

Direct moxibustion is used for the chronic diseases like cough, cold, asthma, chronic diarrhoea and indigestion. Direct moxibustion leads to pain and burning of skin leading to blisters. This is a crude method of treatment, therefore, it has been rejected by various acupuncturists of the world.

2. Indirect moxibustion

In this procedure moxa wool is never brought in direct touch with the skin. A barrier should be kept in-between the skin and the moxa which may be ginger, garlic or salt.

The following methods are being used:

(i) Indirect moxibustion with ginger

In this process ginger is used as a barrier between the moxa wool and skin. Slices of ginger are made by cutting thin pieces of 1 to 2 cm diameter and the moxa wool is kept over them and burnt. The acupuncture point is stimulated by the heat crossing the barrier ginger. This method is continued until the skin becomes red and moist. This can be repeated 3 to 5 times until the therapeutic result is obtained.

(ii) Indirect moxibustion with garlic

This method is the same as the indirect method of moxibustion with ginger except that the barrier ginger is replaced by garlic.

(iii) Indirect moxibustion with salt

This is mainly applied over the umbilicus. The salt (sodium chloride) is filled up in the umbilicus up to the level of skin and a piece of ginger is kept over it and moxa wool is ignited. This method is mainly used in emergency cases like acute diarrhoea and vomiting.

(iv) Moxa ironing (warm cup moxibustion)

In this method moxa powder is kept inside the moxa iron and ignited. The moxa iron is then placed over the acupuncture and Ah-shi points (Fig. 11.3).

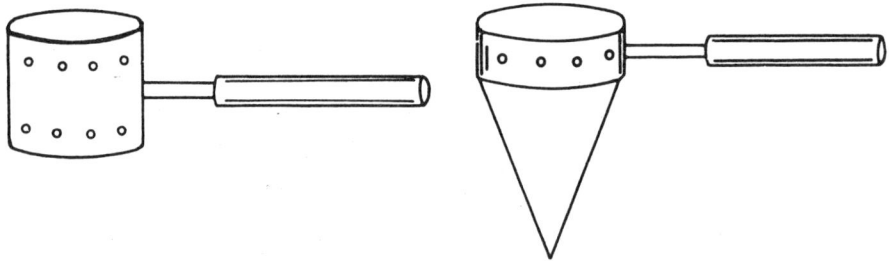

Fig. 11.3 Warm cup moxibustion.

(v) Hot needle with moxa

In this method needles are passed on acupuncture points and a cone of moxa wool is placed over the head of the needle and ignited. This has been found most effective in the cases of acute rheumatic pain (Fig. 11.4).

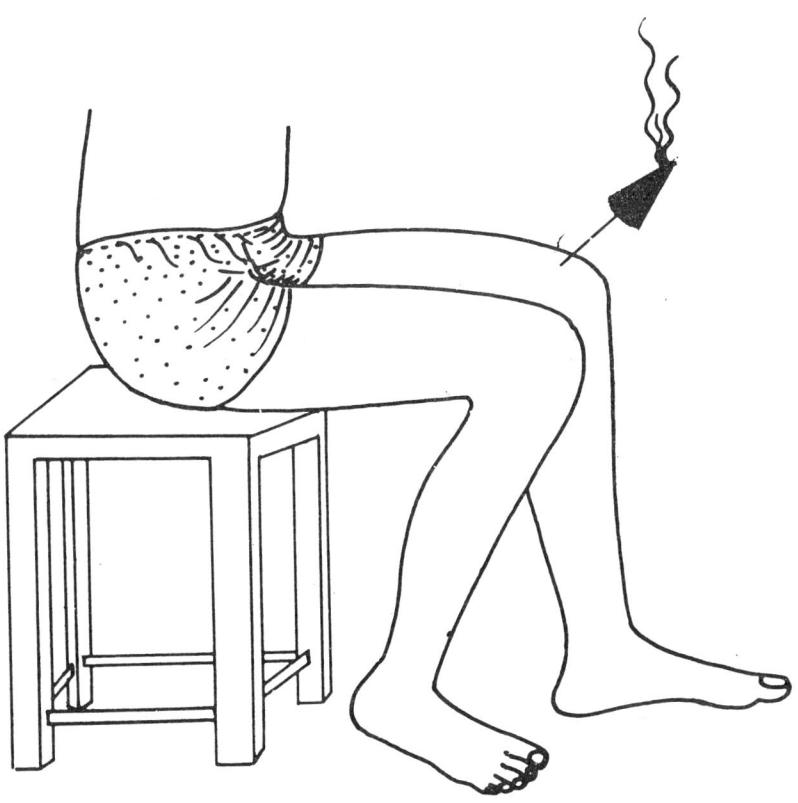

Fig. 11.4 Indirect moxibustion (hot needle moxibustion).

(vi) Indirect moxibustion with moxa roll

Moxa roll is made by moxa powder rolled in paper like cigars. This is ignited and kept 1 inch away from the acupuncture point until heat is intolerable to the patient. This technique can be continued for 5–10 minutes daily on acupuncture points and Ah-shi points.

12

COMPLICATIONS AND CONTRA-INDICATIONS OF ACUPUNCTURE

In the practice of acupuncture, the acupuncturists can encounter a number of complications. These have been discussed here.

Needle dystocia

When the needle is passed on the acupuncture point the muscle may sometimes become stiff due to local spasm and grip the needle tightly. In such a case needle gets fixed into the muscle and even after sufficient pressure it neither can be pushed in nor manoeuvred out. In this peculiar situation the following steps are advocated :

(a) Nothing should be done and the needle should be left in place for some time. Gradually the muscle relaxes and the needle can be easily removed.

(b) A massage around the needle can be given with the finger tips. This will relieve the myospasm and the needle then can be withdrawn.

(c) When a separate needle is inserted 1 to 2 cm away from the first needle, then the spasm will gradually pass away and the needles can be removed.

Bent needle

Needles get bent during insertion owing to the wrong technique of insertion and sometimes owing to muscle twisting during electro-acupuncture. Different techniques to remove the bent needles are advised but it is hardly possible to know the type of the bending inside the muscle with naked eye. We strongly advise that after removing all the needles a uniform pressure should be applied on the acupuncture point so that if a bent needle has punctured some blood vessel inside, the bleeding may be stopped.

Broken needles

Broken needle is a rare complication found in practice because the stainless steel wire needles are strong, unbreakable and can be repeatedly straightened. It is suggested that needles should be discarded after they have been subjected to repeated bending and straightening during the procedure. If at all the needle is broken inside, the best course is to take a skiagram and get the needle surgically removed.

Fainting

This is found more frequently than any other complications because many patients may stand it but some others may not even tolerate the electrical stimulation and strong hand stimulation. Some physiological danger points like Taichong (Liv-3) when used can lead to a sudden hypotension.

To avoid this complication, the patient must always be given a comfortable posture and a constant watch made during the acupuncture therapy. If at all the patient gets an attack of fainting all the needles should be removed immediately and the patient should be given complete rest in lying down position, simple first-aid like loosening of the belts, removal of shoes, washing of the face with cold water should be given. Some Jing-well points can be stimulated if patient does not respond to first-aid.

In our experience almost all the patients can be revived without the need of any adjuvant drugs.

Injury to internal organs

Careless needling on a dangerous point situated near an internal organ can give injuries to that organ. Points situated around the eye, chest and abdomen are more likely victims of this complication. Sometimes due to internal pathological conditions like hepatitis and splenomegaly, the internal organs can be injured. To avoid the complication a complete clinical checkup of the patient and careful needling is advised.

Immediate emergency measures should be taken if the internal viscera are injured.

Bleeding

This is not a very common complication of acupuncture but sometimes when the superficial veins are punctured during the removal of the needle, bleeding can occur. Only a firm pressure on the bleeding spot will stop the bleeding.

Infection

The authors have not encountered any infection during their practice of several years of acupuncture but this complication can occur when the needling is done on infected areas and if the sterilisation is improper.

Forgotten needle

In a busy clinic where a number of patients are receiving the treatment removal of the needles is done by the nursing staff who are likely to forget removing one or two needles due to overwork, carelessness or negligence and the patient may go home along with the needles. These forgotten needles can lead to infection and bleeding, and may become bent. To avoid such an avoidable complication, the practice of making a note of the number of the needles applied on the treatment card of the patient and to recount them at the time of removal is strongly recommended.

CONTRA-INDICATIONS OF ACUPUNCTURE

As such acupuncture does not have any contra-indications but it should not be given in certain physiological and pathological conditions where it may lead to certain adverse effects. Acupuncture in conditions like pregnancy, full stomach, empty stomach, acute cardiac arrythmias and congestive cardiac failure may result in abortion, vomiting, fainting and cardiac arrest, respectively.

It is relatively contra-indicated in cases of malignancy because the same needle may carry the malignant cells to certain depth causing the infection to spread further. If same needle is by chance withdrawn and reinserted on some other spot, it will lead to further metastasis.

13
ACUPUNCTURE POINTS

The entire human body has spots which become tender during physical or mental illness and disappear when the disease is cured. They are endowed with healing effect on the disease when stimulated by needling or moxibustion. These spots are termed as acupuncture points.

Acupuncture points transmit vital energy of the viscera and channel it to the superficial parts of the body. The imbalance between the two contradictory forces, Yin and Yang, results in various diseases and the effect is reflected in some way on these acupuncture points too. Stimulation of various combinations of these points brings again the flow into proper balance and the disease is cured.

An acupuncture point need not necessarily be tender. The disease may manifest itself on the acupuncture points in a variety of ways, such as:

1. There may be spontaneously tender spots. The best example is the point near the external occipital protuberance Fengchi (GB-20) which becomes tender during frontal headache.
2. Spots that show tenderness on pressure.
3. Tiny nodules are hard and indurated areas in a group of muscles. They are palpable like fibrocystic and fibrositic rheumatic nodules (Figs 13.1 and 13.2).
4. Swollen area (Fig. 13.2).
5. Discoloured area (Fig. 13.2).

Many times there are unexplained discoloured areas on the surface of the body. Physicians go on prescribing a number of antiallergic and antiinflammatory drugs to the patients in the hope of curing some hidden allergy or infection in the body without knowing that they are actually witnessing the acupuncture point as the reflection of the disease, and their simple stimulation may provide cure.

NOMENCLATURE

Each acupuncture point can be described in the three different ways. The oldest nomenclature is by the traditional Chinese name, but the Peoples Republic of China has described the points by numbers on the human body model, irrespective of the meridians. In the

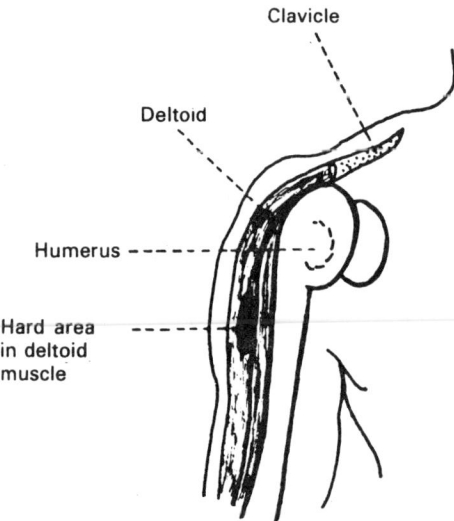

Fig. 13.1   Showing menifestation of the diseases in
            acupuncture.

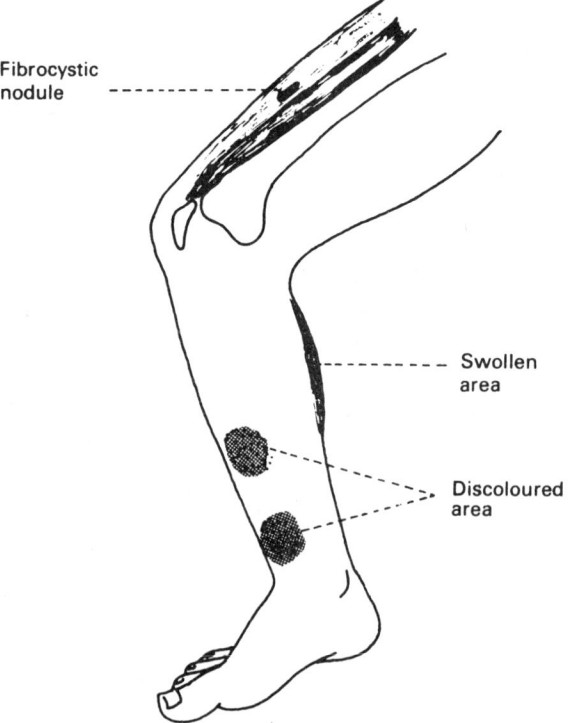

Fig. 13.2   Showing menifestations of the diseases in acupuncture.

European system the numbering of acupuncture points is named after the meridian with a number assigned to that particular point.

From the treatment and prescription point of view, acupuncture points are described as principal (important local points), match (supplementary points) points and auxillary (specific) points. The principal points are the main points for the therapy while the supplementary points are prescribed with the main points during treatment and the procedure is known as the matching. Auxillary points are added to the prescription in order to get specific effects. The acupuncture points can be classified anatomically and functionally. It is useful to remember both the classifications from diagnostic and treatment point of view.

1. Meridian points
The acupuncture points falling on the lines of the classical channels are termed as meridian points. Their number is written along with the short name of the channel and the name itself becomes explanatory, for example Quchi (LI-11) is the name given to the eleventh point on large intestine meridian.

2. Extra meridian points
These are more recently discovered points and do not belong to any of the old traditionally described channels. They exist mainly on the ear, hand, nose and head, and some are found on the trunk.

3. Floating points (Ah-shi points)
As suggested by the name, these points have no specific location. They exist in the vicinity of the diseased part and very often many of them, become sensititive or tender in some diseases. They are termed as Ah-shi points too due to their function as effective stimulation spots (Fig. 13.3).

Functionally acupuncture points are classified into the following groups:

1. Jing-Well points
These are the points which can be used in acute emergencies like shock, convulsions, respiratory failure, cadiac failure, etc. Though grouped functionally, they possess strong anatomical similarities and indicate either the beginning or the end point of twelve meridian channels. Almost all are located on the toes and fingers near the nail beds, except Yongquan (K-1) and Renzhong (GV-26) which are situated on the sole and philtrum of upper-lip respectively. Renzhong (GV-26) enjoys the privilege of not being the terminal point, while there is no Jing-well point on conceptional vessels channel. Examples of the best Jing-well point are Yongquan (K-1) and Renzhong (GV-26) [Figs. 13.4, 13.5 and 13.6].

2. Alarm points
These are the points which function as alarm signals during the diseases of specific organs. They become painful or tender in the disorders of related organs and can be used for diagnosis, treatment and prognosis. Example : Zhongfu (L-1) is an alarm point for lung diseases.

3. The Back-Shu points
These are the points on the urinary bladder channel situated on the back 1.5 t-sun lateral to the posterior mid-line below the spinous process of the corresponding vertebrae. They

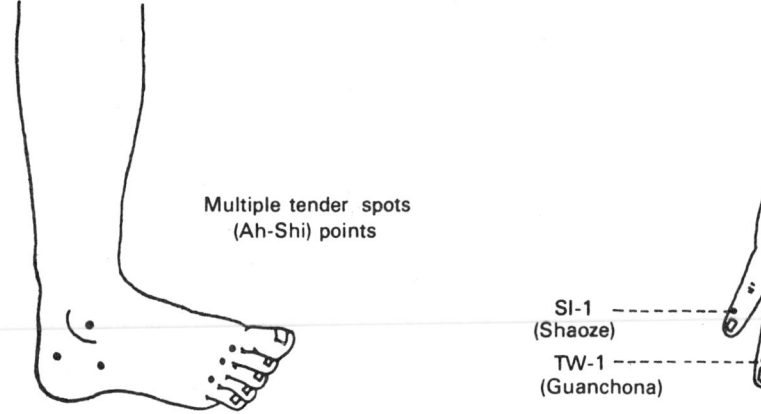

Multiple tender spots
(Ah-Shi) points

Fig. 13.3 Showing Ah-shi points.

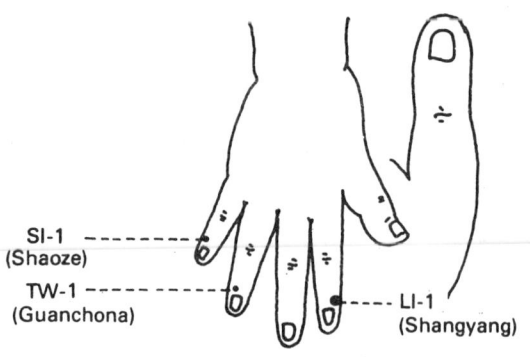

SI-1
(Shaoze)

TW-1
(Guanchona)

LI-1
(Shangyang)

Fig. 13.4 Showing Jingwell points on upper limb.

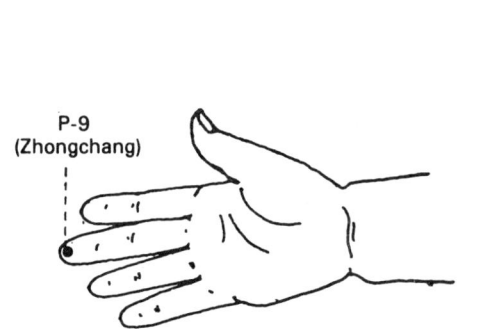

P-9
(Zhongchang)

Fig. 13.5 Showing Jingwell points of upper limb.

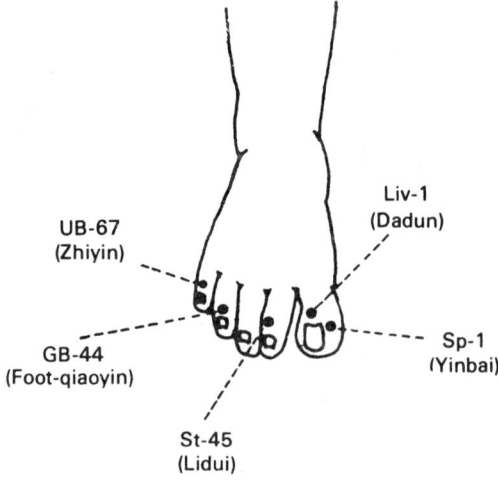

Liv-1
(Dadun)

UB-67
(Zhiyin)

Sp-1
(Yinbai)

GB-44
(Foot-qiaoyin)

St-45
(Lidui)

Fig.13.6 Showing Jingwell points on lower limb.

are similar to the alarm points in their properties and are indicated in the treatment of diseases of their corresponding organs and related special sense organs.

Back-Shu points

Sl. No.	Name	Number	Related organ	Location at the vertebral level	Therapeutic uses
1.	Feishu	UB-13	Lung	T-3	Pulmonary tuberculosis, pneumonia, Bronchial asthma and all lung disorders
2.	Jueyinshu	UB-14	Pericardium	T-4	Pericarditis, hiccough fullness of chest, myalgia chest
3.	Xinshu	UB-15	Heart	T-5	All cardiac and mental disorders
4.	Ganshu	UB-18	Liver	T-9	All liver and eye troubles, disorders of gall bladder and backache
5.	Danshu	UB-19	Gall bladder	T-10	All disorders of gall bladder
6.	Pishu	UB-20	Spleen	T-11	Malaria, allergic disorders, oedema and gastric disorders
7.	Weishu	UB-21	Stomach	T-12	All gastric disorders
8.	Sanjiaoshu	UB-22	Triple warmer	L-1	To maintain homeostesis
9.	Shenshu	UB-23	Kidney	L-2	All renal disorders, ear disorders, genital disorders
10.	Dachangshu	UB-25	Large intestine	L-4	Constipation disorders, low backache and sciatica
11.	Xiaochangshu	UB-27	Small intestine	S-1	Disorders of small intestine sacro-iliac and lumbo sacral joints, enteritis and leucorrhoea
12.	Pangguangshu	UB-28	Urinary bladder	S-2	Retention of urine, enuresis and pain in lumbosacral region

Note : T Thoracic vertebra, L Lumber vertebra, S Sacral vertebra.

4. The Mu-front points

These are the acupuncture points on the front of the chest and abdomen. They are similar to the back-shu points and possess the properties of alarm points. They are most commonly used in the diagnosis and treatment and are listed as below.

The Mu-front points

Sl. No.	Name	Number	Related organ	Location	Therapeutic uses
1.	Zhongfu	L-1	Lung	Interspace between the 1st & 2nd ribs 6 t-sun lateral to midline of chest	Bronchial asthma, cough, dyspnoea, chest pain
2.	Qimen	Liv-14	Liver	Directly below the nipple in 6th intercostal space	Pleuritis, hepatitis and chest pain

Sl. No.	Name	Number	Related organ	Location	Therapeutic uses
3.	Riyue	GB-24	Gall bladder	One rib below Liv-14 (7th intercostal space)	Cholecystitis, hepatitis
4.	Zhangmen	Liv-13	Spleen	Free end of 11th rib	Diarrhoea, pain in subcostal region, abdominal distension splenomegaly, malarial
5.	Jingmen	GB-25	Kidney	Free end of 12th rib	Subcostal pain and Renal disorders
6.	Tianshu	St-25	Large intestine	2 t-sun lateral to the umbilicus	Abdominal distention, gastroenteritis, paralytic ileus, appendicitis, costal pain, diarrhoea
7.	Shanzhong	CV-17	Pericardium	Midway between the two nipples	Bronchial asthma, bronchitis, pain in chest, fullness of chest, hiccough
8.	Jujue	CV-14	Heart	6 t-sun above the umbilicus in midline	Palpitation, anxiety, vomiting and mental disorders, anorexia nervosa
9.	Zhongwan	CV-12	Stomach	Midway between umblicus and xiphoid process	Dyspepsia, vomiting gastralgia, gastroptosis, gastritis and abdominal distention
10.	Shimen	CV-5	Triple warmer	2 t-sun below umbilicus in midline	Dysurea, irregular menstrual cycle, amenorrhoea, oedema, abdominal distension and leucorrhoea
11.	Guanyuan	CV-4	Small intestine	3 t-sun below umbilicus in midline	Impotence, spermatorrhoea, menorrhagia, menstrual dysfuction
12.	Zhongji	CV-3	Urinary bladder	4 t-sun below umbilicus in midline	Spermatorrhoea, impotence, pelvic inflammation, incontinence of urine, retention of urine, leucorrhoea, menstrual disturbances

5. The Yuan (source) points

These points possess maximum energy of the channel. They are prescribed in the treatment of chronic disorders of the pertaining organ. They are located around the wrist and ankle. Each of the twelve channels has one Yuan (source) point.

The Yuan (source) points

Sl. No.	Name of the channel	Name of the point	Number
1.	Lung	Taiyuan	L-9
2.	Pericardium	Daling	P-7
3.	Heart	Shenmen	H-7
4.	Spleen	Taibai	Sp-3
5.	Liver	Taichong	Liv-3
6.	Kidney	Taixi	K-3
7.	Large intestine	Hegu	LI-4
8.	Triple warmer	Yangchi	TW-4
9.	Small intestine	Hand Wangu	SI-4
10.	Stomach	Chong yang	ST-42
11.	Gall bladder	Qiuxu	GB-40
12.	Urinary bladder	Jinggu	UB-64

6. The Luo-connecting points

These acupuncture points form connecting links between Yin and Yang channels. Each of the fourteen channels possess a luo-connecting point but the spleen channel has two. One is called the heart connecting point of the spleen, Dabao (Sp-21). Luo-connecting points are useful in the following ways when prescribed for treatment.

1. Only one point can bring equilibrium in two luo-connected meridians.
2. Only one connecting point controls the energy between the left and right halves of a meridian.
3. Governed by the law of mid-day mid-night; the luo-connecting points control the flow of energy between the organs related to one another.

Thus it can be said that as a matter of fact luo-connecting points form the buffer links between two meridians of the same side and similar meridians of two opposite sides of the body.

7. Dangerous points

The acupuncture points in the close vicinity of vital organs are termed as dangerous points.

Examples : Qiuhou (Ex.-4), Chengqi (St-1) and Jingming (UB-1) are located around the eye and it is likely to be damaged during needling.

8. Influential points

The eight important tissues of the body are influenced by eight different points on the channels and hence the diseases of these tissues can be treated effectively by combining them with other points.

The eight influential points and their related tissues are given in the table below.

Influential points

Sl. No.	Name of the tissue	The influential point	
1.	Solid organs (Zang)	Zhangmen	(Liv-13)
2.	Hollow organs (Fu)	Zhongwan	(CV-12)
3.	Respiratory tissue	Shanzhong	(CV-17)
4.	Blood	Geshu	(UB-17)
5.	Bones	Dashu	(UB-11)
6.	Bone marrow	Xuanzhong	(GB-39)
7.	Muscles and tendons	Yanglingquan	(GB-34)
8.	Blood vessels	Taiyuan	(L-9)

9. Distal points

These points have specific therapeutic properties on the proximal parts of the body and are situated in the specific distal areas on the extremities (Figs. 13.7 and 13.8).

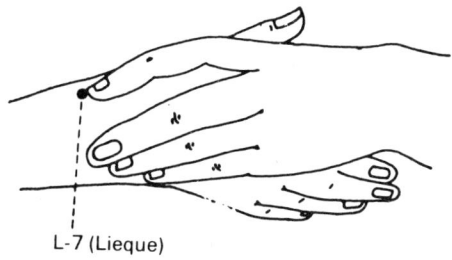

L-7 (Lieque)

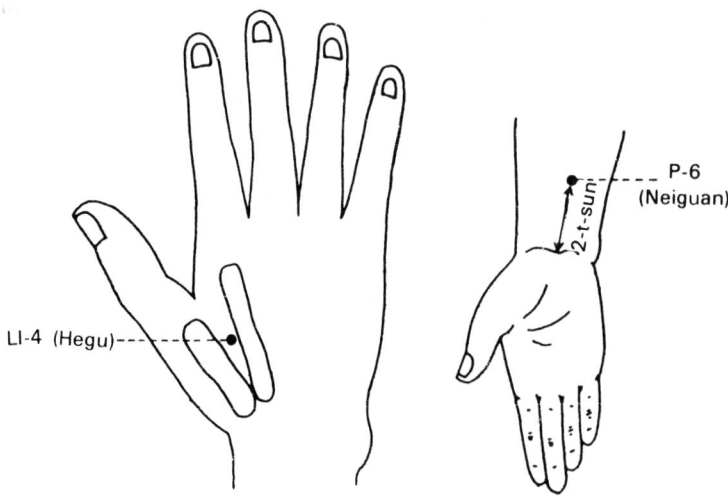

P-6 (Neiguan)

LI-4 (Hegu)

Fig. 13.7 Showing distal points on upper limb.

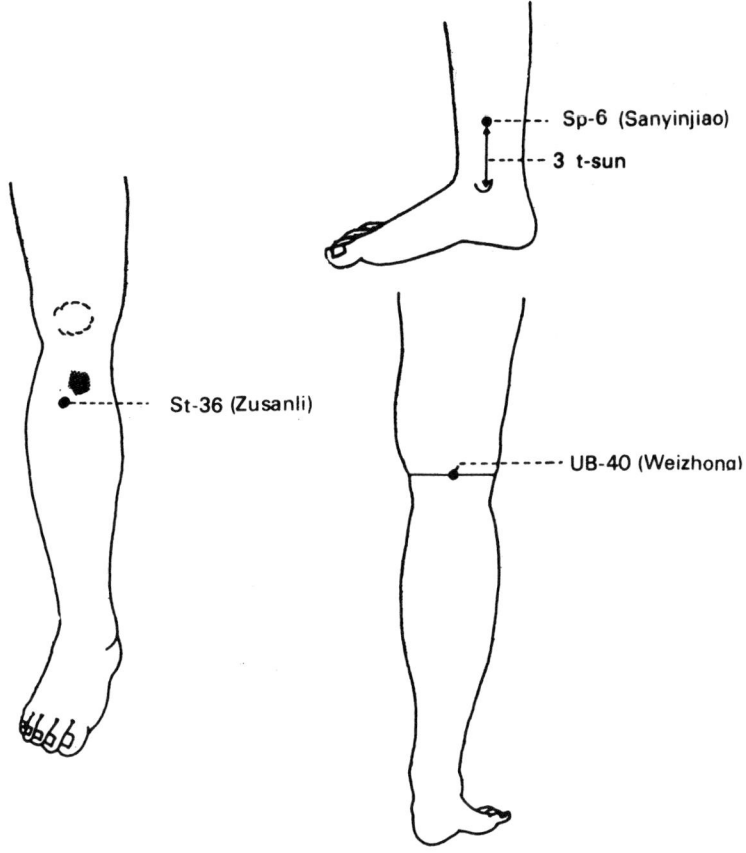

Fig. 13.8 Showing distal points on lower limb.

Distal points

Extremity	Distal point		Area of influence
Upper extremity	Hegu	(LI-4)	Forehead, face, front of neck and special sense organs
	Lieque	(L-7)	Back of head, nape of neck and back of the chest
	Neiguan	(P-6)	Front of chest and abdomen
Lower extremity	Zusanli	(St-36)	Abdominal organs
	Sanyinjiao	(Sp-6)	Genital organs and perineum
	Weizhong	(UB-40)	Lower part of back, kidney and pelvic organs

10.   The Five Shu points

These are the five specific points on each of the twelve meridians, located below elbow and knee on the upper and lower extremities. Each one of these possesses specific properties. They are grouped as follows:

The Five Shu points

Group	Points		Therapeutic uses
I. Jing-well points	Shaoshang	(L-11)	Emergencies irritability, mental disorder, restlessness
	Zhongchong	(P-9)	
	Shaochong	(H-9)	
	Yinbai	(Sp-1)	
	Dadun	(Liv-1)	
	Yongquan	(K-1)	
	Shangyang	(LI-1)	
	Guanchong	(TW-1)	
	Shaoze	(SI-1)	
	Lidui	(St-45)	
	Foot-Qiaoyin	(GB-44)	
	Zhiyin	(UB-67)	
II. Yung-spring	Yuji	(L-10)	Febrile diseases
	Laogong	(P-8)	
	Shaofu	(H-8)	
	Dadu	(Sp-2)	
	Xingjian	(Liv-2)	
	Rangu	(K-2)	
	Erjian	(LI-2)	
	Yemen	(TW-2)	
	Qiangu	(SI-2)	
	Neiting	(St-44)	
	Xiaxi	(GB-43)	
	Tonggu	(UB-66)	
III. Shu-stream	Taiyuan	(L-9)	Rheumatism
	Daling	(P-7)	
	Shenmen	(H-7)	
	Taibai	(Sp-3)	
	Taichong	(Liv-3)	
	Taixi	(K-3)	
	Sanjian	(LI-3)	
	Zhongzhu	(TW-3)	
	Houxi	(SI-3)	
	Xiangu	(St-43)	
	Foot linqi	(GB-41)	
	Shugu	(UB-65)	

Group	Points		Therapeutic uses
IV. Jing-River	Jingqu	(L-8)	Cough, asthma, laryngeal and
	Jianshi	(P-5)	pharyngeal disorders
	Lingdao	(H-4)	
	Shangqiu	(Sp-5)	
	Zhongfeng	(Liv-4)	
	Fuliu	(K-7)	
	Yangxi	(LI-5)	
	Zhigou	(TW-6)	
	Yanggu	(SI-5)	
	Jiexi	(St-41)'	
	Yangfu	(GB-38)	
	Kunlun	(UB-60)	
V. He-Sea	Chize	(L-5)	Gastrointestinal disorders,
	Quze	(P-3)	diseases of Fu organs
	Shaohai	(H-3)	
	Yinlingquan	(Sp-9)	
	Ququan	(Liv-8)	
	Yingu	(K-10)	
	Quchi	(LI-11)	
	Tianjing	(TW-10)	
	Xiaohai	(SI-8)	
	Zusanli	(St-36)	
	Yanglingquan	(GB-34)	
	Weizhong	(UB-40)	

11. The confluent points

These are eight points on the twelve meridians in the extremities. Because of their connection with eight extra channels, they bring about cure in the diseases of regular meridians as well as those of extra channels, when stimulated. The list of confluent points are as follows:

Gongsun	(Sp-4)
Neiguan	(P-6)
Houxi	(SI-3)
Shenmai	(UB-62)
Waiguan	(TW-5)
Foot Linqi	(GB-41)
Lieque	(L-7)
Zhaohai	(K-6)

12. Tonification points

Each one of the twelve meridians possesses a point which when stimulated bring the tonification of the meridian for example. When Shaochong (H-9) is stimulated, tonification of the heart occurs, if it is not already in excess. Following is the list of tonification points:

Tonification points:

Taiyuan	(L-9)
Quchi	(LI-11)
Jiexi	(St-41)
Dadu	(Sp-2)
Shao-chong	(H-9)
Quyuan	(SI-13)
Zhiyin	(UB-67)
Fuliu	(K-7)
Zhongchong	(P-9)
Zhongzhu	(TW-3)
Xiaxi	(GB-43)
Ququan	(Liv-8)

13. Sedation points

In contrast to the points of tonification, these when stimulated bring about sedation of the meridians. It is a set of 14 points, one located on each meridian and two more on large intestine and kidney meridians.

Example : Ligou (Liv-5) being the point of sedation for the liver when it is stimulated it brings the sedation of liver meridian.

List of sedation points

Chize	(L-5)
Erjian	(LI-2)
Sanjian	(LI-3)
Lidui	(St-45)
Shangqiu	(Sp-5)
Xiaohai	(SI-8)
Shugu	(UB-65)
Yongquan	(K-1)
Rangu	(K-2)
Daling	(P-7)
Tianjing	(TW-10)
Yanglingquan	(GB-34)
Xingjian	(Liv-2)

14

SYSTEMIC DESCRIPTION OF MERIDIANS

According to the traditional Chinese descriptions, 12 paired meridians and 2 unpaired meridians (running in the anterior and posterior midlines) are present in the body. Meridians running vertically from below upwards or above downwards are the main meridians. The 12 paired meridians originate from the internal viscera of the body and are named according to the viscera of origin.

1. The Lung Meridian
2. The Large Instestine Meridian
3. The Stomach Meridian
4. The Spleen Meridian
5. The Heart Meridian
6. The Small Intestine Meridian
7. The Urinary Bladder Meridian
8. The Kidney Meridian
9. The Pericardium Meridian
10. The Triple Warmer Meridian
11. The Gall Bladder Meridian
12. The Liver Meridian
13. The Governing Vessels Meridian
14. The Conceptional Vessels Meridian
15. The Eight Extra Meridian

1. THE LUNG MERIDIAN

According to the traditional Chinese description, the lung meridian is a Yin channel associated with the element metal and possesses interior and exterior relationship with the large intestine meridian.

Total number of points : 11.

Starting points   : On the body surface first intercostal space on the front of the chest at the infraclavicular fossa.

Terminal points   : On the lateral side of the thumb, close to the root of the nail.

Pathway   : After originating from the middle warmer (stomach) it descends to connect with the large intestine. It ascends up towards the diaphragm and enters its principal organ, the lung. From here it courses upwards and outwards towards the first intercostal space to become superficial (Fig. 14.1).

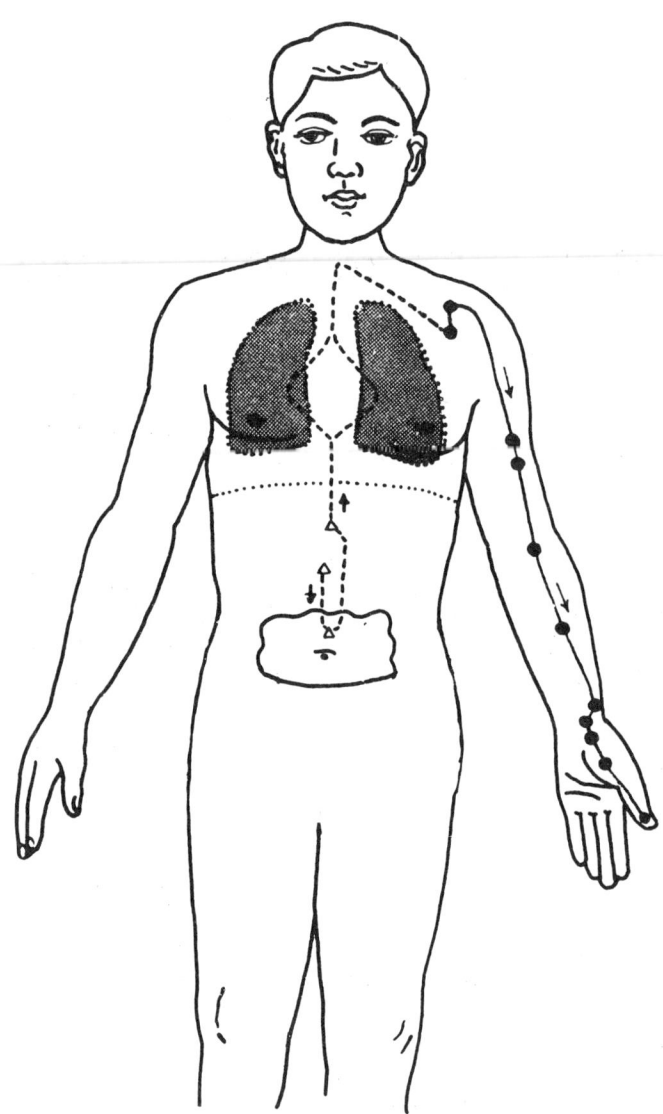

Fig. 14.1   The lung meridian.

Superficial route   : On the skin superficially first it runs along the medial aspect of the upper arm and then courses antero-laterally to reach the lateral border of biceps tendon at cubital fossa. From there it runs on antero-lateral aspect of the forearm on the front of the radius to end on the radial side of the corner of the nail of the thumb (Fig. 14.2).

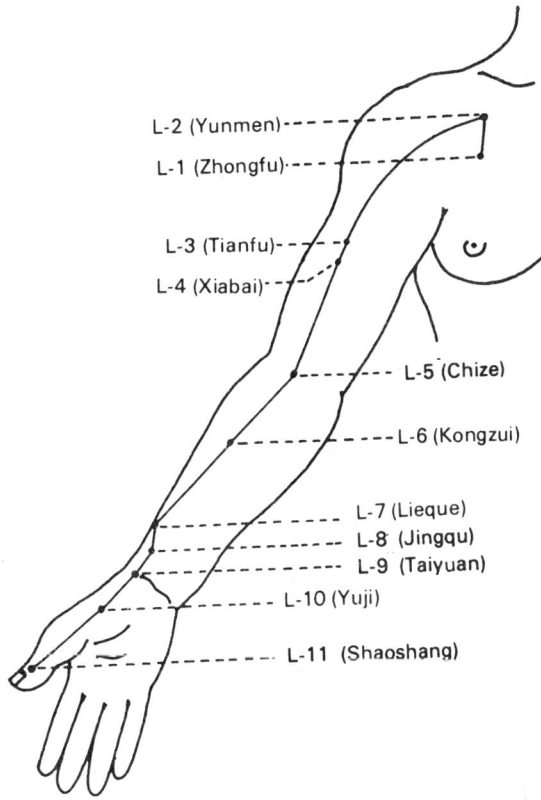

L-2 (Yunmen)
L-1 (Zhongfu)
L-3 (Tianfu)
L-4 (Xiabai)
L-5 (Chize)
L-6 (Kongzui)
L-7 (Lieque)
L-8 (Jingqu)
L-9 (Taiyuan)
L-10 (Yuji)
L-11 (Shaoshang)

Fig. 14.2   The lung meridian.

Branch   : One branch splits from the lung meridian above the wrist at the level of Lieque (L-7) and runs towards the outer side of the tip of the index finger to connect with the large intestine channel.

Therapeutic indications

1. Respiratory disorders : (i) Cough, dyspnoea, haemoptysis, fullness in the chest and chills, (ii) Upper respiratory tract disorders like coryza, nasopharyngitis and tracheitis, (iii) Lung disorders like bronchitis, asthma and pneumonitis.
2. Diseases along the pathway of the meridian like painful conditions of shoulder and elbow joints.
3. Skin disorders.

DESCRIPTION OF THE POINTS

L-1 (52) Zhongfu (Chungfu)

Location	:	6 t-sun lateral to the mid-line in first intercostal space, on the front of the chest near the coracoid process (Fig. 14.3).
Peculiarities	:	It is an alarm point of the lung.
		It is a dangerous point.
		It is a Mu front point.
Indications	:	Cough, dyspnoea, haemoptysis, pain in chest, asthma, pulmonary tuberculosis, fullness in the chest, pneumonia and bronchitis.
		Thoracodynia, intercostal neuralgia, herpes-zoster and fibrositis of the chest wall.
		Arthritis of shoulder joint, and breast disorders.
Needling	:	0.5 t-sun or less, slanting laterally (careless needling can lead to pneumothorax and shock).

L-2 (53) Yunmen

Location	:	In the infraclavicular fossa 6 t-sun lateral to the mid-line (Fig. 14.3).
Indications	:	Cough, asthma and periarthritis of the shoulder joint.
Needling	:	0.5 to 1 t-sun deep slanting outwards.

L-3 (54) Tianfu (Tienfu)

Location	:	3 t-sun below the axilla at the internal side of the biceps muscle (Fig. 14.4).
Indications	:	Dyspnoea, cough, pain in chest, asthma, epistaxis and pain in the inner side of the upper arm.

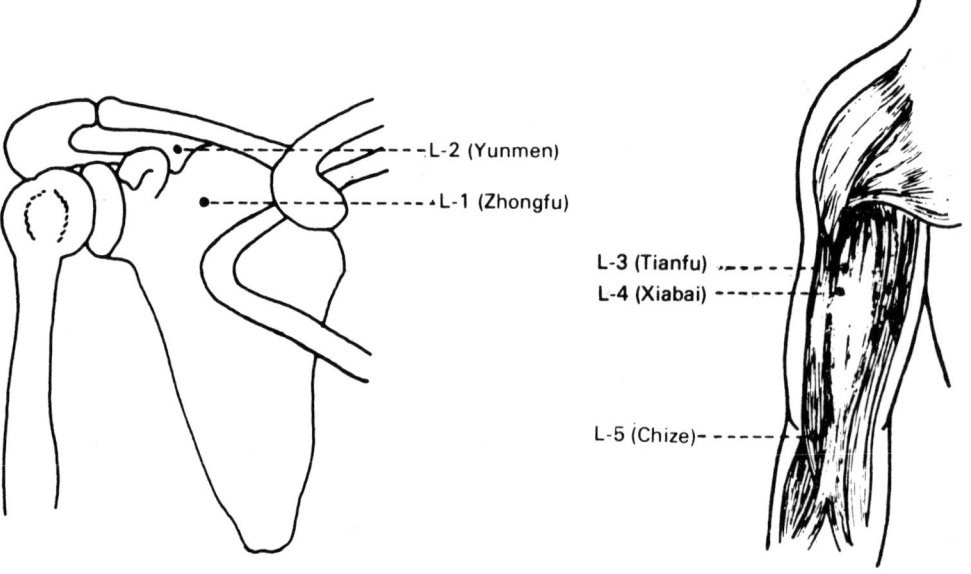

Fig. 14.3   Fig. 14.4

Needling   :   0.5 to 1 t-sun, straight.

L-4 (55) Xiabai (Hsiapai)
Location   :   1 t-sun below Tianfu (L-3) on the medial aspect of the upper arm, antero-lateral to the humerus (Fig. 14.4).
Indications   :   Dyspnoea, cough, pain in the chest and in the inner part of upper arm.
Needling   :   1 to 2 t-sun, straight.

L-5 (56) Chize (Chihtse)
Location   :   On the front of the elbow, in the depression lateral to the tendon of biceps brachii muscle, slightly flexed elbow makes the biceps tendon prominent, rendering localisation of the point easier (Fig. 14.5).

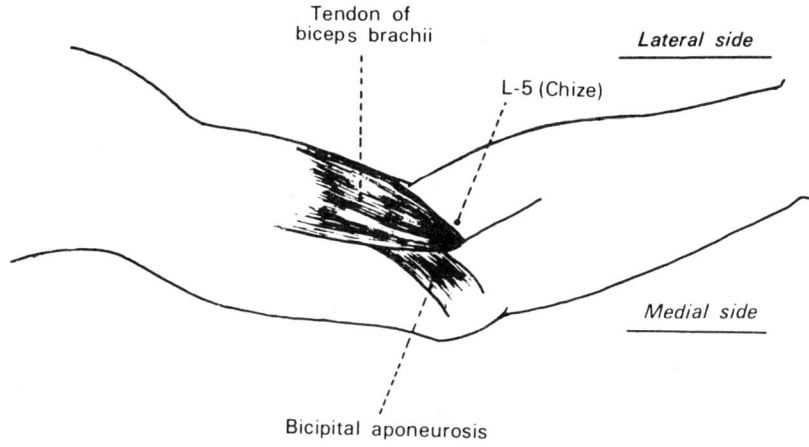

Fig. 14.5

Indications   :   Respiratory diseases like asthma and bronchitis, epistaxis, haemoptysis, cough and sore throat.
                      Diseases of the elbow joint like arthritis and synovitis, swollen and painful arm can also be treated by this point.
                      Paralysis and neuropathies of the upper extremity.
                      Skin disorders like allergy, dermatitis and psoriasis.
                      NOTE : Bleeding at this point may also be helpful in skin disorders.
Needling   :   0.5 to 1.0 t-sun, straight.

L-6 (57) Kongzui (Kungtsui)
Location   :   On the radial side of the forearm 7 t-sun proximal to the distal wrist crease (Taiyuan—L-9).
Peculiarity   :   It is a xi-cleft point.
Indications   :   Acute lung disorders like haemoptysis, asthmatic bronchitis and dyspnoea.
                      Cough.

Tonsillitis.

Myoneuropathies of arm and elbow.

Acupuncture anaesthesia.

Needling   : 1 to 1.5 t-sun, straight.

L-7 (58) Lieque (Liehchueh)

Location   : 1.5 t-sun proximal to the distal wrist crease, on the outer aspect of the forearm. (Alternatively, it is located by linking the two hands of the patient together so that the index finger and thumb of both hands are crossed; where the tip of the index finger touches is the point) [Fig. 14.6].

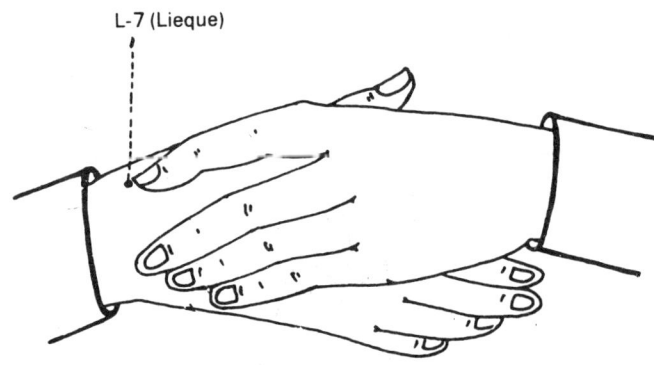

L-7 (Lieque)

Fig. 14.6

Peculiarities   : This is a Luo-connecting point.

This is a distal point for the back of head and neck and back of the chest.

Indications   : Respiratory diseases like bronchial asthma and asthmatic bronchitis.

Local diseases like arthritis of wrist, wrist-drop.

Cervical spondylosis, stiffneck and torticollis.

Bell's palsy.

Headache.

Disorders along the channel like Parkinsonism and paralysis of the upper extremity.

Needling   : 1 to 1.5 t-sun, slanting upwards.

L-8 (59) Jingqu (Chingchu)

Location   : 1 t-sun proximal to distal wrist crease on the medial side of the radial styloid process lateral to the radial artery (Fig. 14.7).

Indications   : Asthma, cough, dyspnoea, pharyngitis, chest pain and painful conditions of wrist and hand.

Needling   : 0.5 to 0.8 t-sun, slanting upwards. (Radial artery should be protected from injury.)

L-9 (60) Taiyuan

Location	: On the lateral end of the distal transverse wrist crease, lateral to the radial artery (Fig. 14.7).
Peculiaritics	: It is an influential point for the vascular diseases and Yuan (source) point of the lung channel.
Indications ·	: Respiratory disorders like asthma, bronchitis chest pain and cough. Diseases of blood vessels like Burger's disease, Raynaud' disease, varicose veins, varicose ulcers and arterio-sclerosis. Painful conditions of the back and shoulder, myoneuropathies of the upper extremity, carpal tunnel syndrome and painful disorders of the wrist and hand.
Needling	: 0.5 t-sun, straight. It is safer to palpate the radial pulse before needling in order to avoid injury to the artery.

L-10 (61) Yuji (Yuchi)

Location	: On the thenar eminence of the palm, over middle of the first metacarpal bone, at the junction of the two colours of the skin (Fig. 14.8).
Indications	: Polyneuropathy, carpal tunnel syndrome, peripheral vascular disorders, pain and numbn. s in the hand, paresis and paresthesia of the hand, respiratory disorders like cough, asthma and haemoptysis and febrile conditions.

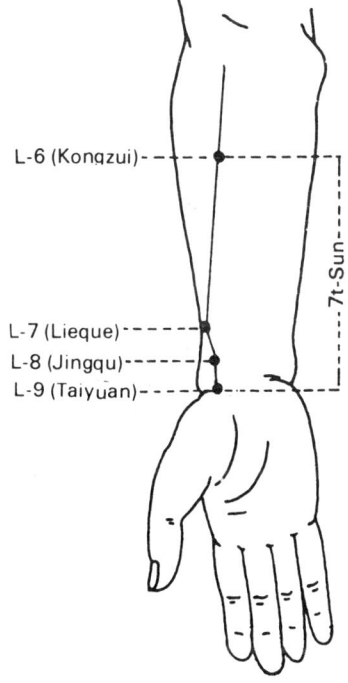

Fig. 14.7

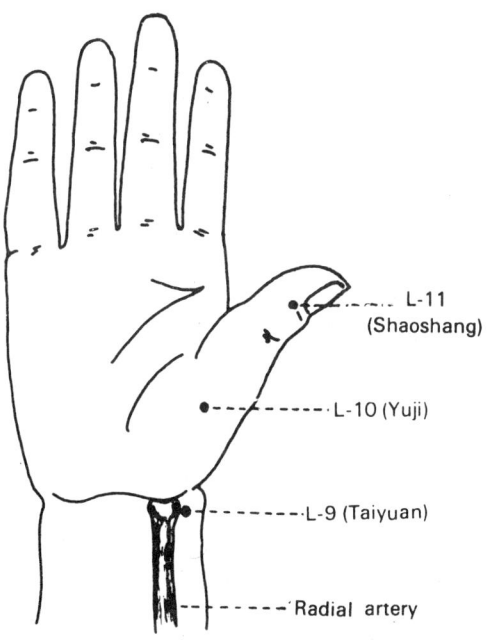

Fig. 14.8

Needling   :   It can be used in nasopharyngitis also.
                      0.3 to 0.5 t-sun, straight.
                      It is a painful point for needling.

L-11 (62) Shaoshang

Location   :   On the lateral side of the thumb 0.1 t-sun proximal to the corner of the nail.
Peculiarities   :   It is a Jing-well point.
Indications   :   Acute emergencies like coma, apoplexy, shock, hyperpyrexia, status epilepticus, respiratory failure and cardiac arrest.
                      Tonsillitis.
Needling   :   0.1 t-sun, obliquely upwards.
                      Point can be made to bleed in acute emergency.

2. THE LARGE INTESTINE MERIDIAN

According to the traditional Chinese description, it is a Yang channel, associated with the element metal and possesses interior and exterior relationship with the lung meridian.

Total number of points :   20.
Starting point   :   Tip of the radial side of the index finger.
Terminal point   :   Between nasolabial groove and ala-nasi.
Pathway   :   After taking origin from the starting point on the radial side of the index finger, this channel passes over the first dorsal inter-metacarpal space to reach the space bound by the tendons of the muscles extensor pollicis longus and brevis (commonly known as anatomical snuff-box). Here it crosses over the scaphoid bone and courses postero-laterally upwards to reach the lateral side of the elbow. Further, it ascends along the anterior border of the outer side of the upper arm to the shoulder joint and anterior border of acromion up to the 7th cervical vertebra. From here it runs towards supraclavicular fossa and then divides into two branches.
Branches   :   At the level of supraclavicular fossa, main trunk splits into a superficial branch for the face and a deep inner branch.
Superficial branch : From supraclavicular fossa it ascends up to the neck, passes over inferior angle of the mandible and ascends over the upper lip to reach opposite ala-nasi to end over there. At the philtrum there is a crossing of the two opposite large intestine channels.
Inner branch   :   It descends down from the supraclavicular fossa to lung and from there it crosses the cardiac orifice of the diaphragm and reaches its principle organ, the large intestine (Figs. 14.9 and 14.10).

Therapeutic indications

1. All the diseases along the pathway of the meridian.
2. Painful disorder of any part of the body.
3. Disorders of the large intestine.

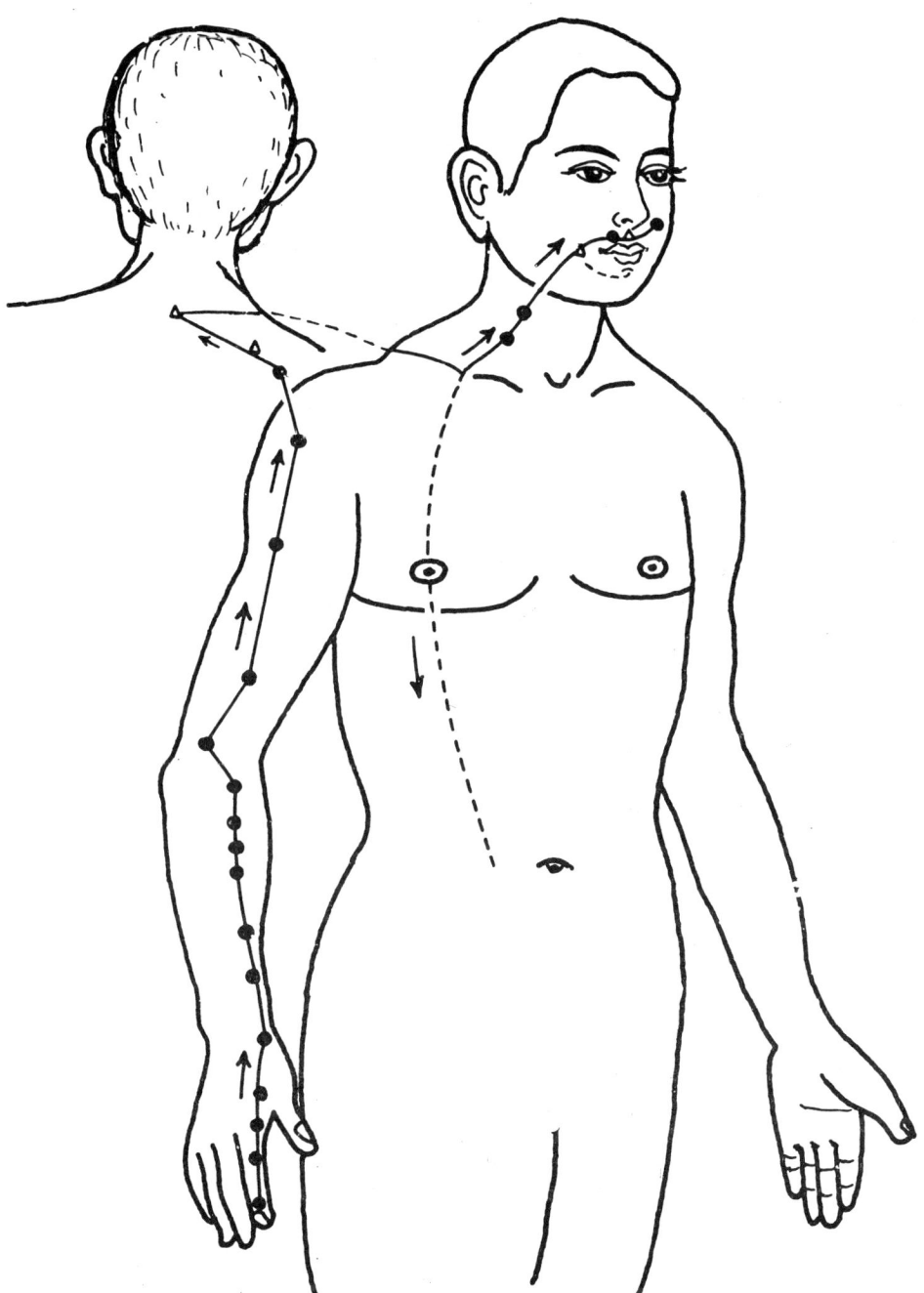

Fig. 14.9   The large intestine meridian.

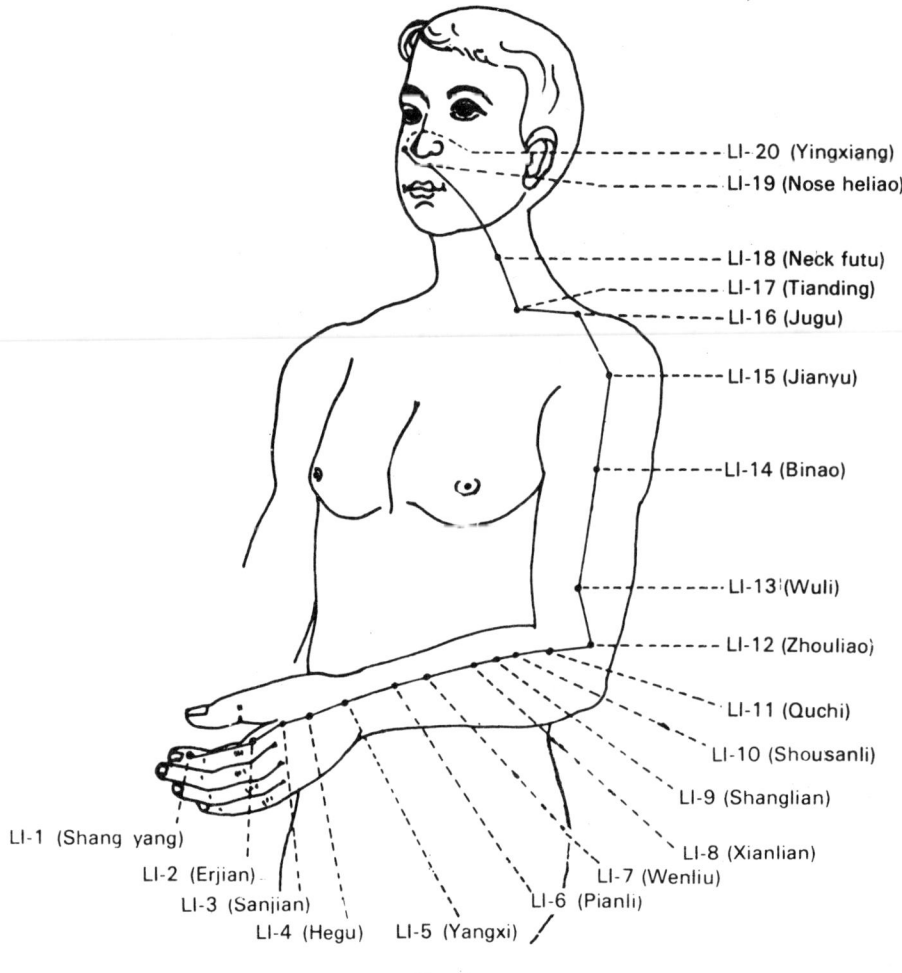

Fig. 14.10

4. Disorders of the related organ lung.
5. Skin disorders.
6. Nasal disorders.
7. Infections.
8. Conditions where homeostatis and immunity improvement is required.
9. Acute emergencies (LI-1, Jing-well point is used).
10. As analgesic points for all acupuncture anaesthesia.

DESCRIPTION OF THE POINTS

LI-1 (81) Shang Yang

Location   : 0.1 t-sun proximal to the corner of the nail of the index finger on the radial side (Fig. 14.11).

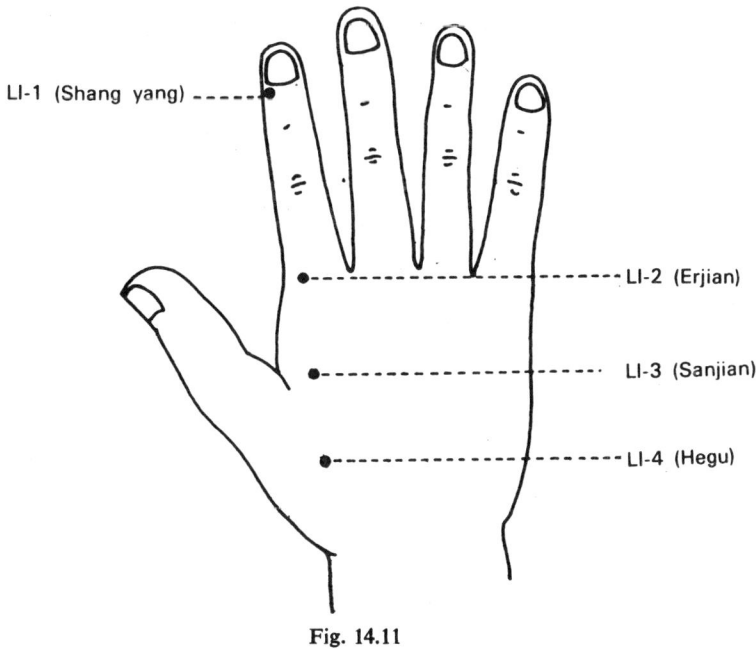

Fig. 14.11

Peculiarity	:	It is a Jing-well point.
Indications	:	Acute emergencies, asthma, fever, deafness, coma, numbness and paraesthesia of the fingers.
Needling	:	1.9 to 0.3 t-sun, straight.
	:	It can be pricked to cause bleeding.

LI-2 (82) Erjian (Erhchien)

Location	:	On the dorsum of the hand at the radial side of the proximal end of the index finger. It is best located by clenching the fist.
Indications	:	Bell's palsy, pyrexia, epistaxis, toothache, pharyngitis, painful conditions of shoulder and back.
Needling	:	Straight 0.2 to 0.3 t-sun.

LI-3 (83) Sanjian (Sanchien)

Location	:	In a depression on the dorsum of the hand proximal and lateral to the head of the second metacarpal bone. Best located by clenching the fist.
Indications	:	Pain in the eyes, trigeminal neuralgia, pharyngitis, sore throat, lower toothache, redness and swelling in the fingers and dorsum of the hand due to various causes.
Needling	:	It is used during acupuncture anaesthesia for dental extraction. 0.5 to 1 t-sun, straight.

LI-4 (84) Hegu (Hoku)

| Location | : | It is located as follows: |

(a) On the highest point of the bulging made by 1st dorsal interosseous muscle when the thumb and index finger are held close together in adduction (Fig. 14.12).

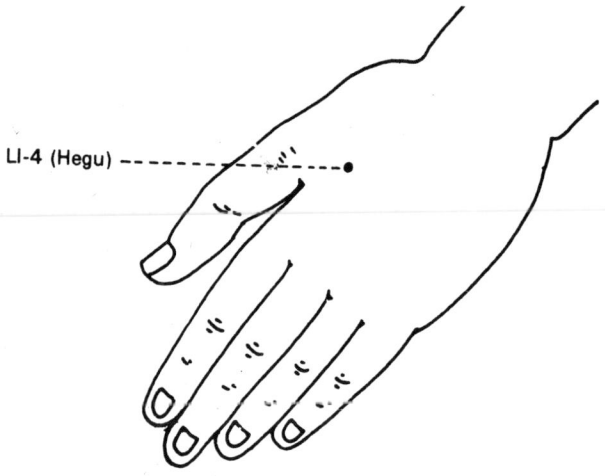

LI-4 (Hegu)

Fig. 14.12

(b) On the dorsum of the hand, at the mid point of 2nd metacarpal bone on the radial aspect (Fig. 14.13).
(c) On the centre of a line joining the mid point of the border of 1st web and junction of the 1st and 2nd metacarpal bones, slightly close to 2nd metacarpal bone (Fig. 14.14).

Peculiarities	:	It is Yuan (source) point of the large intestine channel and a distal point for the face, front of the neck and special sense organs. It is one of the most powerful analgesic point of the body.
Indications	:	Painful conditions of the eye, trigeminal neuralgia, lower toothache, pharyngitis sore-throat, bell's palsy, rhinitis, coryza, pyrexia, and as a supplementary point during any surgical procedure to alleviate pain.
Needling	:	0.5 to 1 t-sun, straight.
Note	:	Analgesia can be induced by using this point. Moxibustion can be given for 10 minutes.

LI-5 (85) Yangxi (Yanghsi)

Location	:	Over the wrist joint, between the tendons of the extensor pollicis brevis and extensor pollicis longus muscles (centre of the anatomical snuff-box) [Fig. 14.15].
Indications	:	Painful conditions of wrist and hand like osteo-arthritis and rheumatoid arthritis, neurological conditions like wrist drop, painful conditions of the eye, toothache, tinnitus aurium and indigestion in infants and children.
Needling	:	0.3 to 0.5 t-sun, straight.

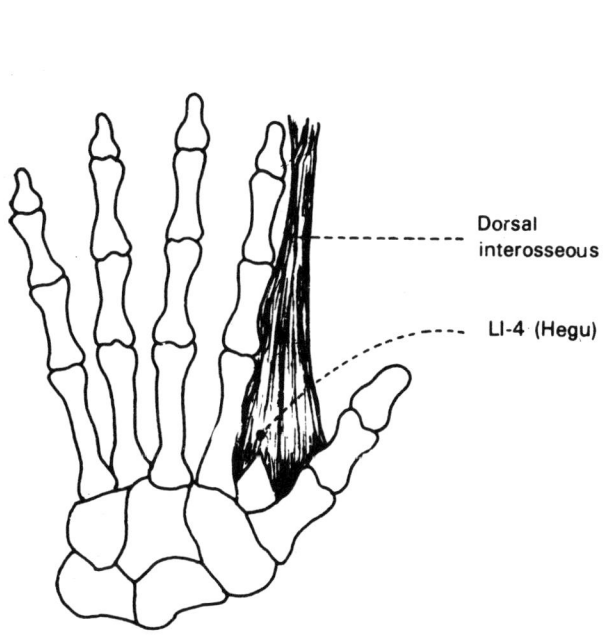

Dorsal
interosseous

LI-4 (Hegu)

Fig. 14.13

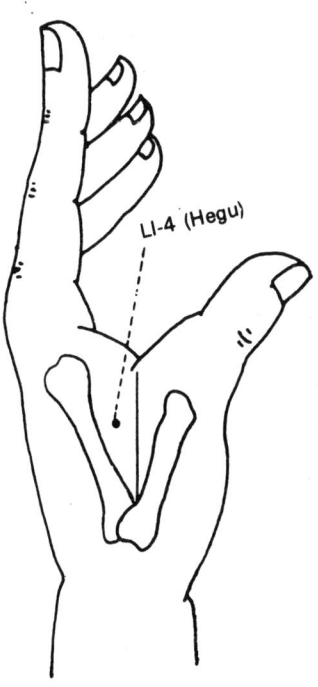

LI-4 (Hegu)

Fig. 14.14

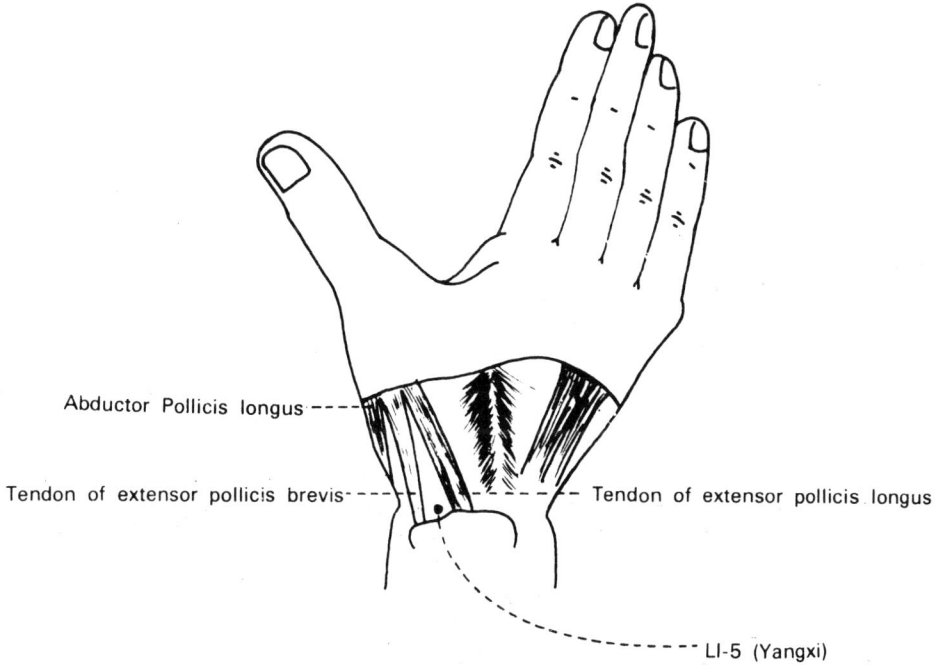

Abductor Pollicis longus

Tendon of extensor pollicis brevis

Tendon of extensor pollicis longus

LI-5 (Yangxi)

Fig 14.15

LI-6 (86) Pianli (Pienli)
Location	:	On the radial side of the back of the wrist 3 t-sun above Yangxi (LI-5).
Peculiarities	:	It is a Luo-connecting point.
Indications	:	Facial paralysis, tonsillitis, epistaxis, pain and swelling in the forearm.
Needling	:	0.5 to 1 t-sun, straight.

LI-7 (87) Wenliu .
Location	:	5 t-sun above Yangxi (LI-5) on a line joining Yangxi (LI-5) and Quchi (LI-11).
Peculiarities	:	It is Xi-cleft point.
Indications	:	Gastro-intestinal disorders, glossitis, stomatitis, parotitis, stiff and painful shoulder, painful arm, cholecystitis, and hepatitis.
Needling	:	0.5 to 1 t-sun, straight.

LI-8 (88) Xialian (Hsialien)
Location	:	4 t-sun distal to Quchi (LI-11).
Indications	:	Painful conditions of elbow and arm, intestinal colic, gas pain and other intra-abdominal disorders, mastitis and fibroadenosis of the breast.
Needling	:	0.5 to 1 t-sun, straight.

LI-9 (89) Shanglian (Shanglien)
Location	:	3 t-sun distal to Quchi (L-11).
Indications	:	Pain, paresis, paralysis and paraesthesia in the upper extremity, pain in shoulder, arm and back, gaseous pain, borborygmy and intestinal colic.
Needling	:	0.5 to 1.5 t-sun, straight.

LI-10 (90) Shousanli (Sanli)
Location	:	2 t-sun distal to Quchi (LI-11).
Indications	:	Hemiplegia, tremors and other involuntary movements of upper extremity, arthritis of elbow, painful shoulder and arm and diarrhoea with griping and other abdominal pain.
Needling	:	1 to 1.5 t-sun, straight.
Note	:	Acupressure for 10 to 15 minutes can be applied on this point for the relief from acute headache.

LI-11 (91) Quchi (Chuchih)
Location	:	a. Mid point of the line connection Chize (L-5) and lateral epicondyle of humerous (Fig. 14.16). b. Semiflex the elbow and take the lateral end of the elbow crease.
Peculiarities	:	It is one of the best immunity improving point, tonification and homeostatic point.
Indications	:	Malaise, weakness and neurasthenia, hypertension, paralysis of the arm, shoulder and back pain, urticaria, diabetes, skin disorders like psoriasis and dermatitis.
Needling	:	0.5 to 1 t-sun, straight.

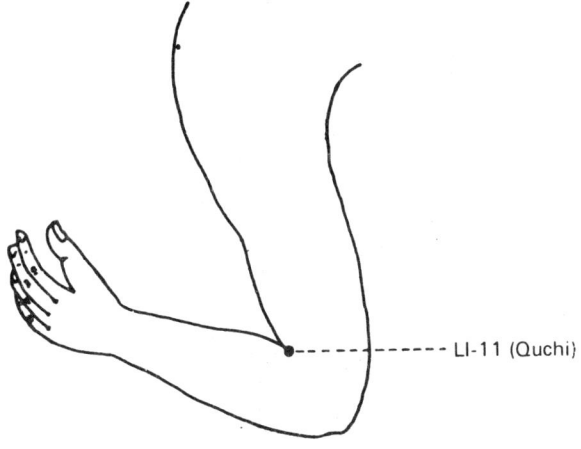

LI-11 (Quchi)

Fig. 14.16

LI-12 (92) Zhouliao (Chouliao)
Location	:	1 t-sun above Quchi (LI-11).
Indications	:	Stiffness, pain and contracture of the elbow.
		Numbness in the elbow.
		Tennis elbow.
		Myositis ossificans around the elbow.
Needling	:	1 to 1.5 t-sun, straight.

LI-13 (93) Wuli
Location	:	3 t-sun above Quchi (LI-11).
Indications	:	Cervical tubercular lymphadenitis, pain and arthritis of the elbow, pain in the arm and pneumonia.
Needling	:	1 to 1.5 t-sun, straight.

LI-14 (94) Binao (Pinao)
Location	:	7 t-sun proximal to the Quchi (LI-11) at the level of insertion of deltoid muscle, on the line joining Quchi (LI-11) and Jianyu (LI-15) [Fig. 14.17].
Peculiarities	:	It is a Ah-shi point for frozen shoulder.
Indications	:	Painful disorder of elbow and shoulder joint, hemiplegia and diseases of the eye.
Needling	:	0.3 to 0.5 t-sun, straight.

LI-15 (95) Jianyu (Chienyu)
Location	:	1. On the depression at antero-inferior border of acromio-clavicular joint when the arm is adducted.
		2. When the arm is held away from the body in adduction, it is situated in the anterior depression of the acromion (Fig. 14.17).

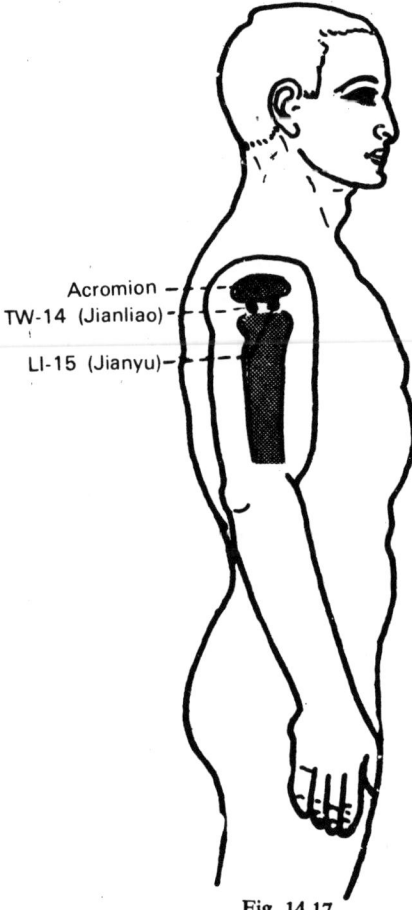

Acromion —
TW-14 (Jianliao)-
LI-15 (Jianyu)-

Fig. 14.17

Indications	:	Periarthritis shoulder (frozen shoulder) paralysis, painful arc syndrome, sprain and strain of the shoulder and all other painful shoulder disorders.
Needling	:	0.5 to 1 t-sun, straight. For the treatment of painful shoulder disorders this point is needled prior to other point.

LI-16 (96) Jugu (Chuku)

Location	:	At the depression between the acromial end of the clavicle and the upper part of the spine of the scapula (just inside the acromio-clavicular joint space).
Indications	:	Periarthritis shoulder, backache and haemoptysis.
Needling	:	1 to 1.5 t-sun, straight.

LI-17 (97) Tianding (Tienting)

Location	:	1 t-sun below Neck Futu (LI-18) at the posterior border of sterno-cleido-mastoid muscle.

Indications   : Pharyngitis, tonsilitis, cervical tubercular lymphadenitis.
Needling   : 0.5 to 1 t-sun, obliquely outwards.

LI-18 (98) Neck Futu (Futu)

Location   : On the neck 3 t-sun lateral to the middle of the laryngeal prominence, between the two heads of the sterno-cleido-mastoid muscle.
Peculiarities   : It is a dangerous point.
Indications   : Excessive expectoration, cough, sore throat, hoarseness of voice, enlarged thyroid, aphasia and stammering.
                : It is used in thyroid surgery as an acupuncture anaesthesia point.
Needling   : 0.5 t-sun or less, obliquely outward.

LI-19 (99) Nose Heliao (Holiao)

Location   : 0.5 t-sun by the side of the Renzhong (GV-26) below the lateral margin of the nostril.
Indications   : Facial paralysis, stuffy nose, trigeminal neuralgia, upper toothache, rhinitis, epistaxis and smoking addiction.
Needling   : 0.3 to 0.5 t-sun, slanting.

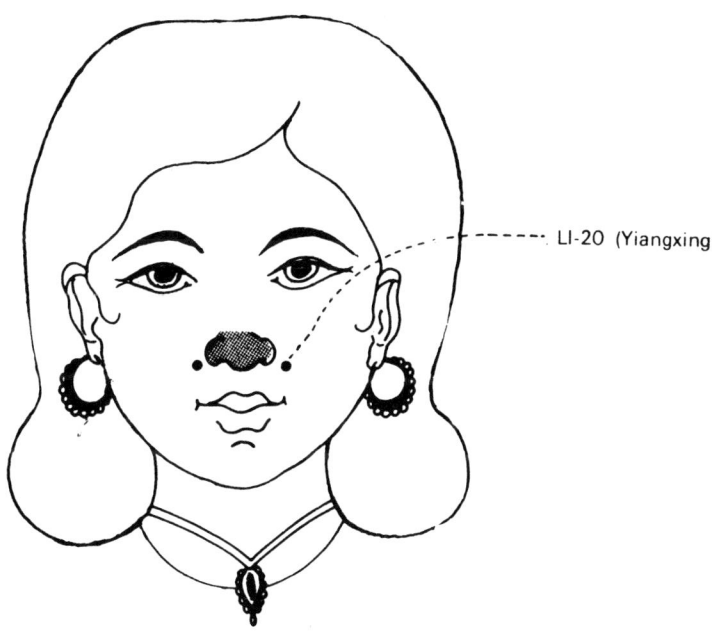

LI-20 (Yiangxing)

Fig. 14.18

LI-20 (100) Yingxiang (Yinghsiang)

Location   : Mid point on the line drawn horizontally from the highest point of the ala-nasi towards naso-labial groove on the opposite side (Fig. 14.18).
Indications   : Trigeminal neuralgia, common cold, upper toothache, maxillary sinusitis, and facial paralysis.
Needling   : 0.3 to 0.5 t-sun, straight.

3. THE STOMACH MERIDIAN

According to the traditional Chinese description it is a Yang channel associated with the element earth and possesses interior and exterior relationship with the spleen meridian.

Total number of points : 45.

Starting point : Below the eye lateral to ala-nasi.

Terminal point : Lateral side of the tip of the second toe near the nail.

Pathway : This channel originates from a point lateral to ala-nasi and ascends to the medial canthus of the eye. Here, after meeting the urinary bladder channel, it courses to the midpoint of the infraorbital margin and descends down straight to the angle of the mouth. It then curves towards the mentolabial sulcus and reaches the angle of the mandible and there it divides into two branches:

1. Ascending branch : From angle of the mandible it ascends up towards the front of the ear and courses further upwards to the angle of the forehead where it joins with the governing vessels channel.

2. Descending branch : It descends down along the lateral side of the neck to reach the supraclavicular fossa and divides again into inner and superficial branches.

   A. Inner branch : This branch passes through the thorax and diaphragm and descends down straight to the inguinal area. At the level of Qichong (St-30) it meets with the superficial branch.

   B. Superficial branch : This branch runs straight downwards from the supraclavicular fossa along the mamillary line to reach the inguinal area where it joins with the inner branch at the level of Qichong (St-30). It further descends down along the front of the thigh up to the knee where it turns laterally to become antero-lateral to the tibia. It descends down directly to the dorsum of the foot where it reaches the lateral side of the tip of the second toe and ends there (Fig. 14.19).

Therapeutic indications

1. Disorders along the pathway:

Points on the face : Used for eye diseases, facial paralysis, trigeminal neuralgia, migraine, toothache and headache.

Points on the chest : Fibrositis of the chest, heaviness and fullness in the chest, chest pain, cardiac disorders and disorders of the mamillary gland like mastitis and deficient lactation.

Points on the anterior abdominal wall : Epigastric pain, gastritis and all other gastrointestinal disorders, pelvic cellulitis and disorders of the menstruation are also treated by these points.

Points in the lower extremity : Arthritis, poliomyelitis, neuropathies and paralysis of the lower limbs.

2. Points below the knee joints are used as distal points for the disorders of the proximal parts of the body. Zusanli (St-36) is the classical example of such a distal point (Fig. 14.20).

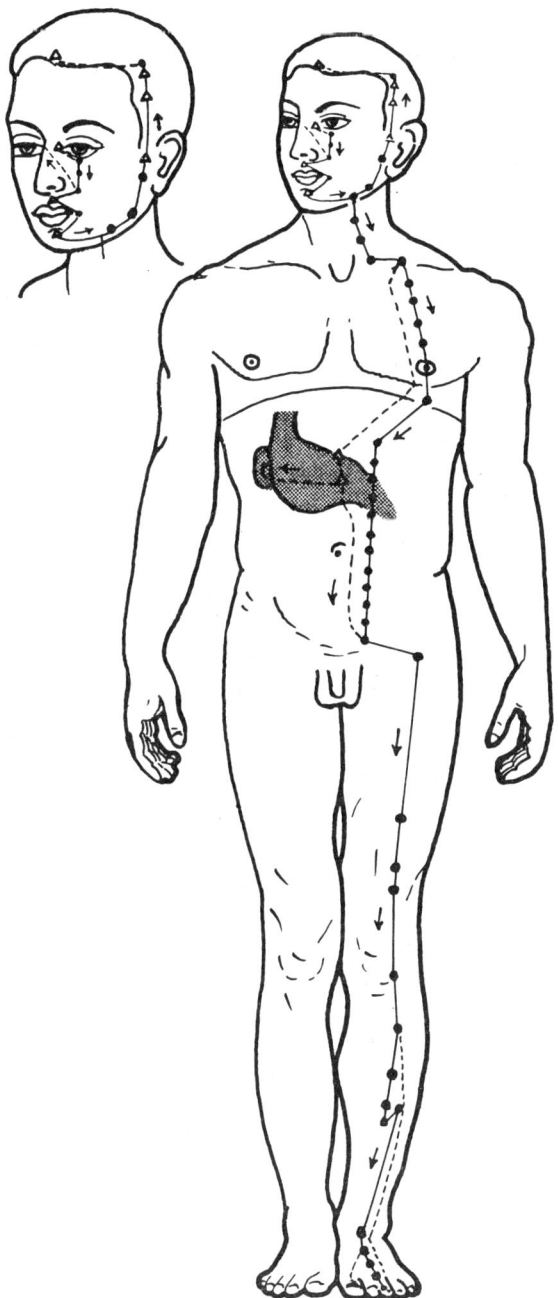

Fig. 14.19 The stomach meridian.

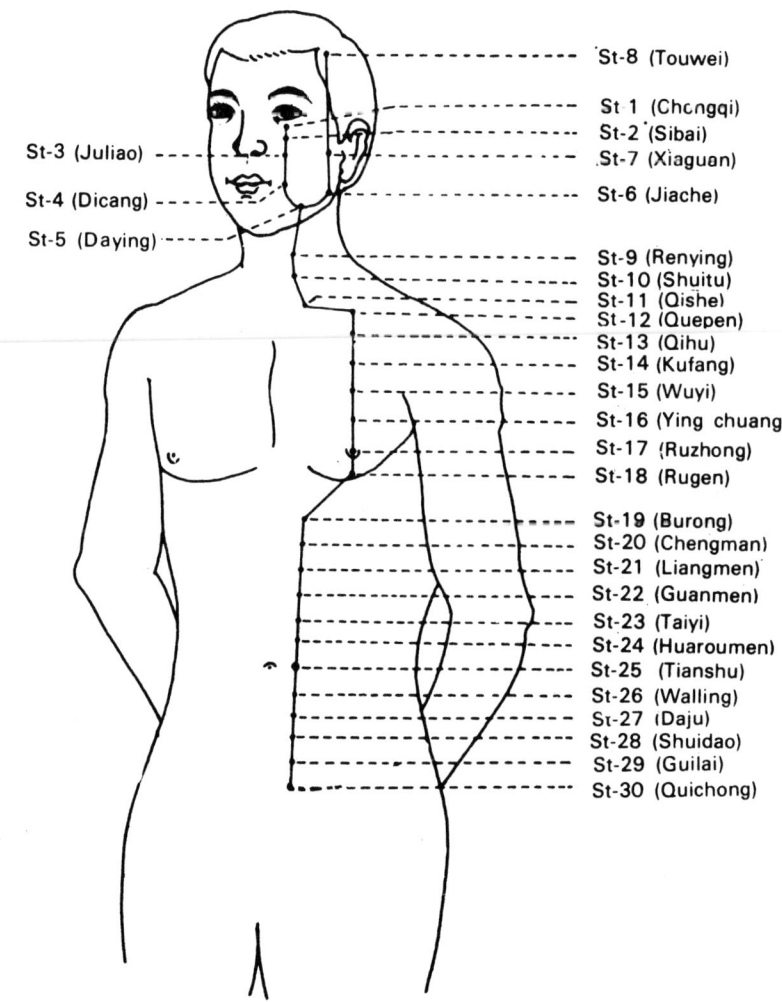

St-8 (Touwei)
St 1 (Chengqi)
St-2 (Sibai)
St-7 (Xiaguan)
St-3 (Juliao)
St-6 (Jiache)
St-4 (Dicang)
St-5 (Daying)
St-9 (Renying)
St-10 (Shuitu)
St-11 (Qishe)
St-12 (Quepen)
St-13 (Qihu)
St-14 (Kufang)
St-15 (Wuyi)
St-16 (Ying chuang)
St-17 (Ruzhong)
St-18 (Rugen)
St-19 (Burong)
St-20 (Chengman)
St-21 (Liangmen)
St-22 (Guanmen)
St-23 (Taiyi)
St-24 (Huaroumen)
St-25 (Tianshu)
St-26 (Walling)
St-27 (Daju)
St-28 (Shuidao)
St-29 (Guilai)
St-30 (Quichong)

Fig. 14.20   The stomach-meridian points on face chest
and abdomen.

DESCRIPTION OF THE POINTS

St-1 (143) Chengqi (Chengchi)

Location   : Below the eye on the mid point of the infraorbital ridge (on the
                 imaginary perpendicular line drawn from the centre of the pupil'
                 [Fig. 14.21].

Peculiarity   : It is dangerous point.

Indications   : Acute and chronic conjunctivitis, epiphora due to wind, myopia,
                 hypermetropia, astigmatism, optic neuritis, retinitis, optic atrophy,
                 cataract, glaucoma and blindness.

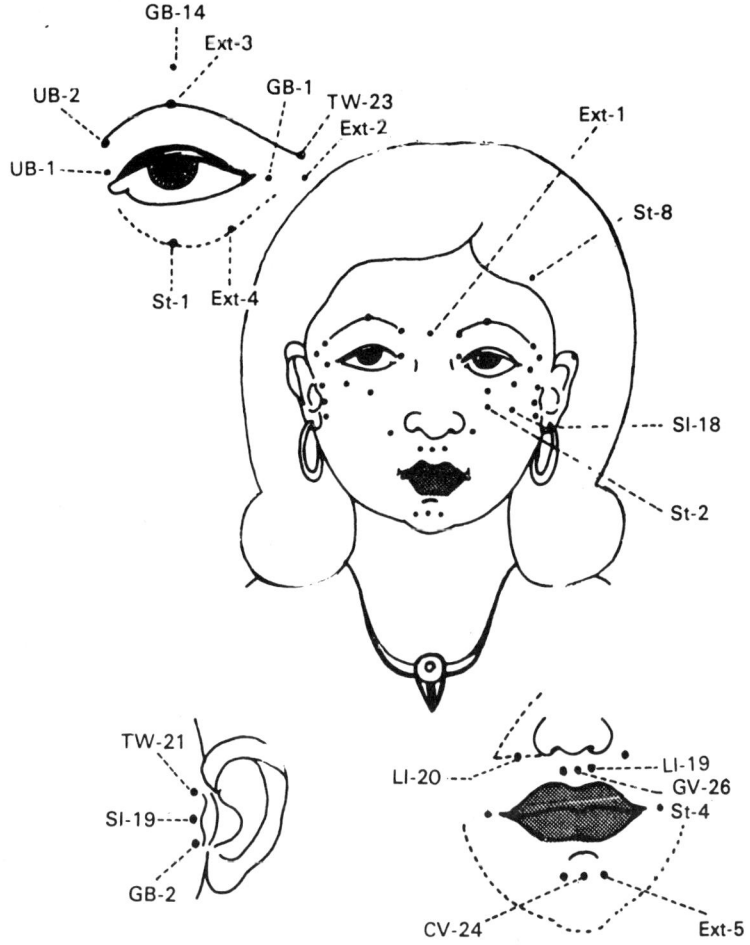

Fig. 14.21 Points on face.

Needling   : 0.5 t-sun or less, straight.
                   Ask the patient to look upwards and then advance the tip of the needle
                   along the inferior border of the orbit.

St-2 (144) Sibai (Szupai)

Location   : 0.7 t-sun below the Chengqi (St-1) in the depression at the infraorbital
                   foramen, vertically below the centre of the pupil.
Indications   : Facial nerve paralysis, trigeminal neuralgia maxillary sinusitis,
                   headache and all eye problems including spasms of eye lids.
Needling   : 0.5 t-sun slanting towards infra-orbital foramen.

St-3 (145) Juliao (Chuliao)

Location   : Directly below the middle of the eye, at a level with the inferior border
                   of the ala-nasi.

Indications   : Facial nerve paralysis, trigeminal neuralgia, toothache, swollen and painful cheeks and lips and nasal disorders like rhinitis and epistaxis.

Needling   : 0.2 to 0.5 t-sun, straight.

St-4(146) Dicang (Tit sang)

Location   : 0.4 t-sun lateral to the angle of the mouth inside the nasolabial sulcus.

Indications   : Excessive salivation, aphasia, facial nerve paralysis and trigeminal neuralgia.

Needling   : 0.3 to 1 t-sun, slanting.

St-5 (147) Daying (Taying)

Location   : In front of the angle of the mandible on the antero-inferior border of the masseter muscle behind the facial artery. It is helpful to palpate the artery on the mandible to locate the point or ask the patient to clench the teeth.

Indications   : Trismus, swollen cheeks, toothache, trigeminal neuralgia, and facial nerve paralysis. It is an anaesthetic point for the tonsillectomy and tooth extraction.

Needling   : 0.5 to 1 t-sun, slanting.

St-6 (148) Jiache (Chiache)

Location   : Over the masseteri muscle anterior to the angle of the mandible. Ask the patient to clench the teeth for better location of the point.

Indications   : Toothache, parotitis, facial nerve paralysis, painful impacted wisdom tooth and acupuncture anaesthesia for tooth extraction and tonsillectomy.

Needling   : 0.3 to-1 t-sun, straight. Transverse, point to point with Dicang (St-4).

Note   : In case of children this point can be pressed strongly by the finger for the extraction of teeth.

St-7 (149) Xiaguan (Hsiakuan)

Location   : In the centre of the depression of the lower margin of zygomatic arch, anterior to temporomandibular joint (Fig. 14.22).
It can be located by keeping the jaw slightly open or by asking the patient for opening and closing the mouth and keeping the finger in front of the ear for palpating the movements of temporomandibular joint or by taking a point 1 t-sun above the Jiache (St-6).

Indications   : Facial nerve paralysis, arthritis or dislocation of temporo-mandibular joint, toothache, deafness, tinnitus aurium, inflammation of the mandible, tetanus and trigeminal neuralgia.
Acupuncture anaesthesia for tooth extraction of upper jaw.

Needling   : 0.5 to 0.8 t-sun, straight.

St-8 (150) Touwei

Location   : At the angle of the forehead 0.5 t-sun inside the natural anterior hairline (Fig. 14.22).

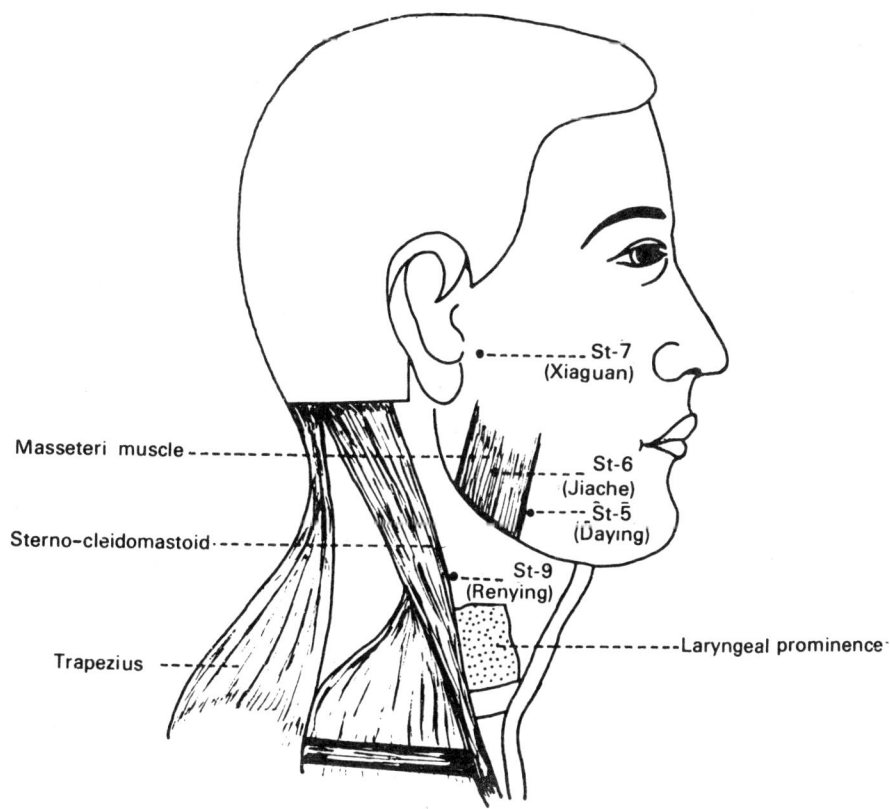

Fig. 14.22

| Indications | : | Headache migraine, giddiness, eye disorders and ophthalmagia, frontal sinusitis and lacrimation.
It is a specific point for paralysis of eye muscles together with **Feiyang** (UB-58). |
| Needling | : | 0.5 to 0.8 t-sun, straight. |

St-9 (151) Renying (Jenying)

Location	:	By the side of the laryngeal prominence behind common carotid artery.
Indications	:	Hypertension, asthma, swollen and painful oropharynx, dysarthria and aphasia.
Needling	:	0.3 to 0.5 t-sun, straight.

St-10 (152) Shuitu

Location	:	On the front of the sterno-cleido-mastoid muscle, midway between Renying (St-9) and Qishe (St-11).
Indications	:	Asthma and sore throat.
Needling	:	Straight 0.3 to 0.5 t-sun.

St-11 (153) Qishe (Chishe)

Location	:	On the superior border of the medical end of the clavicle, in between the two' heads of the sterno-cliedo-mastoid muscle directly below Renying (St-9).
Indications	:	Swollen and painful oropharynx, chest pain and stiff neck.
Needling	:	0.3 to 0.5 t-sun, straight.

St-12 (154) Quepen (Chuehpen)

Location	:	In the middle of the supraclavicular fossa vertically above the nipple.
Indications	:	Pharyngitis, asthma, pleuritis and intercostal neuralgia.
Needling	:	0.3 to 0.5 t-sun, straight.
Note	:	Keep away from the blood vessels.

St-13 (155) Qihu (Chihu)

Location	:	Mid point of the infraclavicular region.
Indications	:	Bronchitis, asthma, and dyspnoea.
Needling	:	0.5 t-sun or less, oblique.
Note	:	Deep insertion should be avoided for all points over the thorax.

St-14 (156) Kufang

Location	:	Under the first rib on the mamillary line.
Indications	:	Bronchitis, heaviness in chest, pain in chest and asthma.
Needling	:	0.5 to 0.8 t-sun, slanting.

St-15 (157) Wuyi

Location	:	Under the second rib on the mamillary line.
Indications	:	Bronchitis, heaviness and pain in the chest and asthma.
Needling	:	0.5 to 0.8 t-sun, slanting.

St-16 (158) Ying Chuang

Location	:	Under the third rib on the mamillary line.
Indications	:	Bronchitis, cough, asthma, pain in ribs, hyperperistalsis, diarrhoea and mastitis.
Needling	:	0.5 to 0.8 t-sun, slanting.

St-17 (159) Ruzhong (Juchung)

Location	:	Centre of the nipple.
Indications	:	Cough, asthma, chest pain, hyperperistalsis, diarrhoea and mastitis.
Peculiarity	:	Though it is useful in the indication given above, it is forbidden point and no needling should be done. It is used only for surface marking.

St-18 (160) Rugen (Juken)

Location	:	Mid-clavicular line, in fifth intercostal space, below the nipple (Fig. 14.23).
Indications	:	Lactational deficiency, mastitis, heart disorders, heaviness and pain in chest and intercostal neuralgia.
Needling	:	0.5 t-sun or less, obliquely outwards.

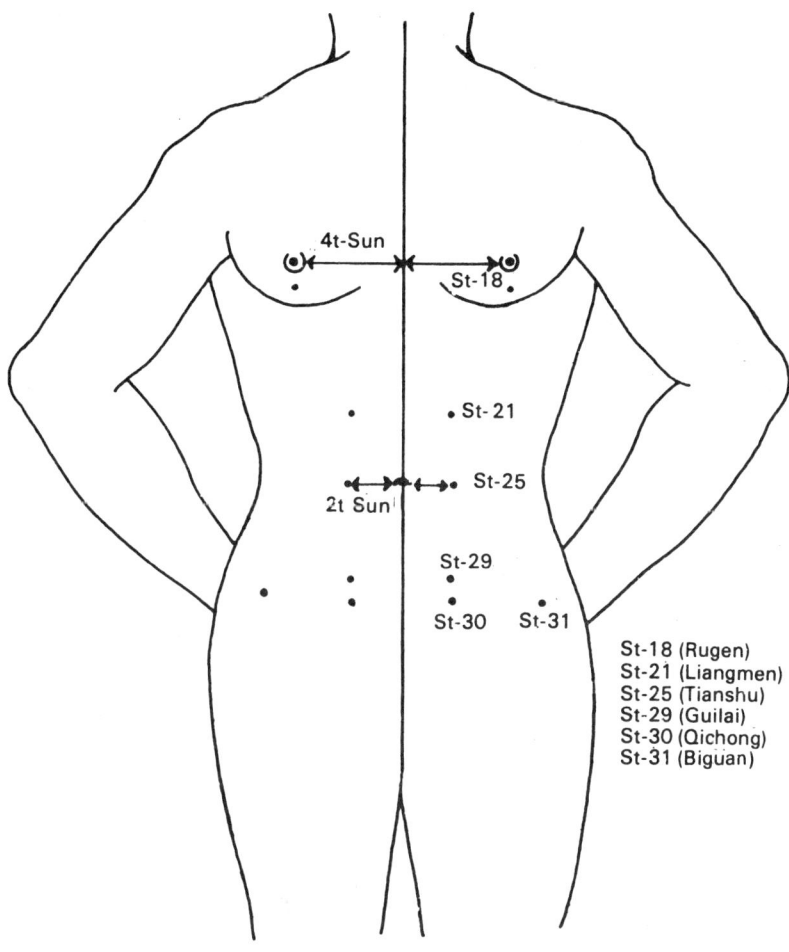

St-18 (Rugen)
St-21 (Liangmen)
St-25 (Tianshu)
St-29 (Guilai)
St-30 (Qichong)
St-31 (Biguan)

Fig. 14.23

St-19 (161) Burong (Pujung)
Location	:	6 t-sun above the umbilicus and 2 t-sun lateral to the midline.
Indications	:	Abdominal pain, intercostal neuralgia, herniation of the bowel, enuresis and insanity.
Needling	:	0.5 to 1 t-sun, straight.

St-20 (162) Chengman
Location	:	5 t-sun above the umbilicus and 2 t-sun lateral to the midline.
Indications	:	Acute and chronic gastritis and epigastric pain.
Needling	:	0.5 to 1.0 t-sun, straight.

St-21 (163) Liangmen
Location	:	4 t-sun above the umbilicus and 2 t-sun lateral to the midline.

Indications   : Gastric ulcer, acute and chronic gastritis, gastroneurosis, duodenal ulcer, gall bladder colic, visceroptosis, umblical and incisional hernia and dyspnoea and Acupuncture anaesthesia.

Peculiarity   : Right side Liangmen (St-21) is a dangerous point because of its position over gall bladder.

Needling   : Right side : 0.5 t-sun or less, slanting.
                     Left side   : 0.5 to 1 t-sun, straight.

St-22 (164) Guanmen (Kuanmen)

Location   : 3 t-sun above the umbilicus and 2 t-sun lateral to the midline.

Indications   : Abdominal pain, distended abdomen, anorexia, hyperperistalsis, diarrhoea and oedema.

Needling   : 0.5 to 1 t-sun, straight.

St-23 (165) Taiyi

Location   : 2 t-sun above the umbilicus and 2 t-sun lateral to the midline.

Indications   : Abdominal pain, herniation of the bowel, enuresis, psychoneurosis and other mental disorders.

Needling   : 0.5 to 1 t-sun, straight.

St-24 (166) Huaroumen (Huajoumen)

Location   : 1 t-sun above the umbilicus and 2 t-sun lateral to the midline.

Indications   : Vomiting, epigastric pain and gastralgia, psychoneurosis and other mental disorders.

Needling   : 0.5 to 1 t-sun, straight.

St-25 (167) Tianshu (Tienshu)

Location   : 2 t-sun lateral to umbilicus over rectus abdominis muscle.

Indications   : Acute and chronic gastroenteritis, dysentery, constipation, paralysis or laxity of the abdominal musculature or visceroptosis, vomiting, chorera, paralytic ileus, appendicitis and menstrual irregularities amongst females.

Peculiarity   : It is a Mu front point and also an alarm point for large intestine.

Needling   : 0.5 to 1 t-sun, straight.

St-26 (168) Walling (Wailing)

Location   : 1 t-sun below the Tianshu (St-25) and 2 t-sun lateral to midline.

Indications   : Gastralgia, intestinal colic, dysmenorrhoea and other menstrual disorders.

Needling   : 0.5 to 1 t-sun, straight.

St-27 (169) Daju (Tachu)

Location   : 2 t-sun below Tainshu (St-25).

Indications   : Gastritis, intestinal colic, gastralgia, spermatorrhoea and nocturnal seminal ejaculation.

Needling   : 0.5 to 1 t-sun, straight.

St-28 (170) Shuidao (Shuitao)

Location   : 3 t-sun below Tainshu (St-25) 2 t-sun lateral to midline.

Indications   : Cystitis, retention of urine, nephritis and orchitis.

Needling   : 0.5 to 1 t-sun, straight.

St-29 (171) Guilai (Kuilai)

Location   : 4 t-sun below Tianshu (St-25) and 2 t-sun lateral to midline.

Indications   : All acute and chronic disorders of urogenital organs, i.e. functional uterine bleeding menorrhagia, amenorrhoea, spasmodic dysmenorrhoea and leucorrhoea, prolapse of uterus and pelvic cellulitis in females, orchitis and epididymitis in males and urinary disorders in both sexes.

Needling   : 0.5 to 1 t-sun, straight.

Note   : Lower bowel disorders can also be treated with this point.

St-30 (172) Qichong (Chichung)

Location   : 5 t-sun below Tianshu (St-25) and 2 t-sun lateral to midline in the inguinal region.

Indications   : Hernia and disorders of urogenital organs, lower bowel disorders.

Needling   : 0.5 to to 1 t-sun, straight.

St-31 (173) Biguan (Pikuan)

Location   : In the line of the lower border of the pubic symphysis, directly below the anterior superior iliac spine.

Indications   : Hemiplegia, paraplegia, poliomyelitis, inguinal lymphadenitis, lumbago, pain of urethritis and disorders of the hip.

Needling   : 1 to 1.5 t-sun, straight.

St-32 (174) Femur Futu (Futu)

Location   : 6 t-sun above the upper margin of the patella between rectus femoris and vatus lateralis on antero-lateral aspect of the thigh (Fig. 14.24).

Indications   : Hemiplegia, paraplegia, poliomyelitis, arthritis of the knee, urticaria, wasting of the quadriceps muscle.

Needling   : 1 to 2 t-sun, straight.

St-33 (175) Yinshi (Yinshih)

Location   : 3 t-sun above the upper and outer margin of the patella.

Indications   : Painful knee and paralysis of the lower extremity.

Needling   : 1 to 2 t-sun, straight or obliquely upwards.

St-34 (176) Liangqiu (Liang Chiu)

Location   : In a depression on the front of thigh 2 t-sun above the upper and outer edge of the patella, vertically above the lateral foramen of patella or Dubi (St-35).

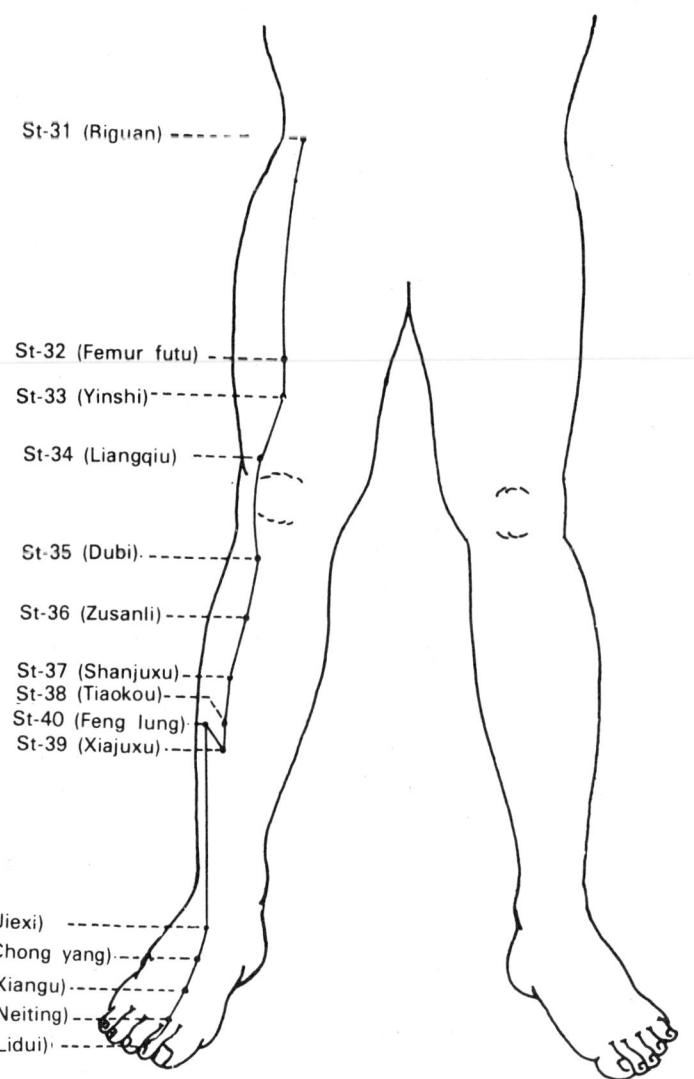

St-31 (Riguan)

St-32 (Femur futu)

St-33 (Yinshi)

St-34 (Liangqiu)

St-35 (Dubi)

St-36 (Zusanli)

St-37 (Shanjuxu)
St-38 (Tiaokou)
St-40 (Feng lung)
St-39 (Xiajuxu)

St-41 (Jiexi)
St-42 (Chong yang)
St-43 (Xiangu)
St-44 (Neiting)
St-45 (Lidui)

Fig. 14.24

Peculiarity	:	It is a Xi-cleft point of the stomach channel.
Indications	:	Diseases of the knee joint, epigastric pain, gastralgia, diarrhoea, mastitis and facial neuralgia.
Needling	:	1 to 1.5 t-sun, straight.

St-35 (177) Dubi (Tupi)

Location : Below the patella lateral to the ligamentum patella. It is best located with the knee slightly flexed and the depression over the lateral foramen of the patella (centre of the lateral knee eye).

Indications   : Arthritis and other diseases of the knee joint, poliomyelitis and weakness of the leg muscle.
Needling   : 0.5 to 1 t-sun, straight or slanting towards medial foramen of the patella Xiyan (Extra 32).

St-36 (178) Zusanli (Tsusanli)   (Tsusanli)

Location   : One finger breadth lateral to the lower border of the tibial tuberosity or 3 t-sun below Dubi (St-35).
Indications   : Immunity improving and tonification of the body in debility, fatigue, weakness and hypotension.
                    Poliomyelitis, polyneuropathy, weakness and myopathies of the leg.
                    Epigastric pain, gastralgia, gastritis, anorexia, nausea, vomiting, diarrhoea, dysentery, constipation, flatulence, paralytic ileus and appendicitis.
                    Hypertension, diabetes, and thromboangitis obliterance, elephantiasis and varicose veins.
Needling   : 1 to 1.5 t-sun, straight.

St-37 (179) Shanjuxu (Shangchuhsu)

Location   . 6 t-sun below Dubi (St-35) one finger breadth lateral to the anterior border of the tibia on the lateral aspect of the leg.
Indications   : Abdominal pain, hemiplegia and acute diarrhoea.
Needling   : 1 to 1.5 t-sun, straight.

St-38 (180) Tiaokou

Location   : 5 t-sun below Zusanli (St-36).
Indications   : Arthritis of the knee joint, periarthritis, paralysis of lower extremities and epigastric pain.
Needling   : 1 to 1.5 t-sun, straight.
Note   : This is a specific point for frozen shoulder.

St-39 (181) Xiajuxu (Hsiachuhsu)

Location   : 6 t-sun below Zusanli (St-36).
Indications   : Paralysis of the lower limbs, acute diarrhoea and epigastric pain.
Needling   : 1.0 to 1.5 t-sun, straight.

St-40 (182) Feng Lung

Location   : 5 t-sun below Zusanli (St-36) and 2 finger breadth lateral to the anterior border of the tibia.
Note   : Feng Lung (St-40) and Tiaokou (St-38) are at the same level.
Peculiarity   : It is a Luo-connecting point of the stomach channel with the spleen channel.
Indications   : Cough with expectoration, hemiplegia paralysis of lower extremities, vertigo, epilepsy and schizophrenia.
Needling   : 1.5 to 2 t-sun, straight.
Note   : This is a specific point for bronchial asthma.

St-41 (183) Jiexi (Chiehhsi)

Location	:	On the dorsum of the foot at the midpoint of the transverse crease of ankle.
Indications	:	Pain and arthritis of the ankle joint, foot drop, chronic non-healing ulcers, varicose veins and hemiplegia.
Needling	:	0.5 to 1 t-sun, straight.

St-42 (184) Chong Yang (Chungyang)

Location	:	On the highest spot of the dorsum of the foot 1.5 t-sun distal to the Jiexi (St-41) by the side of dorsalis pedis artery.
Indications	:	Painful conditions and paralysis of the lower limb, toothache and epilepsy.
Needling	:	0.3 to 0.5 t-sun, straight. Protect the vessels.

St-43 (185) Xiangu (Hsienku)

Location	:	Between the second and third metatarsal bones, on the dorsum of the foot.
Indications	:	Ascites, oedema of face, oedema of the foot, painful conditions of the dorsum of the foot, polyneuropathy, abdominal pain, headache and toothache.
Needling	:	0.5 to 1 t-sun, straight.

St-44 (186) Neiting

Location	:	On the dorsal aspect of the foot 0.5 t-sun proximal to the web space between the second and third toes.
Indications	:	Arthritis of the ankle and small joints of the foot; paralysis and polyneuropathy of the lower extremity.
Note	:	It is one of the best analgesic points and can be used for treating painful conditions of the lower extremity. It is used as a distal point for treating painful disorders of the proximal parts like headache and toothache.
Needling	:	0.2 to 0.5 t-sun, straight or slanting upwards.

St-45 (187) Lidui (Litui)

Location	:	0.1 t-sun proximal to the lateral side of the corner of the nail of the second toe.
Peculiarity	:	It is a Jing-well point.
Indications	:	Acute emergencies, hyperpyrexia and epilepsy.
Needling	:	0.3 to 0.5 t-sun, straight.

4. THE SPLEEN MERIDIAN

According to the traditional Chinese description it is a Yin channel associated with the element earth and possesses interior and exterior relationship with the stomach meridian.

Total number of points : 21.

Starting point	:	Medial side of the great toe.
Terminal point	:	Sixth intercostal space in the mid-axillary line.
Pathway	:	After taking origin from a point at the medial side of the great toe it runs along the junction of the two colours (red and white) of the skin on medial aspect of the foot and courses upwards in front of the medial malleolus. From there it runs along the medial aspect of the leg and posterior aspect of the tibia and reaches anterio-medial aspect of the knee and the thigh to enter into the pelvis. Here it divides into two branches : (i) superficial branch, and (ii) inner branch.
Superficial branch	:	It ascends up from the anterior surface of the abdomen and runs 4 t-sun lateral to the midline up to the chest and at the level of Dabao (Sp-21) it goes deep to meet with the inner branch. It ends in the sixth intercostal space in mid-axillary line.
Inner branch	:	It enters into the abdominal cavity and reaches its principal organ spleen and communicates with the stomach. It ascends up through the diaphragm and courses along the oesophagus to reach the base of the tongue and ends there (Fig. 14. 25).

Therapeutic indications

1. All the disorders along the pathway of the channel.
2. Diseases of the stomach, spleen and pancreas.
3. Allergic disorders and skin diseases.
4. Diseases of the reticuloendothelial system.
5. Gastro-intestinal diseases like epigastric pain, gastritis, emesis and jaundice.
6. Genito-urinary disorders.
7. Oedema and ascites due to various causes.

DESCRIPTION OF THE POINTS

Sp-1 (299) Yinbai (Yinpai)

Location	:	On the inner side of the great toe 0.1; t-sun poximal to the medial corner of tne nail.
Peculiarity	:	This is a Jing-well point.
Indications	:	Acute emergencies, abdominal distension, menstrual disorders and sleep disturbances.
Needling	:	0.1 to 0.3 t-sun, straight.

Sp-2 (300) Dadu (Tatu)

Location	:	On the inner side of the big toe, antero-inferior to the 1st metatarso-phalangeal joint.
Indications	:	Hyperpyrexia, hyperhydrosis, distension of abdomen and epigastric pain.
Needling	:	0.3 to 0.5 t-sun, straight.

Sp-3 ((301) Taibai (Taipai)

Location	:	On the inner aspect of the foot postero-inferior to the head of the 1st metatarsal bone at the junction of the two colours of the skin.

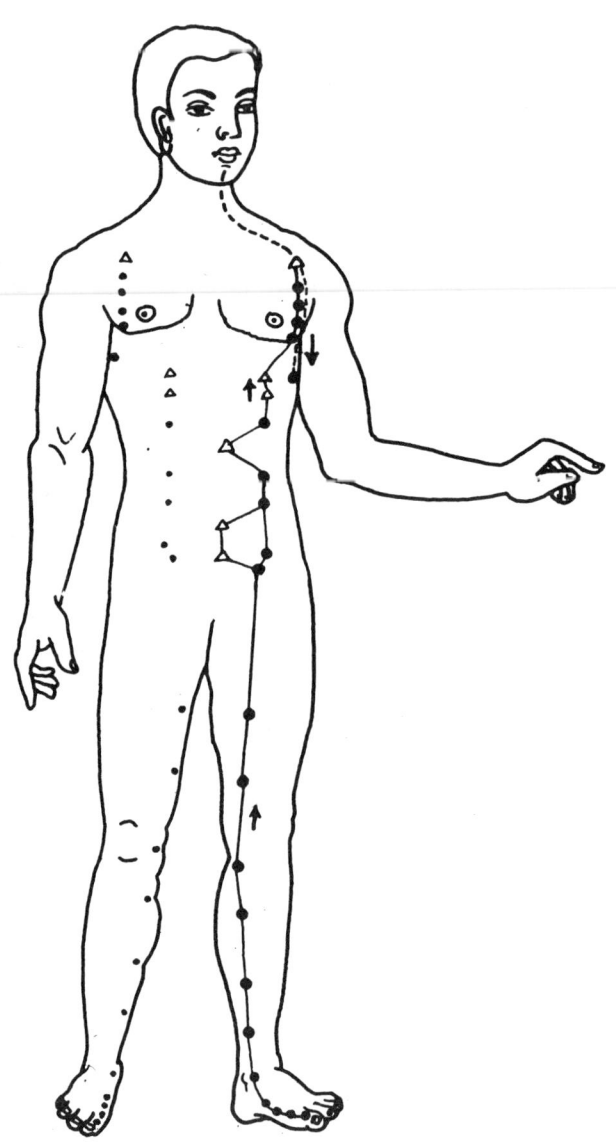

Fig. 14.25   The spleen meridian.

Peculiarity : This is a Yuan (source) point.

Indications : Epigastric pain, gastritis, gastralgia, flatulence, abdominal distension, emesis, bowel disturbances like diarrhoea, dysentry, constipation.

Needling : 0.3 to 0.5 t-sun, straight.

Sp-4 (302) Gongsun (Kungsun)

Location : On the inner aspect of the foot in the proximal end of the 1st metatarsal bone at the junction of the two colours of the skin.

Peculiarity : It is the Luo-connecting point of the spleen channel.

Indications : Epigastric pain, gastralgia, emesis, anorexia, dyspepsia, bowel disturbances like diarrhoea and constipation, menorrhagia and functional uterine bleeding.

Needling : 0.5 to 1 t-sun, straight.

Sp-5 (303) Shang Qiu (Shang Chiu)

Location : At the crossing of the two lines drawn along the anterior and inferior borders of the medial malleolus, respectively.

Indications : Gastritis, arthritis, pain and sprain of ankle joint, planter fascitis.

Needling : 0.3 to 0.5 t-sun, straight.

Sp-6 (304) Sanyinjiao (Sanyinchiao)

Location : 3 t-sun proximal to the tip of medial malleolus just behind the medial border and posterior surface of the tibia (Fig. 14.26).

Peculiarities : It is the distal point for urogenital disorders and diseases of the pelvic cavity.

Kidney, liver and spleen channels meet on this spot in their course (Word *san* means three and *jiao* means channels).

Indications : Bowel disturbances like diarrhoea, abdominal distension, indigestion and lower abdominal pain.

Diseases of the genito-urinary organs in both sexes.

Dysmenorrhoea, amenorrhoea and leucorrhoea in females.

Impotence, spermatorrhoea epididymo-orchitis and phosphaturia in males.

Retention of urine, frequency of micturition, dysuria and enuresis in both sexes.

Diseases of the liver, spleen and kidney.

Diseases of the skin like allergies, psoriasis, eczematoid dermatitis and infections.

Diabetes mellitus (endocrine disorders).

Diseases along the pathway of the channel.

Hemiplegia, polyneuropathy, foot drop and myopathies.

For the general tonification effect in debility, fatigue, weakness and low blood pressure.

Vascular disorders like Buerger's disease and varicose ulcers.

Diseases of the reticulo-endothelial system.

Painless child birth (acupuncture delivery).

Needling : 1.5 to 2 t-sun, straight.

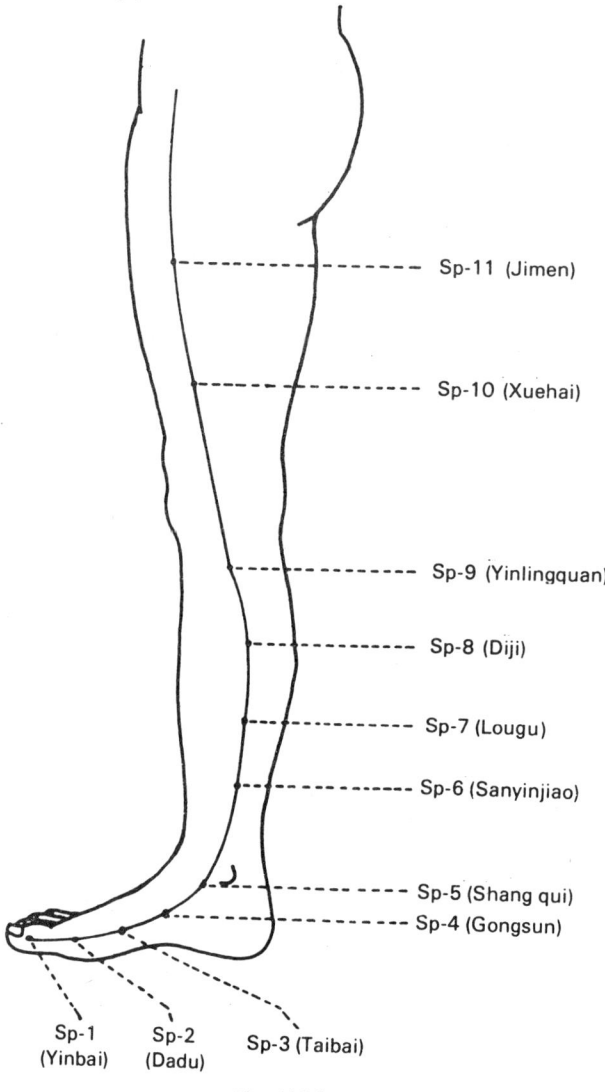

Sp-11 (Jimen)

Sp-10 (Xuehai)

Sp-9 (Yinlingquan)

Sp-8 (Diji)

Sp-7 (Lougu)

Sp-6 (Sanyinjiao)

Sp-5 (Shang qui)
Sp-4 (Gongsun)

Sp-1   Sp-2   Sp-3 (Taibai)
(Yinbai)   (Dadu)

Fig. 14.26

Sp-7 (305) Lougu (Louku)

Location	:	6 t-sun above the apex of the medial malleolus behind the tibia.
Indications	:	Numbnees of the leg and knee, distended abdomen and hyperperistalsis.
Needling	:	1 to 1.5 t-sun, straight.

Sp-8 (306) Diji (Tichi)

Location	:	3 t-sun below Yinling quan (Sp-9).
Peculiarity	:	It is a Xi-cleft point.

Indications : Menstrual disturbances, distended abdomen and pain in the loins and lumbago.

Note : It is a specific point for dysmenorrhoea.

Needling : 1 to 2 t-sun, straight.

Sp-9 (307) Yinlingquan (Yinlingchuan)

Location : In the groove of the lower border of the medial condyle of the tibia in a level with the lower border of the tuberosity of the tibia, same level as that of Yanglingquan (GB-34) (Fig. 14.27).

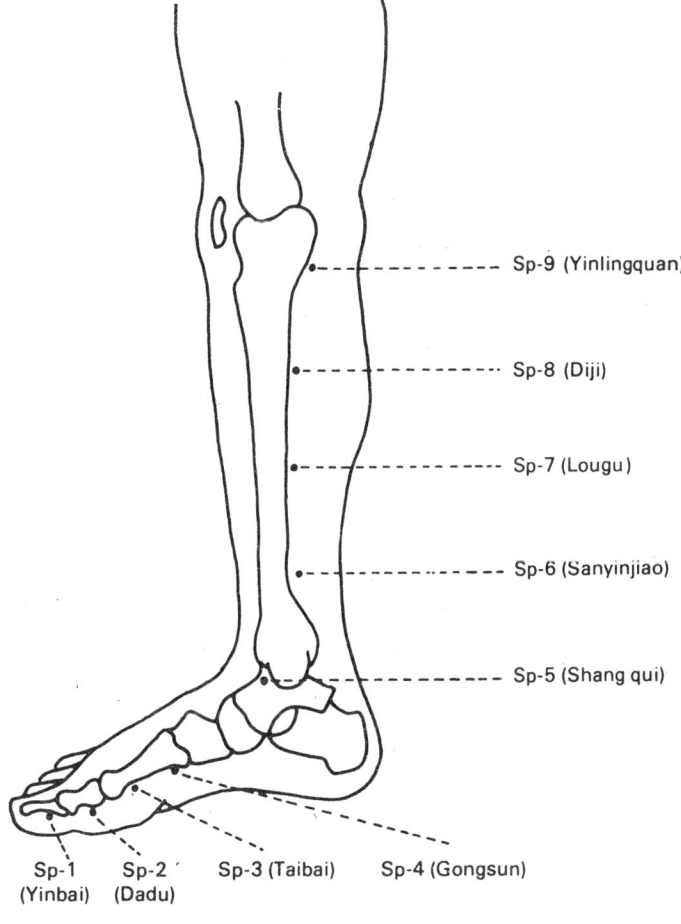

Sp-9 (Yinlingquan)

Sp-8 (Diji)

Sp-7 (Lougu)

Sp-6 (Sanyinjiao)

Sp-5 (Shang qui)

Sp-1 (Yinbai) Sp-2 (Dadu) Sp-3 (Taibai) Sp-4 (Gongsun)

Fig. 14.27

Indications : Abdominal pain, dysuria, enuresis, nocturnal pollution, menstrual disturbances, dysentery, ascites, elephantiasis and oedema anywhere in the body.

It is used in the arthritis of the knee as a local point.

Needling : 1.5 to 2 t-sun straight.

Sp-10 (308) Xuehai (Hsuehhai)

Location   : 2 t-sun proximal to the superior border of the patella on the antero-
medial aspect of the thigh. [It can be easily located by putting the palm
of your opposite hand on the patient's patella when the point is indicated by the tip of the thumb which actually lies on the most prominent
point on the bulge of the vastue medialis muscle (Fig. 14.28). It is
advised to sit in front of the patient while locating the point.]

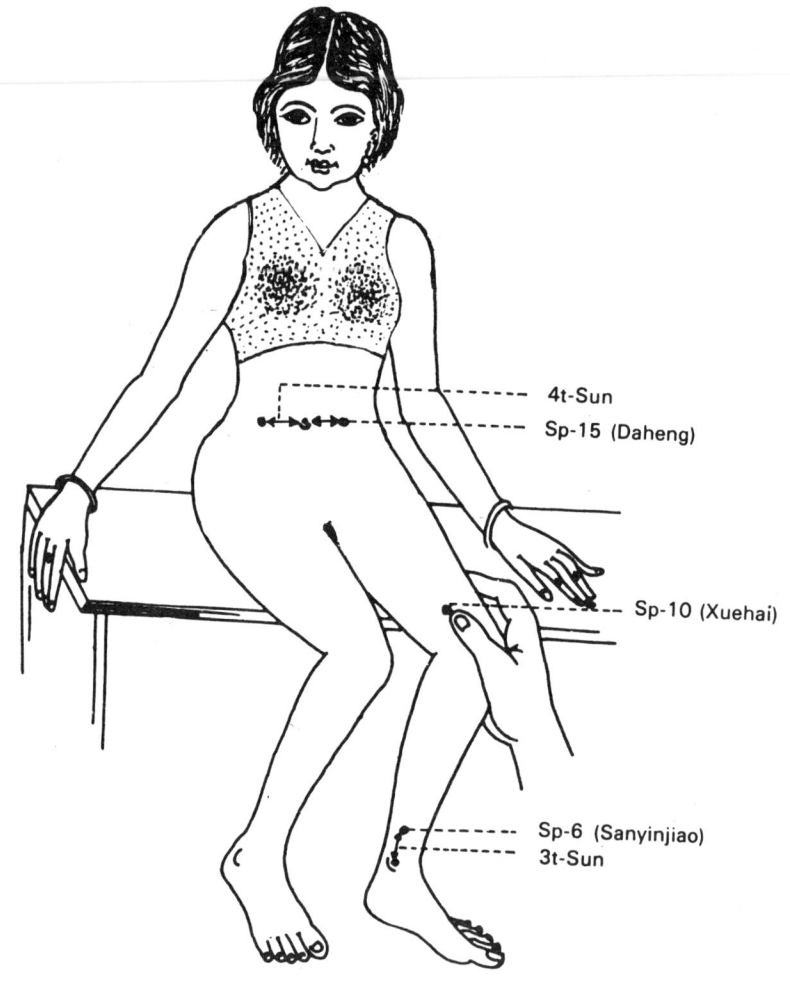

Fig. 14.28

Indications   : Disorders of the knee joint, menstrual disturbances, urticaria, psoriasis,
skin infections, tropical eosinophilia, pneumonitis, various allergic
disorders and diseases of genito-urinary organs.

Needling   : 1 to 1.5 t-sun, straight.

Sp-11 (309) Jimen (Chimen)

Location   : 8 t-sun above the antero-medial border of patella, medial to the sartorius muscle.

Indications   : Frequency of micturition, enuresis, dysuria and inguinal lymphadenitis.

Needling   : 1 to 2 t-sun, straight.

Sp-12 (310) Chongmen (Chungmen)

Location   : 3.5 t-sun lateral to the mid-point of the upper border of the symphysis pubis, just lateral to the femoral artery.

Indications   : Endometritis, orchitis, seminal vesiculitis funiculitis, and hernia.

Needling   : 0.7 to 1 t-sun, straight.
                 Protect the femoral artery.

Sp-13 (311) Fushe

Location   : 4 t-sun lateral to the midline of the anterior abdominal wall, 0.7 t-sun above Chongmen (Sp-12).

Indications   : Appendicitis and appendicular dyspepsia, pain in abdomen, hernia and constipation.

Needling   : 0.5 to 1 t-sun, straight.

Sp-14 (312) Fujie (Fuchieh)

Location   : 4 t-sun lateral to the mid-line and 1.5 t-sun below the umbilicus.

Indications   : Umbilical hernia, inguinal hernia, paraumbilical pain and diarrhoea.

Needling   : 0.5 to 1 t-sun, straight.

Sp-15 (313) Daheng (Taheng)

Location   : Vertically below the nipple 4 t-sun lateral to the umbilicus.

Indications   : Paralytic ileus. diarrhoea, constipation, intestinal parasitosis and epigastric pain.

Needling   : 0.5 to 1 t-sun, straight.

Sp-16 (314) Fuai

Location   : 3 t-sun above Daheng (Sp-15) 4 t-sun lateral to midline (Fig. 14.29).

Indications   : Bowel disturbances like diarrhoea, dysentry, constipation, dyspepsia and abdominal pain.

Needling   : 0.5 to 1 t-sun, straight.

Sp-17 (315) Shidou (Shihtou)

Location   : 5th intercostal space, 6 t-sun lateral to the midline.

Indications   : Heavyness in chest, fibrositis of the chest wall, pain in chest and pain in subcostal region.

Needling   : 0.5 t-sun, slanting.

Sp-18 (316) Tianxi (Tienhsi)

Location   : 4th intercostal space 6 t-sun lateral to the midline.

Indications   : Lactational disorders, mastitis, fibroadenosis of the breast, cough, pain in chest and intercostal neuralgia.

Needling   : 0.5 to 0.8 t-sun, slanting.

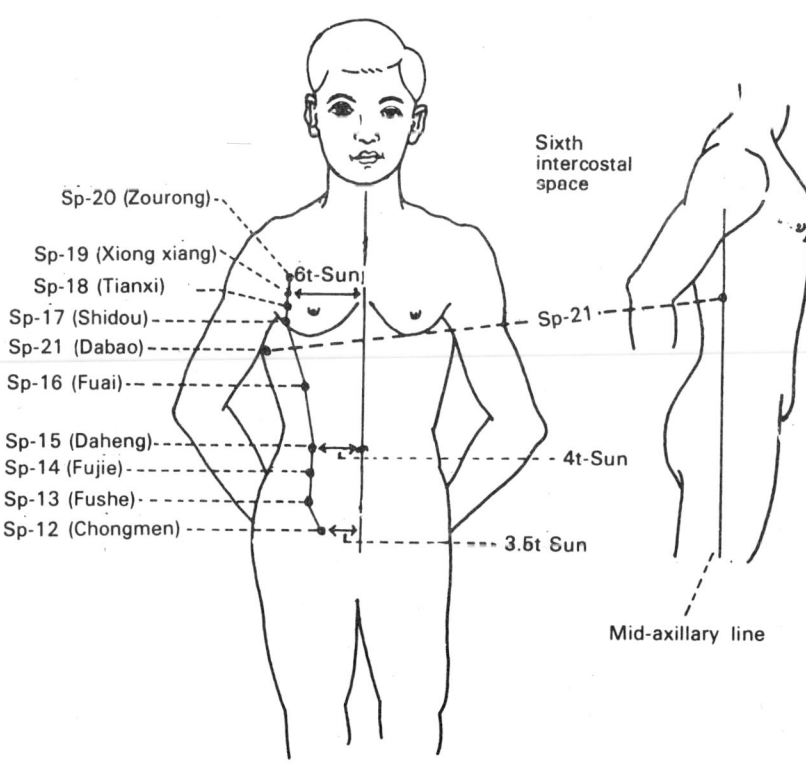

Fig. 14.29

Sp-19 (317) Xiong Xiang (Hsiung-Hsiang)
Location	: 3rd intercostal space, 6 t-sun lateral to midline.
Indications	: Constricting sensation in the chest, heavyness and pain in the chest, subcostal and costal pain.
Needling	: 0.5 to 0.8 t-sun, slanting.

Sp-20 (318) Zhourong (Choujung)
Location	: 2nd intercostal space, 6 t-sun lateral to the midline.
Indications	: Thoracalgia, cough, costal and subcostal pain.
Needling	: 0.5 to 0.8 t-sun, slanting.

Sp-21 (319) Dabao (Tapao)
Location	: 6th intercostal space in the mid-axillary line.
Peculiarity	: It is Luo-connecting point between the stomach and the spleen channel.
Note	: Spleen channel has the previlege of having two Luo-connecting points, the other point being Gongsun (Sp-4).
Indications	: Thoracalgia, dyspnoea, general bodyache, neurasthenia and costal pain.
Needling	: 0.5 to 0.8 t-sun, slanting.

5. THE HEART MERIDIAN

According to the traditional Chinese description it is a Yin channel associated with the element fire and possesses interior and exterior relationship with the small intestine meridian.

Total number of points : 9.

Starting point	:	Centre of the axilla.
Terminal point	:	Lateral side of the little finger proximal to the corner of the nail.
Pathway	:	This channel starts from the heart and it has three branches : (i) inner descending branch, (ii) inner ascending branch, and (iii) superficial branch.
Inner descending branch	:	It descends through the diaphragm and connects with the small intestine.
Inner ascending branch	:	It ascends upwards to the trachea and oropharynx and then further upwards to the eye and brain.
Superficial branch	:	It emerges on the body surface at the centre of the axilla in the mid-axillary line and descends down along the antero-medial aspect of the upper arm, cubital fossa and forearm up to the capitate bone, proximal to the palm and then it terminates on the lateral side of the corner of the nail of the little finger (Fig. 14.30).

Therapeutic Indications

1. Mental disorders : Psychosis, hysteria, palpitation, speech disorders, neurasthenia, anxiety, addiction.
2. Cardiac disorders : Coronary thrombosis, angina pectoris.
3. Sleep disturbances : Insomnia, frequent dreams.
4. Neurological disorders : Schizophrenia, epilepsy, coma, apoplexy, syncope.
5. Autonomic disturbances : Night sweats, hyperhydrosis, erythromelalgia.
6. Disorders along the pathway of the channel : Arthritis of elbow, tennis-elbow, arthritis of the wrist, costalgia, branchial neuralgia, paralysis of the upper extremity, fibrositis around the shoulder, diseases of the shoulder, writer's cramps.
7. Deficient lactation.

DESCRIPTION OF THE POINTS

H-1 (72) Jequan (Chichuan)

Location	:	Centre of the axilla, medial to the axillary artery.
Peculiarity	:	It is a dangerous point.
Indications	:	Costalgia, brachial neuralgia, pain in the arm, paralysis of the upper extremity, deficient lactation, diseases of the shoulder and fibrositis around the shoulder.
Needling	:	0.5 t-sun or less, straight.

H-2 (73) Qingling (Chingling)

Location	:	On the antero-medial aspect of the arm in a groove medial to the muscle biceps branchii ·3 t-sun above the elbow.
Indications	:	Costal and subcostal pain, painful shoulder and arm.
Needling	:	0.5 to 1 t-sun, straight.

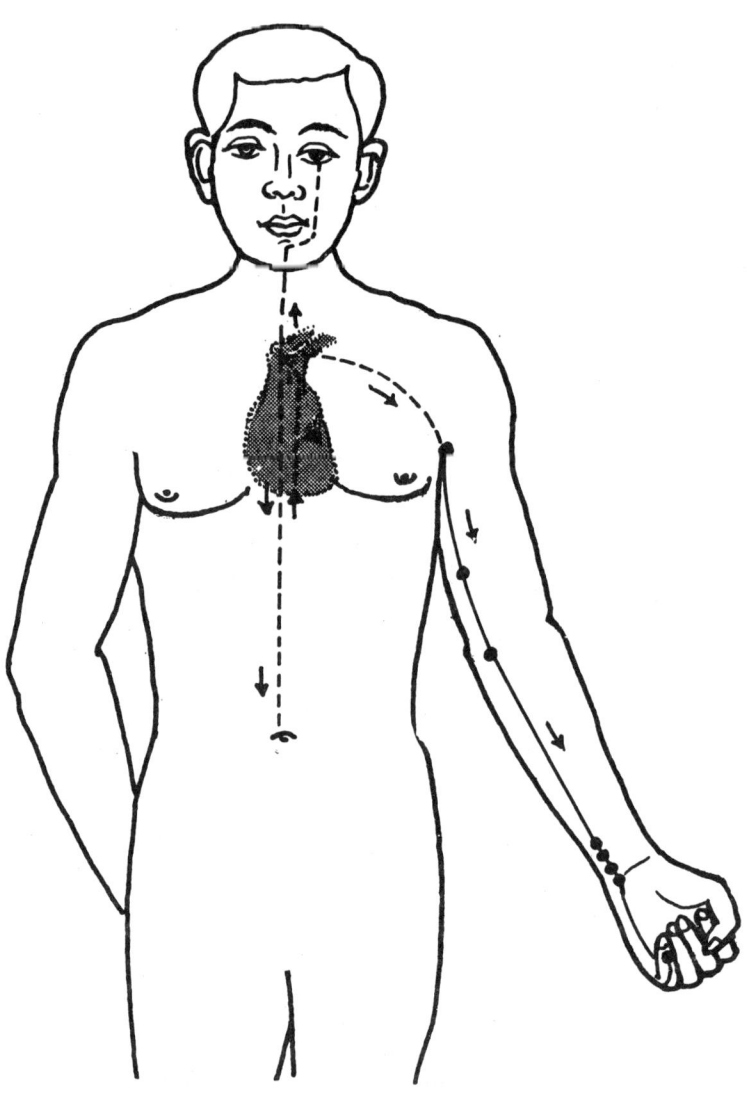

Fig. 14.30   The heart meridian

H-3 (74) Shaohai

Location   :   At the midpoint of the line joining medial end of the transverse cubital crease and medial epicondyle of the humerus when the elbow is kept in the flexed position (Fig. 14.31).

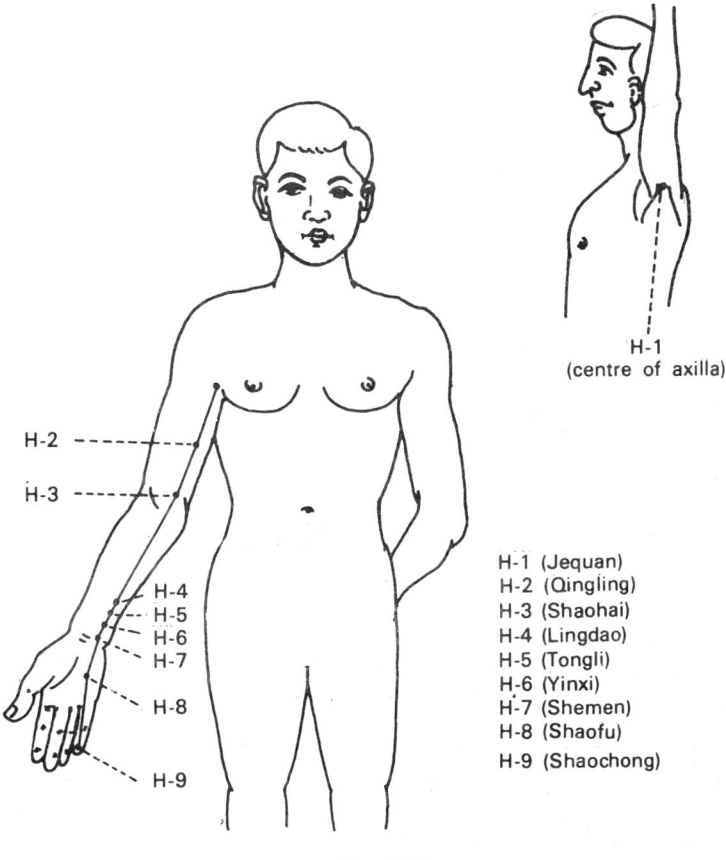

H-1
(centre of axilla)

H-1 (Jequan)
H-2 (Qingling)
H-3 (Shaohai)
H-4 (Lingdao)
H-5 (Tongli)
H-6 (Yinxi)
H-7 (Shemen)
H-8 (Shaofu)
H-9 (Shaochong)

Fig. 14.31

Indications   :   Writer's cramps, arthritis of the elbow joint, tremor and numbness of the arm, tennis-elbow, angina pectoris and coronary thrombosis.

Needling   :   0.5 to 1 t-sun, straight.

H-4 (75) Lingdao (Lingtao)

Location   :   On the medial aspect of the forearm, 1.5 t-sun above the posterior border of the pisiform bone, lateral to the tendon of muscle flexor carpi ulnaris [1.5 t-sun above Shenmen (H-7)].

Indications   :   Arthritis of the wrist, psychosis, hysteria, ulna neuralgia and angina pectoris.

Needling   :   0.5 to 1 t-sun, straight.

H-5 (76) Tongli (Tungli)

Location	: 1 t-sun above the posterior border of the pisiform bone lateral to the tendon of the flexor carpi ulnaris [on the ulnar side of the wrist 1 t-sun above Shenmen (H-7)].
Peculiarity	: It is a Luo-connecting point of the heart channel.
Indications	: Speech disorders like-aphasia, hoarseness of voice, stammering, palpitation, psychosis and other mental disorders, insomnia and painful arm and wrist.
	NOTE : This is a specific point for speech disorders.
Needling	: 0.5 to 1 t-sun, straight.

H-6 (77) Yinxi (Yinhsi)

Location	: On the front of the wrist, 0.5 t-sun proximal to the posterior border of the pisiform bone lateral to the tendon of the muscle flexor carpi ulnaris.
Peculiarity	: It is Xi-cleft point.
Indications	: Psychoneurosis, neurasthenia, palpitation, night sweats, angina-pectoris and myocardial infarction.
Needling	: 0.5 to 1 t-sun, straight.

II-7 (78) Shenmen

Location	: On the inner side of the wrist, just proximal to the pisiform bone, in a groove lateral to the tendon of muscle flexor carpi ulnaris. [The medial end of the most distal wrist crease on the anterior aspect (Fig. 14.31)].
Peculiarity	: It is the Yuan (source) point of the heart channel.
Indications	: Anxiety, insomnia, palpitation, hysteria, mental disorders, frequent dreams, hyperhydrosis, alcohol addiction, schizophrenia and epilepsy. It is one of the best tranquilising points.
Needling	: 0.5 t-sun or less, straight or slanting.

H-8 (79) Shaofu

Location	: On the palm between the 4th and 5th metacarpal bones. Close the fist and mark the point between the tips of the little and ring fingers.
Indications	: Arthritis of the carpal joints.
	Carpal tunnel syndrome.
	Palpitation.
	Neuropathies of the hand.
	Erythromelalgia, Raynaud's diseases.
	Chest pain, costalgia.
	Enuresis and dysuria.
	Pruritis vulvae.
Needling	: 0.5 t-sun or less, straight.
	Moxa heat for 5 minutes.

H-9 (80) Shaochong (Shaochung)

Location	: On the lateral side of the little finger about 0.1 t-sun proximal the lateral corner of the nail.

Peculiarity   : It is a Jing-well point.
Indications   : All acute emergencies, coronary thrombosis, palpitation, chest pain, coma, syncope, apoplexy.
Needling   0.1 to 0.3 t-sun, straight.
                   Sometimes trinagular needle is used until bleeding.

6. THE SMALL INTESTINE MERIDIAN

According to the traditional Chinese description it is a Yang channel associated with the element fire and possesses interior and exterior relationship with the heart channel.
Total number of points : 19.

Starting point   : Corner of the nail of the little finger.
Terminal point   : A point in front of the centre of the tragus and tempromandibular joint.
Pathway   : After taking origin from the ulnar side of the tip of the little finger, the meridian passes along the medial side of the palm and wrist and emerges from the styloid process of the ulna. It then courses upwards along the posteromedial aspect of the forearm, midpoint of the olecranon and medial epicondyle, posteromedial aspect of the upper arm upto the shoulder joint. It takes a turn around the shoulder joint and reaches supraclavicular fossa, where it divides into two branches. In its course it meets the governing vessels channel at the level of Dazhui (GV-14).

Branches

Inner branch   : It reaches the heart along the oesophagus from where it courses through the cardiac orifice to reach the stomach and then further down to end in the principal organ, small intestine.
Superficial branch : It reaches the angle of the mandible and again divides into two sub-branches :
Zygomatic branch   : It ends in the zygomatic area after taking a turn from the medial canthus of the eye.
Auricular branch   : It passes to the lateral canthus of the eye and then turns back to reach the front of the ear and ends there (Fig. 14.32).

Therapeutic Indications

1. All the disorders along the pathway of the channel, i.e. myopathies, neuropathies, paralysis, wrist-drop, arthritis, etc.
2. Diseases of the small intestine.
3. Ear disorders: Deafnees, tinnitus aurium, vertigo.
4. Eye diseases: Corneal opacity, diminished vision.
5. Stiffness of the neck and cervical region.
6. Heart disorders.
7. Neurological and psychosomatic disorders: Convulsions, hysteria, epilepsy, mental disorders.
8. Speech disorders: Aphonia, hoarseness of voice, aphasia.

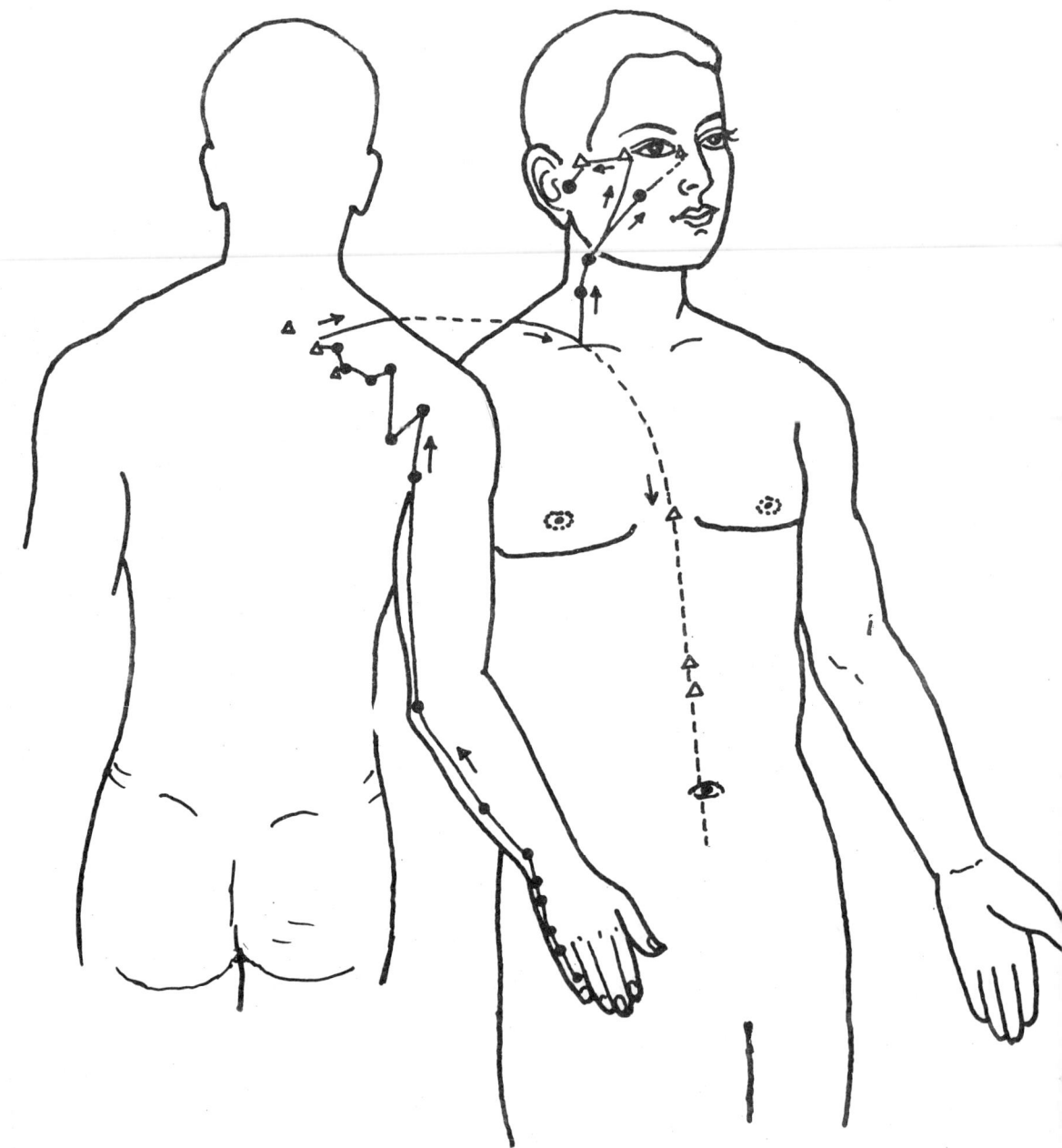

Fig. 14.32   The small intestine meridian

DESCRIPTION OF THE POINTS

SI-1 (124) Shaoze (Shaotse)

Location : 0.1 t-sun proximal to the corner of the nail of the little finger on its medial side (Fig. 14.33).

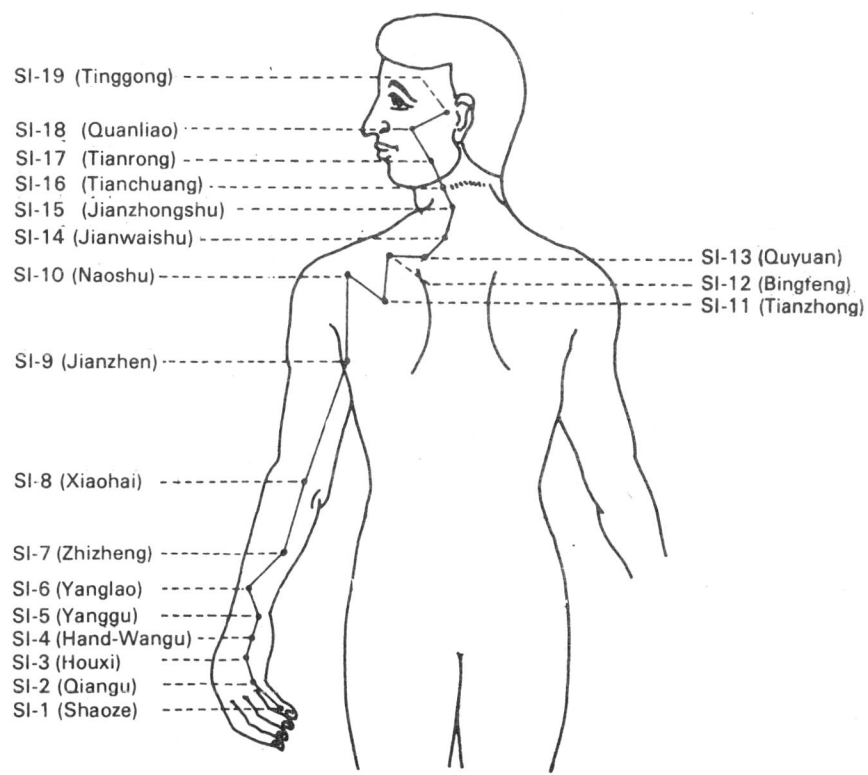

SI-19 (Tinggong)
SI-18 (Quanliao)
SI-17 (Tianrong)
SI-16 (Tianchuang)
SI-15 (Jianzhongshu)
SI-14 (Jianwaishu)
SI-10 (Naoshu)
SI-13 (Quyuan)
SI-12 (Bingfeng)
SI-11 (Tianzhong)
SI-9 (Jianzhen)
SI-8 (Xiaohai)
SI-7 (Zhizheng)
SI-6 (Yanglao)
SI-5 (Yanggu)
SI-4 (Hand-Wangu)
SI-3 (Houxi)
SI-2 (Qiangu)
SI-1 (Shaoze)

Fig. 14.33

Peculiarity : It is a Jing-well point.
Indications : All acute emergencies like cordiac and respiratory arrest, convulsions, shock, hysteria and epilepsy.
: It is used in combination with Shangzhong (CV-17) in case of deficient lactation.
Neddling : 0.1 t-sun, straight upwards, or until bleeding with trinagular needle.

SI-2 (125) Qiangu (Chienku)

Location : On the ulnar side of the metacarpophalangeal joint of the little finger.
Indications : Painful arm, tingling and numbness of the fingers, pyrexia, corneal opacity, diminished vision, paralysis of pharyngeal muscles and pharyngitis.
Needling : 0.3 to 0.5 t-sun, straight.

SI-3 (126) Houxi (Houhsi)

Location	:	At the medial end of the main transverse palmar crease, on the ulnar border of the hand proximal to the 5th metacarpophalangeal joint.
Indications	:	Cervical spondylosis, stiffness of the neck torticollis, occipital headache, paralysis of upper extremities, epilepsy, tinnitus aurium and deafness.
Needling	:	0.2 to 0.3 t-sun, straight.
Note	:	This is a very painful point and must be used only when it is unavoidable to use it.

SI-4 (127) Hand-Wangu (Wanku)

Location	:	On the ulnar side of the hand between the 5th metacarpal bone and the hamate bone.
Peculiarity	:	It is a Yuan (source) point.
Indications	:	Stiff fingers, arthritis of the wrist joint and metacarpophalangeal and interphalangeal joints, headache, cholecystitis, tinnitus and wrist drop.
Needling	:	0.3 to 0.5 t-sun, straight.

SI-5 (128) Yanggu (Yangku)

Location	:	On the medial aspect of the wrist in a groove between the pisiform bone and the ulnar styloid process.
Indications	:	Painful arm and wrist (lateral aspect), pain and swelling in the cervical region, cervical spondylosis, psychoneurosis, insanity, deafness and tinnitus.
Needling	:	0.3 to 0.5 t-sun, straight.

SI-6 (129) Yanglao

Location	:	On the posterior aspect of the wrist in a groove lateral to the ulnar styloid process, proximal to the inferior radio-ulnar joint.
Peculiarity	:	This is a Xi-cleft point.
Indications	:	Paralysis of the upper extremity, arthritis of the wrist joint, wrist-drop.
	:	Cervical spondylosis, stiff neck.
	:	Status asthmaticus in association with Shanzhong (CV-17).
Needling	:	0.5 to 1 t-sun, straight or slanting upwards.

SI-7 (130) Zhizheng (Chihcheng)

Location	:	On the ulnar side of the foreram 5 t-sun proximal to Yanggu (SI-5).
Peculiarity	:	It is a Luo-connecting point.
Indications	:	Cervical spondylosis, stiffness of neck, stiff finger, psychological disturbances.
Needling	:	0.5 to 0.8 t-sun, straight.

SI-8 (131) Xiaohai (Hsiaohai)

Location	:	In a depression on the back of the elbow between olecranon and medial epicondyle.
Note	:	Ulnar nerve is in the close proximity of the needle.
Indications	:	Stiff neck, painful elbow and shoulder, back ulnar neuritis swollen cheeks, epilepsy and psychoneurosis.

Needling   :   0.3 to 0.5 t-sun, straight.

SI-9 (132) Jianzhen (Chiencheng)

Location   :   1 t-sun above the lower margin of the posterior axillary fold (arm being kept in full adduction).

Indications   :   Periarthritis of the shoulder joint, paralysis and polyneuropathy of the upper extremity.

Needling   :   0.5 to 1 t-sun, straight.
                        Moxa heat for 10 minutes.

SI-10 (133) Naoshu

Location   :   Vertically above Jianzhen (SI-9) just below the spine of the scapula.

Indications   :   Periarthritis of shoulder, paralysis of upper extremity, other painful conditions of the shoulder and arm.

Needling   :   1 to 2 t-sun, straight.

SI-11 (134) Tianzhong (Tientsung)

Location   :   At the level with the spinous process of the 4th thoracic vertebra, in the centre of infra-scapular fossa (Fig. 14.34).

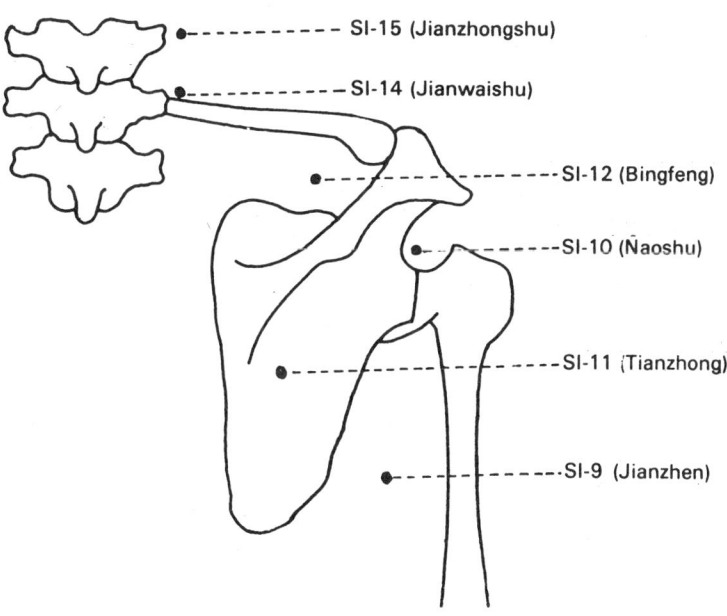

Fig. 14.34

Indications   :   Painful conditions of the elbow, arm and shoulder.

Needling   :   0.5 to 1 t-sun, straight.

SI-12 (135) Bingfeng (Pingfeng)

Location   :   At the centre of infrascapular fossa (Fig. 14.34).

Indications : Painful conditions of the shoulder, numbness in upper extremity, pain in arm elbow and finger.

Needling : 0.5 to 1 t-sun, straight.

SI-13 (136) Quyuan (Chuyuan)

Location : In the suprascapular fossa, near the medial border of the scapula midway between the spinous process of second thoracic vertebra and Naoshu (SI-10).

Indications : Restricted movements, pain and contracture of the shoulder joint.

Needling : 0.5 to 1 t-sun, slanting.

SI-14 (137) Jianwaishu (Chienwaishu)

Location : 3 t-sun lateral to the inferior border of the spinous process of the 1st thoracic vertebra.

Indications : Pain in the back of the shoulder and scapula, stiffness of the neck, pain in the nape of the neck and cervical spondylosis.

Needling : 0.3 to 1 t-sun, straight.

SI-15 (138) Jianzhongshu (Chienchungshu)

Location : 2 t-sun lateral to the inferior border of the spinous process of the seventh cervical vertebra.

Indications : Painful conditions of the shoulder and back like frozen shoulder, fibrositis, myositis and muscle cramps.

: Stiffness of the neck.

: Asthmatic bronchitis, bronchial asthma, eosinophilic lung.

Needling : 0.5 to 1 t-sun, straight.

SI-16 (139) Tianchuang

Location : On the posterior border of the sterno-cleido-mastoid muscle at the level with the laryngeal prominence.

Indications : Deafness, tinnitus aurium, stiffness of the neck, cervical spondylosis, sore throat, aphasia, painful tonsils and diseases of the thyroid.

Needling : 0.5 to 1 t-sun, straight.

SI-17 (140) Tianrong (Tienjung)

Location : Behind the angle of the jaw, on the anterior border of the sterno-cleido-mastoid muscle.

Peculiarity : It is a dangerous point.

Indications : Sore throat, tonsillitis, thyroiditis, aphonia, aphasia.

Needling : 0.5 to 1 t-sun, straight.

SI-18 (141) Quanliao (Chuanliao)

Location : Just below the inferior border of the zygomatic bone at a level vertically below the outer canthus of the eye.

Indications : Trigeminal neuralgia, Bell's palsy, pain in the upper teeth, spasm of the facial muscles.

It is also used as an anaesthetic point for brain surgery and tooth extraction.

Needling   : 0.5 to 1 t-sun, slanting.

SI-19 (142) Tinggong (Tingkung)

Location   : In the depression between the tragus of the ear and temporomandibular joint when the mouth is slightly open.

Indications   : Otitis media, tinnitus, deafness, labyrinthitis, Meniere's disease, motion sickness and arthritis of the temporomandibular joint.

Needling   : 0.5 to 1 t-sun, straight.
                  : Mouth should be slightly opened to locate the point.
                  Moxa heat for 5 minutes.

7. THE URINARY BLADDER MERIDIAN

According to the traditional Chinese description it is a Yang channel associated with the element water and possesses interior and exterior relationship with the kidney meridian.

Total number of points : 67

Starting point   : Medial canthus of the eye.

Terminal point   : Lateral side of the tip of the little toe.

Pathway   : This is the longest channel. It starts from the medial canthus of the eye, runs over the forehead and head close to the midline. At vertex it connects with the governing vessels channels. At this level a small branch splits off and goes to the ear (this branch has no point) while the main branch goes to the occiput and at the nape of the neck, 0.5 t-sun above the natural hairline [Tianzhu (UB-10)] it divides into the medial and lateral branches. These two branches descend down up to the back of the popliteal fossa where they unite in the centre to form a single branch again. The single main branch runs down on the back of the leg and lateral border of the foot and ends at the lateral aspect of the tip of the little toe.

Branches

Medial branch   : This branch runs on the back of the trunk 1.5 t-sun lateral to the midline. It descends down up to the fourth sacral foramen, makes a Z-turn to reach back to the first dorsal sacral foramen and then again descends down over the buttock, hip joint, back of thigh to reach the popliteal fossa where it meets the lateral branch. At the level of the lower border of spinous process of the second lumbar vertebra [Shenshu (UB-23)] an inner branch goes to the kidney and urinary bladder.

Lateral branch   : This branch runs parallel to the medial branch 3 t-sun lateral to the midline on the back of the trunk. It courses over the buttock and back of the thigh and joins the medial branch on the back of the popliteal fossa at the level of Weizhong (UB-40) (Fig. 14.35).

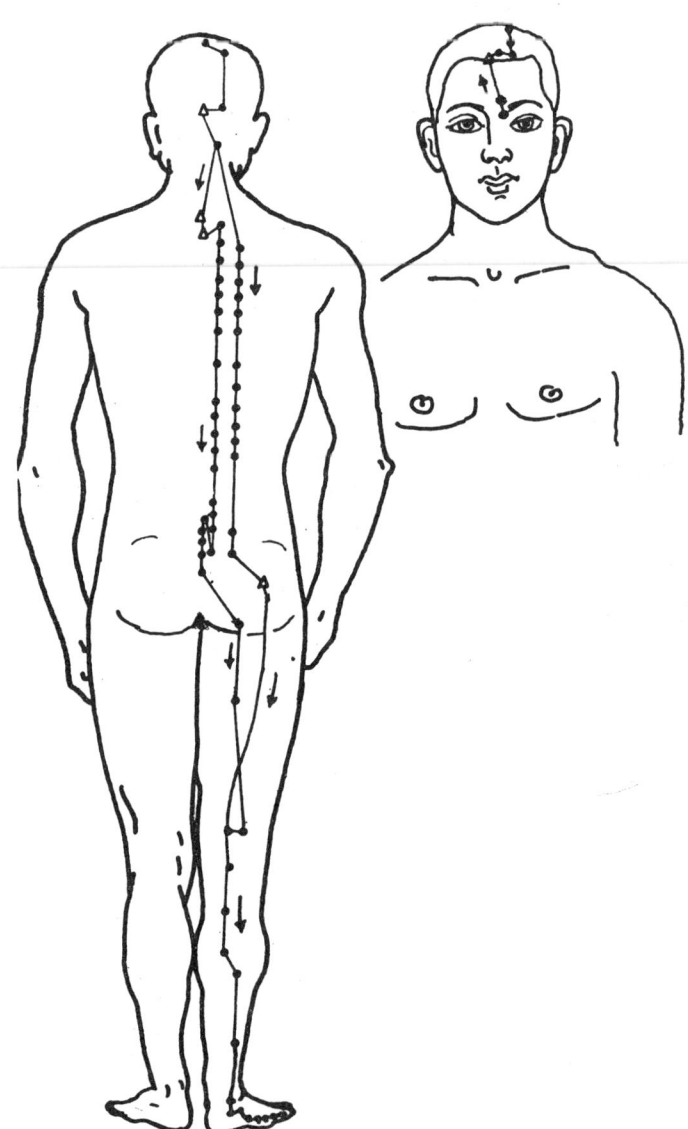

Fig. 14.35 The urinary bladder meridian

Therapeutic Indications

1. Disorders along the pathway of the channel : Urinary bladder channel being the longest of all the channels and covering almost the entire length of the body enjoys the privilege of having plenty of therapeutic indications like eye diseases, sinus disease, migraine, trigeminal neuralgia diseases of the neck and cervical spine are treated by using the channel points.

2. Points on the medial branch represent vital internal organs and they play the important role in the treatment of the diseases of the corresponding organs. Commonly known as backshu points, these all are the alarm points for the corresponding organs.

3. The points on the lumber region are mainly used for low backache and urogenital disorders.

4. The points on the lower extremity are used for myopathies, hemiplegia, sciatica, muscle cramps, arthritis and other local disorders.

DESCRIPTION OF THE POINTS

UB-1 (232) Jingming (Chingming)

Location	:	On the margin of the orbit 0.1 t-sun above the medial canthus (Fig. 14.36).
Peculiarity	:	It is a dangerous point.
Indications	:	Conjunctivitis, myopia, hypermetropia, optic atrophy, visual defects, blindness and facial paralysis.

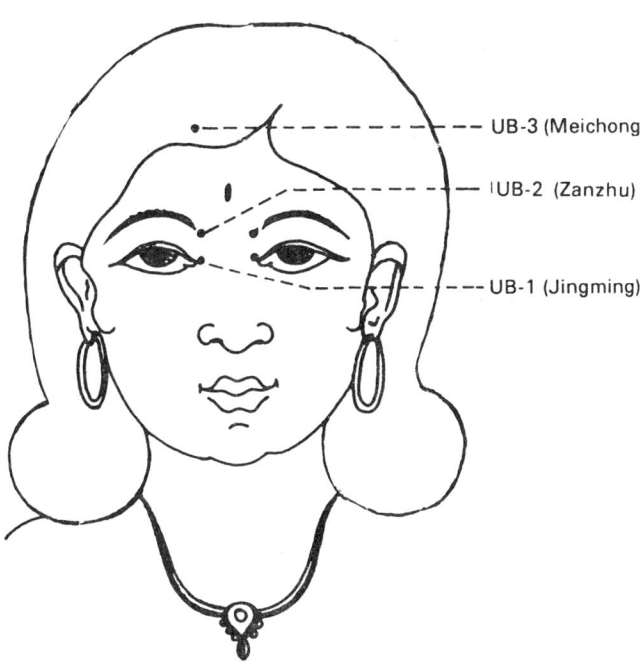

Fig. 14.36

Needling   : 0.2 to 0.3 t-sun into the anterior border of the orbit.
Note   : No rotation should be done with the needle. It should be inserted very slowly and taken out gently and quickly.

UB-2 (233) Zanzhu (Tsanchu)

Location   : At the inner end of the eyebrow directly above the inner canthus of the eye.
Indications   : Frontal headache, frontal sinusitis, trigeminal neuralgia, blurring of the vision, epiphora, diseases of the eye and nose.
Needling   : Subcutaneous route, horizontally downwards or laterally 0.2 to 0.3 t-sun deep.

UB-3 (234) Meichong

Location   : Above Zangzhu (UB-2), 0.5 t-sun inside the natural hair line (Fig. 14.37).

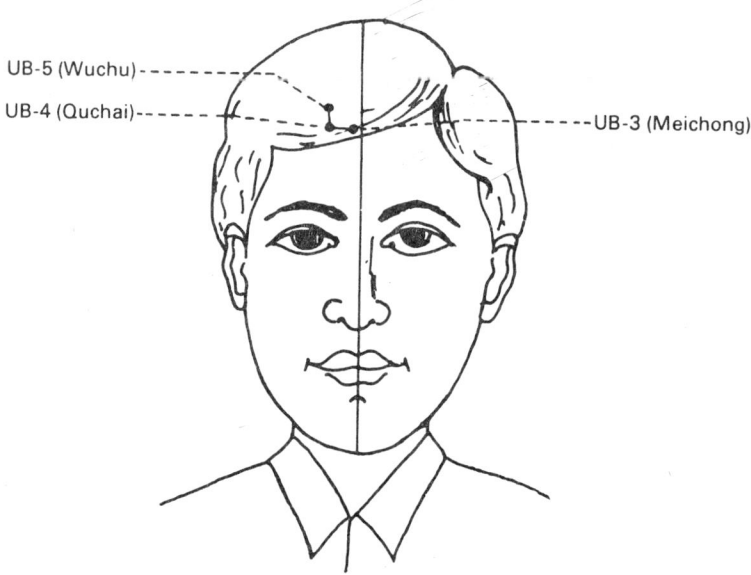

Fig. 14.37

Indications   : Headache, lacrimation and blurring of the vision.
Needling   : 0.3 to 0.5 t-sun, slanting.

UB-4 (235) Quchai (Chucha)

Location   : 1.5 t-sun lateral and 0.5 t-sun inside the midpoint of the anterior natural hair line (Fig. 14.38).
Indications   : Frontal headache and sinusitis, nasal congestion and epistaxis.
Needling   : 0.3 to 0.5 t-sun, slanting downward.

UB-5 (236) Wuchu

Location   : 1 t-sun above anterior natural hair line directly above Quchai (UB-4).

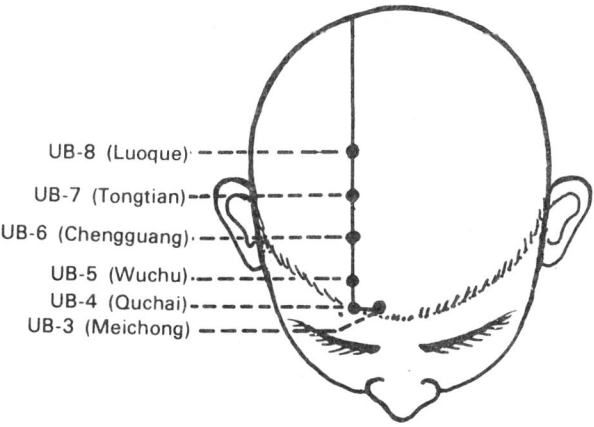

UB-8 (Luoque)
UB-7 (Tongtian)
UB-6 (Chengguang)
UB-5 (Wuchu)
UB-4 (Quchai)
UB-3 (Meichong)

Fig. 14.38

| Indication | : | Headache, frontal sinusitis, epilepsy. |
| Needling | : | 0.3 to 0.5 t-sun, slanting. |

UB-6 (237) Cheng Guang (Cheng Kuang)

Location	:	1.5 t-sun behind Wuchu (UB-5).
Indication	:	Headache, dizziness and coryza.
Needling	:	0.3 to 0.5 t-sun, slanting.

UB-7 (238) Tongtian (Tungtien)

Location	:	3 t-sun behind Wuchu (UB-5).
Indications	:	Headache, coryza, sinusitis.
Needling	:	0.3 to 0.5 t-sun, slanting.

UB-8 (239) Luoque (Lochueh)

Location	:	4.5 t-sun behind Wuchu (UB-5).
Indications	:	Coryza, nasal congestion, bleeding from the nose, vertical headache, sinusitis.
Needling	:	0.3 to 0.5 t-sun, slanting.

UB-9 (240) Yuzhen (Yuchen)

Location	:	1.3 t-sun lateral to the midpoint of the superior border of the external occipital protuberance.
Indications	:	Vertical and occipital headache, myopia, giddiness and unsteadiness.
Needling	:	1.3 to 0.5 t-sun, slanting.

UB-10 (241) Tianzhu (Tienchu)

| Location | : | On the lateral side of the trapezius muscle, 0.5 t-sun above the natural hair line, 0.3 t-sun lateral to the midline between the first and second cervical vertebrae (Fig. 14.39) |

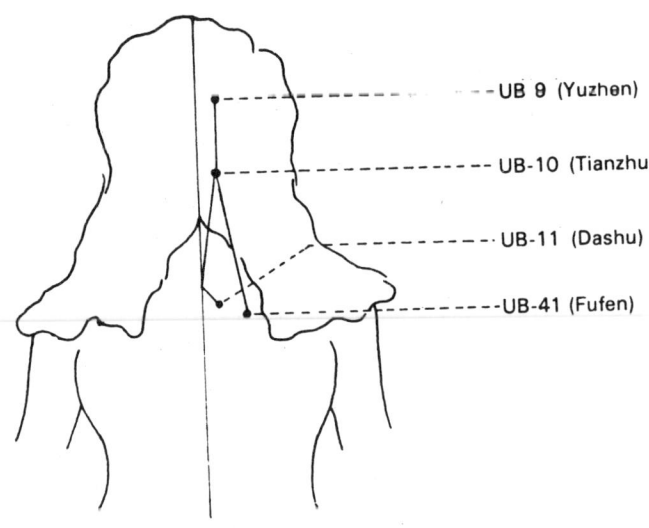

Fig. 14.39

Peculiarities	.	1 It is a dangerous point.
		2. Urinary bladder channel divides into two at this point.
Indications	:	Hysteria, epilepsy, schizophrenia, neurosthenia, insomnia, occipital headache, stiffness of the neck and disorders of the eye.
Needling	:	0.5 to 1 t-sun, straight.

UB-11 (242) Dashu (Tachu)

Location	.	On tne back, 1.5 t-sun lateral to the tip of the spinous process of the 1st thoracic vertebra (Fig. 14.39).
Peculiarity	:	It is an influential point for the bone and arthritis.
Indications	:	Bronchitis, pneumonia, asthma, pleurisy, neck pain, backache, shoulder pain, tuberculosis of the bone, arthritis and numbness of the limbs.
Needling	:	0.5 to 1 t-sun, slanting.

UB-12 (243) Fengmen (Fengmen)

Location	:	On the back, 1.5 t-sun lateral to the tip of the spinous process of the 2nd thoracic vertebra.
Indications	:	Allergic rashes, coryza and bronchitis.
Needling	:	0.3 to 0.5 t-sun, straight, or 0.3 to 0.5 t-sun, slanting.

UB-13 (244) Feishu

| Location | : | On the back, 1.5 t-sun lateral to the tip of the spinous process of the third thoracic vertebra and on a level with the spine of the scapula (Fig. 14.40). |
| Peculiarity | : | It is an alarm point for the lung. |

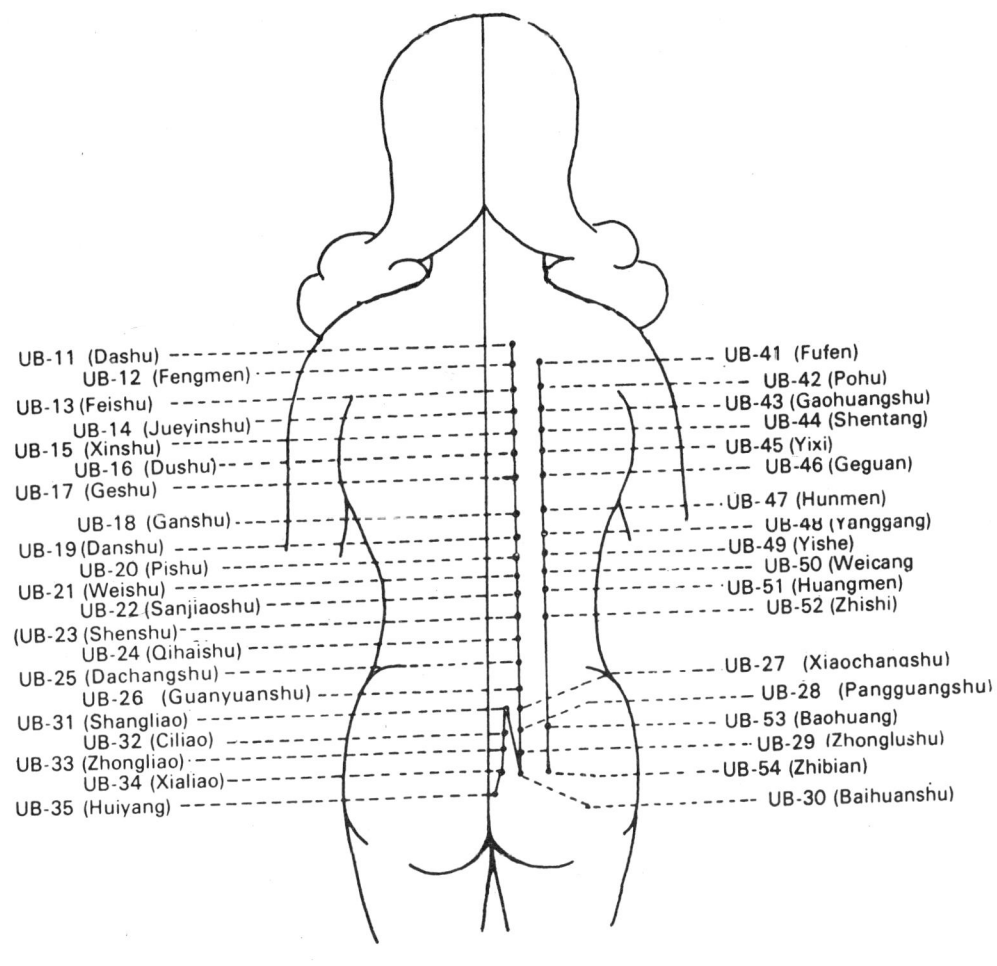

UB-11 (Dashu) -
UB-12 (Fengmen) - - - - - - - - - - - - - - - - - -
UB-13 (Feishu) - - - - - - - - - - - - - - - - - - -
UB-14 (Jueyinshu) - - - - - - - - - -
UB-15 (Xinshu) - - - - - - - - - - - - -
UB-16 (Dushu) - - - - - - - - - -
UB-17 (Geshu) - - - - - - - - - - - -
UB-18 (Ganshu) - - - - - - - - - - - - -
UB-19 (Danshu) - - - - - - - - - - - - -
UB-20 (Pishu) - - - - - - - - - - - - - - -
UB-21 (Weishu) - - - - - - - - - - - - -
UB-22 (Sanjiaoshu) - - - - - - - - - - -
(UB-23 (Shenshu) - - - - - - - - - - -
UB-24 (Qihaishu) - - - - - - - - - - - -
UB-25 (Dachangshu) - - - - - - - - - -
UB-26 (Guanyuanshu) - - - - - - -
UB-31 (Shangliao) - - - - - - - - - - -
UB-32 (Ciliao) - - - - - - - - - - - -
UB-33 (Zhongliao) - - - - - - - - - - -
UB-34 (Xialiao) - - - - - - - - - - -
UB-35 (Huiyang) - - - - - - - - - - -

UB-41 (Fufen)
UB-42 (Pohu)
UB-43 (Gaohuangshu)
UB-44 (Shentang)
UB-45 (Yixi)
UB-46 (Geguan)
UB-47 (Hunmen)
UB-48 (Yanggang)
UB-49 (Yishe)
UB-50 (Weicang)
UB-51 (Huangmen)
UB-52 (Zhishi)
UB-27 (Xiaochangshu)
UB-28 (Pangguangshu)
UB-53 (Baohuang)
UB-29 (Zhonglushu)
UB-54 (Zhibian)
UB-30 (Baihuanshu)

Fig. 14.40

| Indications | : | Bronchitis, pneumonia, pulmonary tuberculosis, asthma, cough, common cold, low back pain and soft tissue diseases of the back like fibrositis of the thoracic wall, hiccough, vertical headache. |
| Needling | : | 0.3 to 0.5 t-sun straight or slanting. |

UB-14 (245) Jueyinshu (Chuehyinshu)

Location	:	On the back, 1.5 t-sun lateral to the tip of the spinous process of the 4th thoracic vertebra.
Peculiarity	:	It is an alarm point for pericardium.
Indications	:	Neurasthenia, pressure on the chest, chest pain, vertex pain, pericarditis, hiccough, palpitation, mental disorders.
Needling	:	0.5 to 1 t-sun slanting.

UB-15 (246) Xinshu (Hsinshu)

Location	:	On the back, 1.5 t-sun lateral to the tip of the spinous process of the 5th thoracic vertebra.
Peculiarity	:	It is an alarm point for heart.
Indications	:	Palpitation, cardiac arrthythmias, hysteria, epilepsy, neurasthenia, schizophrenia and loss of memory.
Needling	:	0.5 to 1 t-sun, slanting.

UB-16 (247) Dushu (Tushu)

Location	:	On the back, 1-5 t-sun lateral to the tip of the spinous process of the 6th thoracic vertebra.
Indications	:	Hyperperistalsis, abdominal pain, alopecia, endocarditis and itching.
Needling	:	0.5 to 1 t-sun, slanting and straight.

UB-17 (248) Geshu (Keshu)

Location	:	On the back, 1.5 t-sun lateral to the tip of the spinous process of the 7th thoracic vertebra, at the level with the inferior angle of the scapula.
Peculiarities	:	1. Influential point for blood. 2. It is a diaphragm point.
Indications	:	Hiccough, paralysis of the diaphragm, eventration of the diaphragm, anorexia nerveosa, neurotic vomiting, anaemia, blood dyscrasias, haemorrhagic disorders and allergic rashes.
Needling	:	0.5 to 1 t-sun, slanting towards midline.

UB-18 (249) Ganshu (Kanshu)

Location	:	On the back, 1.5 t-sun lateral to the tip of tne spinous process of the 9th thoracic vertebra.
Peculiarity	:	Alarm point for the liver.
Indications	:	Hepatitis, hepatic cirrhosis, alcoholic liver, sluggish liver, cholecystitis, diseases of the eye and neurasthenia.
Needling	:	0.5 to 1 t-sun, slanting towards midline.

UB-19 (250)Danshu (Tanshu)

Location	:	On the back, 1.5 t-sun lateral to the tip of the spinous process of the 10th thoracic vertebra.
Peculiarity	:	Alarm point for the gall bladder.
Indications	:	Cholecystitis and other gall bladder diseases, hepatitis.
Needling	:	0.5 to 1 t-sun, slanting towards midline.

UB-20 (251) Pishu

Location	:	On the back, 1.5 t-sun lateral to the tip of the spinous process of the 11th thoracic vertebra (Fig. 14.41).
Peculiarity	:	1. Alarm point for the spleen. 2. Specific point for oedema.
Indications	:	Malarial spleen and fever, oedema, gastritis, gastric ulcer, hepatitis, enteritis, debility.
Needling	:	0.5 to 1 t-sun, slanting towards midline.

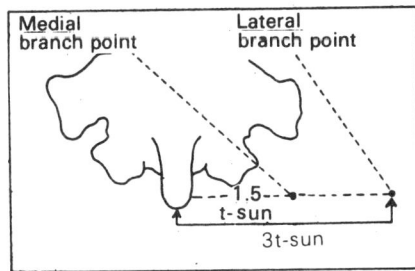

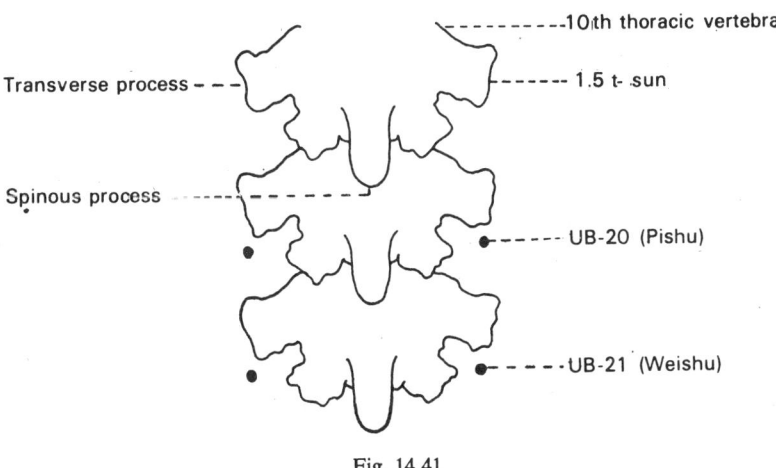

Fig. 14.41

UB-21 (252) Weishu
Location	:	On the back, 1.5 t-sun lateral to the tip of the spinous process of the 12th thoracic vertebra.
Peculiarity	:	It is an alarm point for the stomach.
Indications	:	Gastritis, gastro-enteritis, gastric ulcer, epigastric pain, gastroptosis, dyspepsia, anorexia, emesis, hepatitis, hiatus hernia.
Needling	:	0.5 to 1 t-sun, slanting towards midline.

UB-22 (253) Sanjiaoshu (Sanchiaoshu)
Location	:	On the back of abdomen, 1.5 t-sun lateral to the tip of the spinous process of the first lumber vertebra.
Peculiarity	:	It is an alarm point for the triple warmer.
Indications	:	Epigastric pain, gastritis, anorexia, vomiting, enteritis, nephritis, lumbago, incontinence of the urine.
Needling	:	1 to 1.5 t-sun, straight.

UB-23 (254) Shenshu
Location	:	On the back of abdomen 1.5 t-sun lateral to the tip of the spinous process of the second lumbar vertebra.
Peculiarity	:	It is an alarm point for the kidney.

Indications   : Lumbago, nocturnal pollutions, impotence, irregular menstruation, chronic pelvic cellutitis, nephritis, neurasthenia, genital disorders.
Needling   : 0.5 to 1.5 t-sun, slanting towards the midline.

UB-24 (255) Qihaishu (Chihaishu)

Location   : On the back of abdomen, 1.5 t-sun lateral to the tip of the spinous process of the 3rd lumbar vertebra.
Indications   : Haemorrhoids, prolapsed rectum, lumbago.
Needling   : 0.5 to 1 t-sun, slanting towards the midline.

UB-25 (256) Dachangshu (Tachangshu)

Location   : On the back of abdomen, 1.5 t-sun lateral to the tip of the spinous process of the 4th lumbar vertebra.
Peculiarity   : It is an alarm point for large intestine.
Indications   : Enteritis, dysentery, constipation, lumbago, sciatica, paralysis of the lower extremities.
Needling   : 0.5 to 1 t-sun, slanting towards the midline.

UB-26 (257) Guanyuanshu (Kuanyuanshu)

Location   : On the back of the abdomen, 1.5 t-sun lateral to the lower end of the tip of the 5th lumbar vertebra.
Indications   : Enteritis, cystitis, lumbago, parametritis, urinary incontinence.
Needling   : 0.5 to 1 t-sun, slanting towards the midline.

UB-27 (258) Xiaochangshu (Hsiaochangshu)

Location   : On the back of abdomen, 1.5 t-sun lateral to the midline at the level of sacroiliac joint.
Peculiarity   : It is an alarm point for the small intestine.
Indications   : Sciatica, lumbago, nocturnal pollution, urinary incontinence, pelvic peritonitis.
Needling   : 0.5 to 1 t-sun, slanting towards midline.

UB-28 (259) Pangguangshu (Pangkuangshu)

Location   : 1.5 t-sun lateral to the posterior midline over the sacroiliac joint at the level with the 2nd sacral vertebra.
Peculiarity   : Alarm point for the urinary bladder.
Indications   : Cystitis, pain in the lumbo-sacral region, sciatica, diarrhoea, constipation and diabetes.
Needling   : 1 to 1.5 t-sun, straight.

UB-29 (260) Zhonglushu (Chunglushu)

Location   : At the level with the third sacral vertebra, 1.5 t-sun lateral to the posterior midline.
Indications   : Sciatica, sacroiliac strain, lumbosacral strain and pain in the lumbo-sacral region, enteritis.
Needling   : 1 to 1.5 t-sun, straight.

UB-30 (261) Baihuanshu (Paihuanshu)

Location   : 1.5 t-sun lateral to the posterior midline at the level with the hiatus sacralis.
Indications   : Sciatica, sacral neuralgia and endometritis.
Needling   : 0.5 to 1 t-sun, straight.

UB-31 (262) Shangliao

Location   : On the first posterior sacral foramen midway between the posterior midline and the posterior superior iliac spine (Fig. 14.42).
Indications   : Epididymo-orchitis, haemorrhoids, prolapsed rectum, menstrual disturbances, dysurea, diseases of the urinary and generative organs, neurasthenia and lumbago.
Needling   : 1 to 1.5 t-sun, straight.

UB-32 (263) Ciliao (Tzuliao)

Location   : On the second posterior sacral foramen midway between the lower part of the posterior superior iliac spine and the posterior midline (Fig. 14.42).

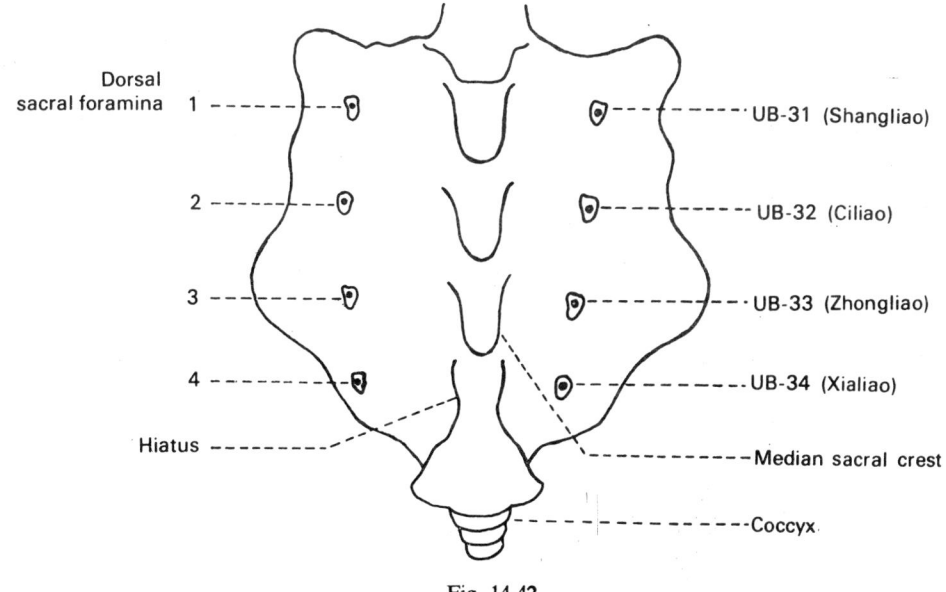

Fig. 14.42

Indications   : Urogenital disorders, menstrual disorders, haemorrhoids, lumbago, sciatica.
Needling   : 1 to 1.5 t-sun, straight.

UB-33 (264) Zhongliao (Chungliao)

Location   : On the third posterior sacral foramen.
Indication   : Same as Ciliao (UB-32).
Needling   : 1 to 1.5 t-sun, straight.

UB-34 (265) Xialiao (Hsialiao)

Location	:	On the 4th posterior sacralforamen.
Indications	:	Same as Ciliao (UB-32).
Needling	:	1 to 1.5 t-sun, straight.

UB-35 (266) Huiyang

Location	:	0.5 t-sun lateral to the posterior midline at the level of tip of the coccyx.
Indications	:	Menstrual disorders, backache during menstrual period, lumbar pain, leucorrhoea, impotence, diarrhoea and haemorrhoids.
Needilng	:	1.5 t-sun, straight.

UB-36 (267) Chengfu

Location	:	Midpoint of the gluteal sulcus.
Indications	:	Low back pain, sciatica, paralysis of the lower extremities, arthritis of the hip joint, perthese disease and haemorrhoids.
Needling	:	1.5 to 3 t-sun, straight.

UB-37 (268) Yinmen

Location	:	6 t-sun below Chengfu (UB-36) in the centre of the back of the thigh (Fig. 14.43).
Indications	:	Low backache, poliomyelitis, sciatica and paralysis.
Needling	:	1.5 to 2 t-sun, straight.

UB-38 (269) Fuxi (Fuhsi)

Location	:	On the lateral side of the popliteal fossa 1 t-sun above Weiyang (UB-39).
Indications	:	Poliomyelitis, paralysis of outer aspect of the lower limbs, cystitis and constipation.
Needling	:	1 to 2 t-sun, straight.

UB-39 (279) Weiyang

Location	:	On the lateral end of the popliteal crease, medial to the tendon of the biceps femoris muscle.
Indications	:	Cramps of the calf muscles, low backache, paralysis of the lower extremities.
Needling	:	0.5 to 1 t-sun, straignt.

UB-40 (271) Weizhong (Weichung)

Location	:	Midpoint of the popliteal fossa.
Peculiarity	:	It is the distal point for kidney, low backache, sciatica and urogenital disorders.
Indications	:	Low back pain, sciatica, lumbago, paralysis of the lower extremities, poliomyelitis, genitourinary disorders, menstrual disorders, impotence, arthritis of knee joint.
Needling	:	1 to 1.5 t-sun, straight.

UB-41 (272) Fufen

Location	:	On the back 3 t-sun lateral to the tip of the spinous process of the 2nd thoracic vertebra.

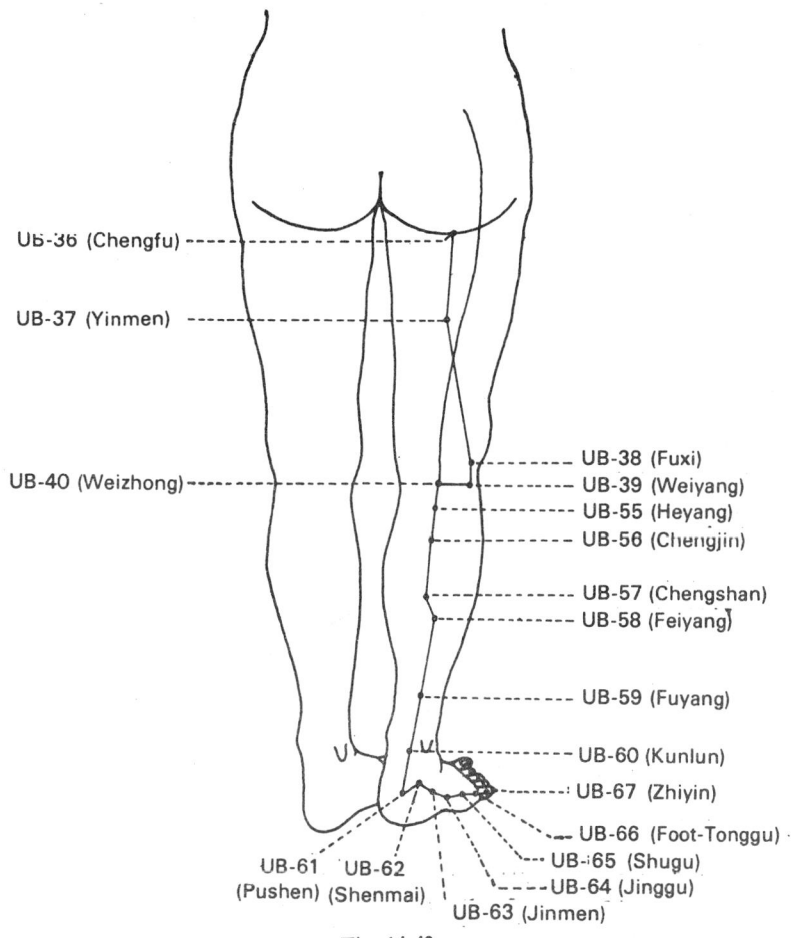

UB-36 (Chengfu)

UB-37 (Yinmen)

UB-40 (Weizhong)

UB-38 (Fuxi)
UB-39 (Weiyang)
UB-55 (Heyang)
UB-56 (Chengjin)

UB-57 (Chengshan)
UB-58 (Feiyang)

UB-59 (Fuyang)

UB-60 (Kunlun)
UB-67 (Zhiyin)
UB-66 (Foot-Tonggu)
UB-65 (Shugu)
UB-64 (Jinggu)

UB-61   UB-62
(Pushen) (Shenmai)
UB-63 (Jinmen)

Fig. 14.43

Indications   : Painful disorders of the shoulder, intercostal neuralgia, numbness in
                    the elbow and the arm.
Needling   : 0.5 to 0.8 t-sun, slanting.

UB-42 (273) Pohu
Location   : On the back 3 t-sun lateral to the tip of the spinous process of the 3rd
                    thoracic vertebra.
Indications   : Pulmonary tuberculosis, bronchitis, asthmatic bronchitis, asthma,
                    pneumoconiosis, pleuritis, thickened pleura, emesis, painful shoulder.
Needling   : 0.5 t-sun or less, straight or slanting.

UB-43 (274) Gaohuangshu (Kaohuang)
Location   : On the back 3 t-sun lateral to the tip of the spinous process of the the
                    4th thoracic vertebra.
Indications   : Pulmonary tuberculosis, asthmatic bronchitis, neurasthenia, debility.
Needling   : 0.5 t-sun or less, slanting.

UB-44 (275) Shentang

Location : On the back 3 t-sun lateral to the tip of the spinous process of the 5th thoracic vertebra.

Indications : Heart disorders, asthmatic bronchitis, frozen shoulder, backache.

Needling : 0.5 to 1 t-sun, straight.

UB-45 (276) Yixi (Yihsi)

Location : On the back 3 t-sun lateral to the tip of the spinous process of the 6th thoracic vertebra.

Indications : Intercostal neuralgia, pericarditis, asthmatic bronchitis, asthma, labyrinthitis, vertigo, unsteadyness, vomiting and hiccough.

Needling : 0.5 to 1 t-sun, straight.

UB-46 (277) Geguan (Kekuan)

Location : On the back, 3 t-sun lateral to the tip of the spinous process of the 7th thoracic vertebra.

Indications : Emesis, belching, hiccough, intercostal neuralgia, backache.

Needling : 0.5 to 1 t-sun, slanting towards spine.

UB-47 (278) Hunmen

Location : On the back, 3 t-sun lateral to the tip of the spinous process of the 9th thoracic vertebra.

Indications : Hepatic disorders, gastralgia, epigastric pain, reflex oesophagitis, endocarditis pleuresy.

Needling : 0.5 to 1 t-sun, slanting.

UB-48 (279) Yanggang (Yangkang)

Location : On the back, 3 t-sun lateral to the tip of the spinous process of the 10th tharacic vertebra.

Indications : Hepatic disorders, jaundice, diarrhoea, abdominal pain and hyperperistalsis.

Needling : 0.5 to 1 t-sun, slanting towards spine.

UB-49 (280) Yishe

Location : On the back, 3 t-sun lateral to the tip of the spinous process of the 11th thoracic vertebra.

Indications : Hepatitis, vomiting, backache, flatulence.

Needling : 0.5 to 1 t-sun, slanting towards spine.

UB-50 (281) Weicang (Weitsang)

Location : On the back 3 t-sun lateral to the tip of the spinous process of the 12th thoracic vartebra.

Indications : Epigastric pain, pain in spinal region, flatulence, emesis, constipation.

Needling : 0.5 to 1 t-sun, slanting towards spine.

UB-51 (282) Huangmen

Location : On the back of abdomen, 3 t-sun lateral to the spinous process of the 1st lumbar vertebra.

Indications   : Epigastric pain, hepatosplenomegaly, chronic mastitis, constipation.

Needling   : 1 to 1.5 t-sun, straight.

UB-52 (283) Zhishi (Chihshih)
Location   : On the back of the abdomen 3 t-sun lateral to the tip of the spinous process of the second lumbar vertebra.

Indications   : Nocturnal emissions, phosphaturia, spermatorrhea, impotence, dysurea, oedema, backache.

Needling   : 1 to 1.5 t-sun, straight.

UB-53 (284) Baohuang (Paohuang)
Location   : On the dorsal surface of the sacrum, 3 t-sun lateral to the midpoint of the 2nd sacral vertebra.

Indications   : Urinary retention, backache, flatulence, abdominal distension, enteritis.

Needling   : 0.5 to 1 t-sun, straight.

UB-54 (285) Zhibian (Chihpien)
Location   : 3 t-sun lateral to the posterior midline at the level of the 4th sacral foramen on the dorsal aspect of the sacrum.

Indications   : Low backache, sciatica, sacroiliac strain, haemorrhoids, paralysis of the lower extremities, numbness, tingling and pain in lower extremities, frequency of micturition, cystitis, impotence, arthritis and deformities of the hip joint.

Needling   : 1.5 to 2 t-sun, straight.

UB-55 (286) Heyang (Hoyang)
Location   : 2 t-sun below Weizhong (UB-40).

Indications   : Leg cramps, low backache, paralysis of the lower extremities, poliomyelitis.

Needling   : 1 to 2 t-sun, straight.

UB-56 (287) Chengjin (Cheng Chin)
Location   : Midway between Heyang (UB-55) and Chengshan (UB-57).

Indications   : Leg cramps, lumbago, low backache, haemorrhoids.

Needling   : 1 to 2 t-sun, straight.

UB-57 (288) Chengshan
Location   : On the calf, where the two bellies of the gastrocnemius unite, midway between Weizhang (UB-40) and the heel (upper border of the (calcaneum).

Indications   : Sciatica, paralysis of the leg, leg cramps planter fascitis, poliomyelitis, frontal headache, prolapsed rectum.

Needling   : 1 to 3 t-sun, straight.

UB-58 (289) Feiyang
Location   : 7 t-sun above Kunlun (UB-60).

Peculiarity   : It is Luo-connecting point.

| Indications | : | Ophthalmoplegia, sciatica, nephritis. |
| Needling | : | 1 to 2 t-sun, straight. |

UB-59 (290) Fuyang
Location	:	3 t-sun above Kunlun (UB-60).
Indications	:	Lumbosacral strain, headache, strain and arthritis of the ankle joint.
Needling	:	1 to 2 t-sun straight.

UB-60 (291) Kunlun
Location	:	Central point of the groove between the tendo-achilis and posterior border of the lateral malleolus of the fibula, at the level of its tip.
Indications	:	Poliomyelitis, paralysis of the lower extremity, foot drop, sciatica, low backache, calcaneal spur, painful disorders of the ankle joint and soft tissue around it, retained placenta.
Needling	:	0.5 to 1.0 t-sun, straight.
Note	:	Authors have observed very good results in interstitial neuritis of the leg, thrombophlebitis and stiff ankle by using Chengshan (UB-57) and Feiyang (UB-58) in combination with Yanglingquan (GB-34).

UB-61 (292) Pushen
Location	:	1.5 t-sun below Kunlun (UB-60).
Indications	:	Calcaneal spur, planter fascitis, painful heel, weakness and paralysis of lower extremities, painful disorders of the ankle joint.
Needling	:	0.3 to 0.5 t-sun, straight.

UB-62 (293) Shenmai (Shenmo)
Location	:	On the outer aspect of the ankle, 0.5 t-sun below the tip of the lateral malleolus.
Peculiarity	:	It is a very potent sedative point of the body.
Indications	:	Painful disorders of the ankle joint, low backache, paralysis of the leg, foot drop, headache, epilepsy, apoplexy, psychological disturbances, insomnia.
Needling	:	0.3 to 0.5 t-sun, straight.

UB-63 (294) Jinmen (Chinmen)
Location	:	Anterio-inferior to Shenmai (UB-62), proximal to the tuberosity of the 5th metatarsal bone.
Peculiarity	:	It is a Xi-cleft point.
Indications	:	Epilepsy, infantile convulsions, painful disorders of the ankle joint.
Needling	:	0.3 to 0.5 t-sun, straight.

UB-64 (295) Jinggu (Chingku)
Location	:	On the outer aspect of the foot, inferior to the tuberosity of the 5th metatarsal bone, at the junction of the two colours of the skin.
Peculiarity	:	It is a Yuan (source) point.
Indications	:	Epilepsy, headache, leg pain, unsteadyness.
Needling	:	0.3 to 0.5 t-sun, straight.

UB-65 (296) Shugu

Location	:	On the lateral border of the foot, behind and below the 5th metatarso-phalangeal joint.
Indications	:	Epilepsy, headache, unsteadyness, vertigo, leg cramps, pain along the lateral border of the foot, lumbago.
Needling	:	0.5 t-sun or less, straight.

UB-66 (297) Tonggu (Tungku)

Location	:	On the lateral border of the foot, antero-inferior to the 5th metatarso-phalangeal joint.
Indications	:	Headache, stiff neck fainting, epistaxis, indigestion.
Needling	:	0.3 to 0.5 t-sun straight.

UB-67 (298) Zhiyin (Chihyin)

Location	:	0.1 t-sun behind and lateral to the corner of the nail of the little toe.
Peculiarity	:	It is a Jing-well point.
Indications	:	All acute emergencies, difficult labour, malposition of the foetus.
Needling	:	0.1 t-sun, straight. Moxa heat for 5 minutes.

8. THE KIDNEY MERIDIAN

According to the traditional Chinese description it is a Yin channel associated with the element water and possesses interior and exterior relationship with the urinary bladder meridian.

Total number of points : 27.

Starting point	:	At the junction of anterior one-third and posterior two-third of the sole in the hollow between 2nd and 3rd metatarso-phalangeal joints.
Terminal point	:	Infraclavicular region.
Pathway	:	After taking origin from the inferior aspect of the little toe, it enters the sole, passes behind the medial malleolus, and ascends on the leg to reach medial side of the popliteal fossa. It reaches pelvis after coursing over the posteromedial aspect of the thigh where it divides into two branches:
1. Inner branch	:	Leads to the principle organ kidney and communicates with urinary bladder. It courses upwards internally to end at the route of the tongue.
2. Superficial branch	:	It ascends to the abdomen and chest, and ends at the infraclavicular region 2 t-sun lateral to the midline (Fig. 14.44).

Therapeutic Indications

1. Disorders along the pathway of the channel.
2. Genito-urinary disorders like cystitis, nephritis, impotence, spermaturia and menstruation disorders.
3. Alopecia.

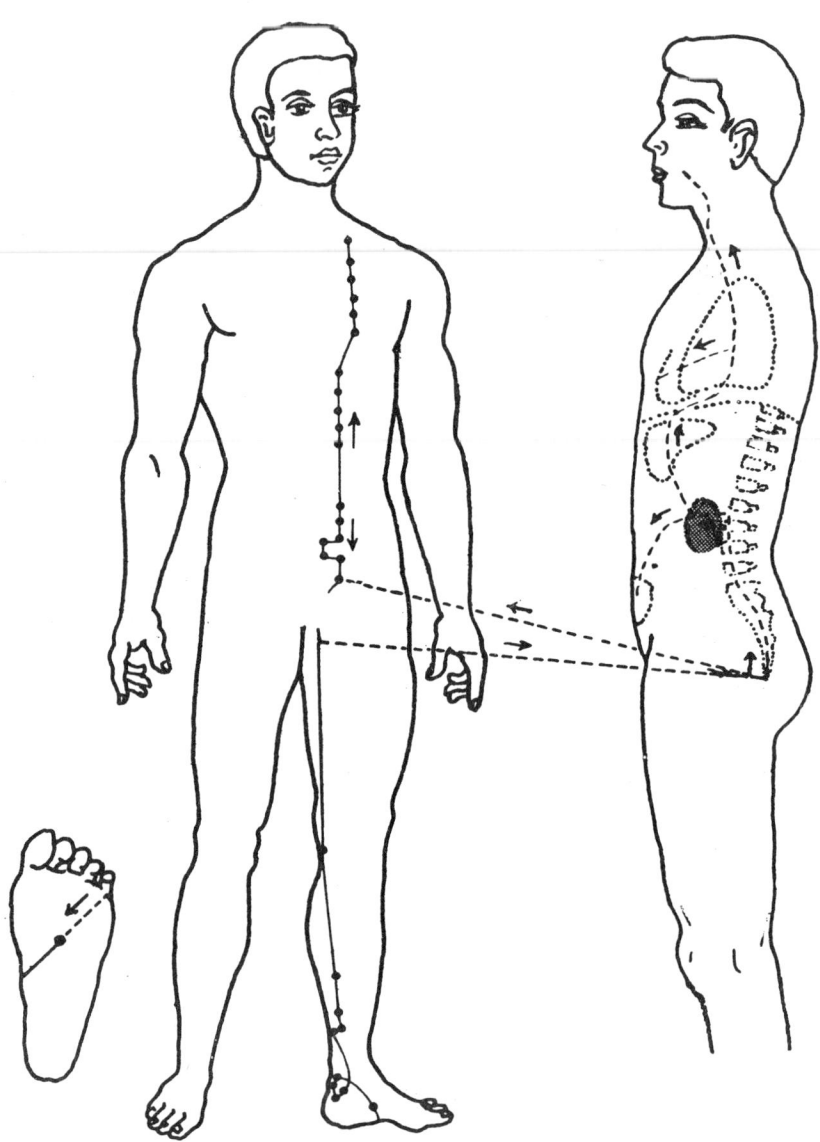

Fig. 14.44   The kidney meridian

4. All ear disorders (kidney opens to the ear).
5. Disorders of the bones.
6. Pulmonary disorders can be treated by using this channel because lung represents metal and water is the son of metal. Water being the element of the channel provides it the therapeutic properties of treating lung disorders.
7. Water destroys fire hence the disorders of heart, brain and small intestine can be treated by using kidney channel.
8. Diseases of liver and gall bladder can be treated by this channel because wood is the son of water.

Indications mentioned above is a classic example of application of the doctrine of five elements in the selection of the points.

DESCRIPTION OF THE POINTS

K-1 (334)Yongquan (Yungchuan)

Location   : In the hollow of the sole at the junction of its anterior one-third and posterior two-third in the depressions between the 2nd and 3rd metatarsophalangeal joints (Fig. 14.45a and b).

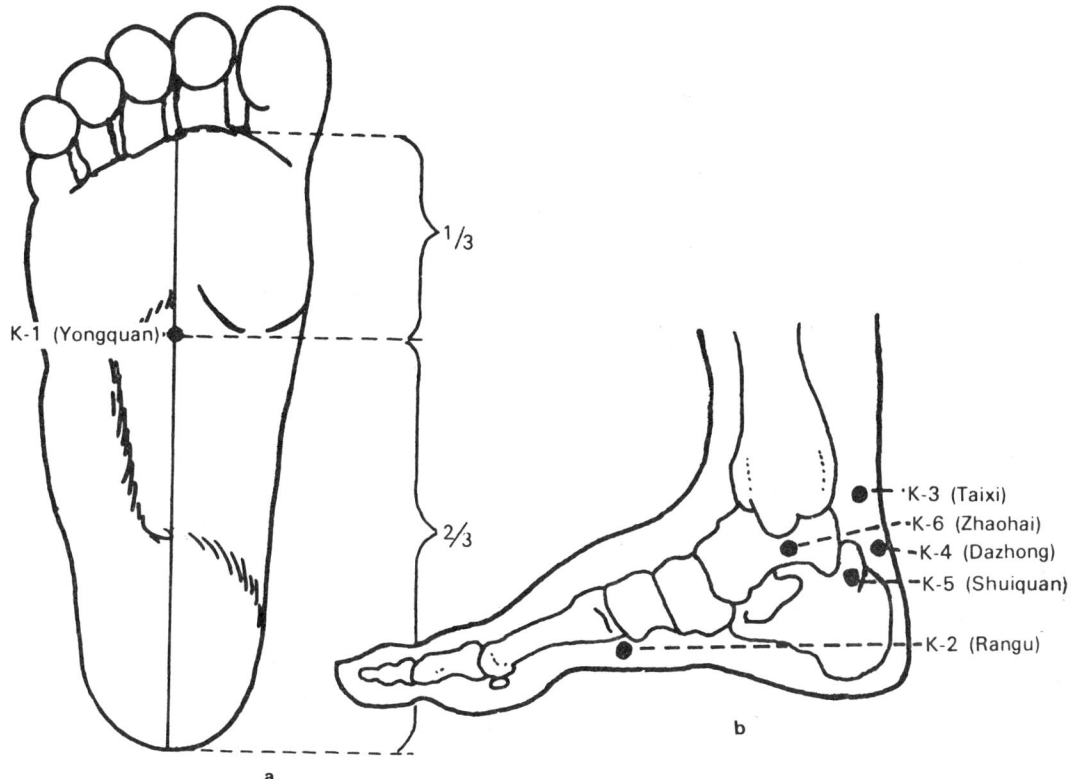

Fig. 14.45

Peculiarity : It is nicely located when the toes are planter flexed.
It is a Jing-well point.

Indications : 1. It is used as a powerful and effective Jing-well point during emergencies.
2. Unconsciouness, epilepsy, infantile convulsions, severe nausea and vomitings, dysurea.
3. Planter fascitis, arthritis of small joints of foot, foot drop.

Needling : 0.5 to 1 t-sun, straight.
: Strong hand stimulation with a thick needle is given.

K-2 (335) Rangu (Janku)

Location : On the medial border of the foot in the depression postero-inferior to the tuberosity of the navicular bone.

Indications : Cystitis, menstrual irregularities like menorrhagia, functional uterine bleeding, planter fascitis, pharyngitis, diabetes mellitus.

Needling : 0.5 to 1 t-sun, straight.

K-3 (336) Taixi (Taihsi)

Location : Midway between the tip of medial malleolus and tendo-achilles, just opposite the Kunlun (UB-60) [Fig.14.46].

Peculiarity : It is Yuan (source) point of the kidney channel.

Indications : 1. Cystitis, nephritis, enuresis, urinary incontinence, spermatorrhoea, impotence, spasmodic dysmenorrhoea.
2. Paralysis of the lower extremities, foot drop.
3. Planter fascitis, arthritis of the ankle joint and foot.
4. Planter fascitis, arthritis of the ankle joint, calcaneal spur, sprains of the ankle joint and foot.

Needling : 0.5 to 1 t-sun straight or point to point with Kunlun (UB-60).

K-4 (337) Dazhong (Tachung)

Location : Posterio-inferior to Taixi (K-3) in front of the tendo-achilles, and above the calcaneus.

Peculiarity : It is the Luo-connecting point.

Indications : Hysteria, hepatitis, asthma, constipation, planter fascitis, calcaneal spur, dysuresis.

Needling : 0.3 to 0.5 t-sun, straight.

K-5 (338) Shuiquan (Shuichuan)

Location : 1 t-sun below Taixi (K-3), on the medial part of the tubercle of the calcaeum.

Peculiarity : It is a Xi-cleft point.

Indications : Renal colic, irregular menstruation, prolapse of the uterus.

Needling : 0.5 to 1 t-sun, straight.

Note : This is a specific point for renal colic. Strong stimulation should be given to this point.

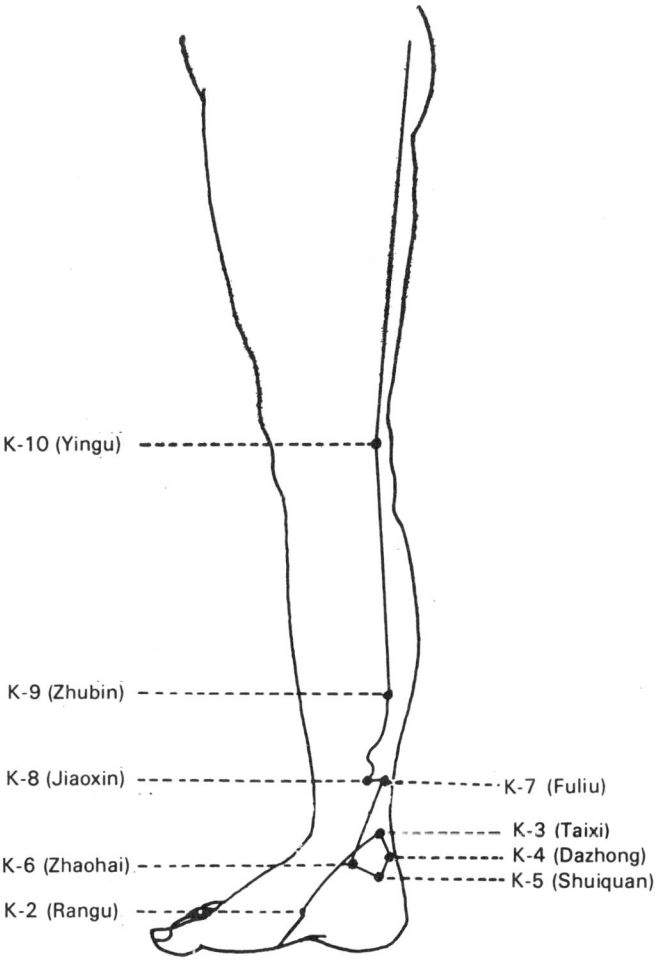

Fig. 14.46.

K-6 (339) Zhaohai (Chaohai)

Location	:	1 t-sun directly below the tip of the medial malleolus, on the medial aspect of the ankle.
Indications	:	Painful disorders of the ankle joint like arthritis and sprains, menstrual disturbances, prolapse of the uterus, epilepsy.
Needling	:	0.5 to 1 t-sun, straight.

K-7 (340) Fuliu

Location	:	2 t-sun above Taixi (K-3).
Indications	:	Hyperhydrosis, nephritis, orchitis, night sweating.
Needling	:	0.5 to 1 t-sun straight.

K-8 (341) Jiaoxin (Chiaohsin)

Location   :   0.5 t-sun anterior to the Fuliu (K-7).
Indications   :   Menstrual disturbances, orchitis.
Needling   :   0.5 to 1 t-sun, straight.

K-9 (342) Zhubin (Chupin)

Location   :   5 t-sun above the Taixi (K-3), 1 t-sun behind the medial border of the tibia or the inner aspect of the leg.
Indications   :   Epilepsy, calf muscle cramps.
Needling   :   1 to 1.5 t-sun, straight.

K-10 (343) Yingu (Yinku)

Location   :   At the medial side of the popliteal fossa, between the tendons of semitendinosus and semi-membranosus muscle (medial end of the transverse popliteal crease of the flexed knee.
Indications   :   Diseases of the genital organs, painful conditions of the knee.
Needling   :   1 to 1.5 t-sun, straight.

K-11 (344) Henggu (Hengku)

Location   :   In the lower abdomen, 0.5 t-sun lateral to Qugu (CV-2) [Fig. 14.47].
Indications   :   Impotence, dysuria, incontinence of urine, spermatorrhoea.
Needling   :   0.5 to 1 t-sun, straight.

K-12 (345) Dahe (Taheh)

Location   :   1 t-sun directly above Henggu (K-11) and 0.5 t-sun lateral to Zhongji (CV-3).
Indications   :   Leucorrhoea, spermatorrhoea, priapism, balanitis, vulvitis.
Needling   :   0.5 to 1 t-sun straight.

K-13 (346) Qixue (Chihsueh)

Location   :   2 t-sun directly above Henggu (K-11) and 0.5 t-sun lateral to Guanyuan (CV-4).
Indications   :   Irritable colon syndrome, diarrhoea, menstrual disturbances.
Needling   :   0.5 to 1 t-sun, straight.

K-14 (347) Siman (Szuman)

Location   :   3 t-sun directly above Henggu (K-11).
Indications   :   Postpartum haemorrhage and pain.
Needling   :   0.5 to 1 t-sun, straight.

K-15 (348) Abdomen-Zhongzhu (Chungchu)

Location   :   0.5 t-sun lateral to Abdomen Yin Jiao (CV-7).
Indications   :   Lower abdominal pain, menstrual disturbances.
Needling   :   0.5 to 1 t-sun, straight.

K-16 (349) Huanghsu

Location   :   0.5 t-sun lateral to the umbilicus.

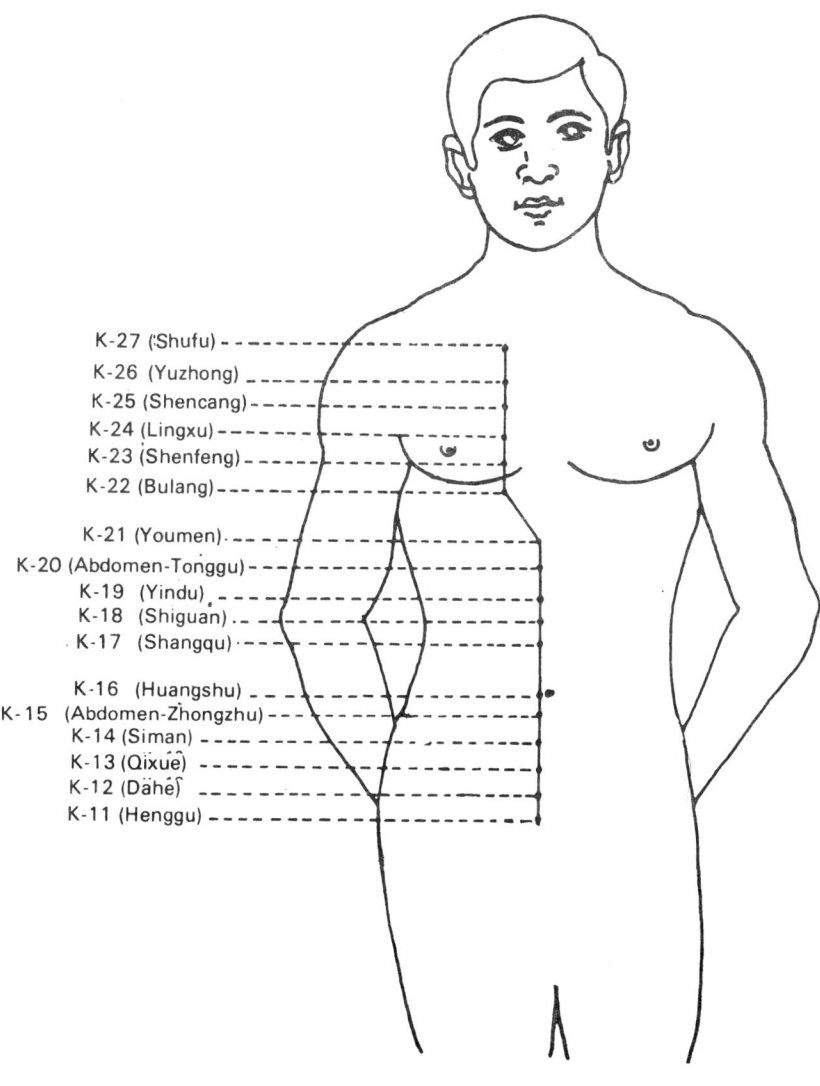

K-27 ('Shufu)
K-26 (Yuzhong)
K-25 (Shencang)
K-24 (Lingxu)
K-23 (Shenfeng)
K-22 (Bulang)

K-21 (Youmen)
K-20 (Abdomen-Tonggu)
K-19 (Yindu)
K-18 (Shiguan)
K-17 (Shangqu)

K-16 (Huangshu)
K-15 (Abdomen-Zhongzhu)
K-14 (Siman)
K-13 (Qixue)
K-12 (Dahe)
K-11 (Henggu)

Fig. 14.47

Indications   : Abdominal pain, jaundice, hepatitis, menstrual disturbances, hernia, constipation.

Needling   : 0.5 to 1 t-sun, straight.

K-17 (350) Shangqu (Shangchu)

Location   : 2 t-sun directly above Huangshu (K-16) and 0.5 t-sun lateral to mid-line.

Indications   : Epigastric pain, ventral hernia, hiatus hernia, anorexia.

Needling   : 0.5 to 1 t-sun, straight.

K-18 (351) Shiguan (Shihkuan)
Location   : 3 t-sun directly above Huangshu (K-16) and 0.5 t-sun lateral to the midline.
Indications   : Epigastric pain, hiccough, postpartum pain, constipation.
Needling   : 0.5 to 1 t-sun, straight.

K-19 (352) Yindu (Yintu)
Location   : 4 t-sun directly above Huangshu (K-16) and 0.5 t-sun lateral to the midline.
Indications   : Hyperperistalsis, epigastric pain.
Needling   : 0.5 to 1 t-sun, straight.

K-20 (353) Abdomen-Tonggu (Tungku)
Location   : '5ǰ t-sun directly above Huangshu (K-16) and 0.5 t-sun lateral to the midline.
Indications   : Epigastric pain, gastralgia, emesis, abdominal distension.
Needling   : 0.5 to 1 t-sun, straight.

K-21 (354) Youmen (Yumen)
Location   : 6 t-sun above Huangshu (K-16) and 0.5 t sun lateral to the midline.
Indications   : Feeling of constriction in the chest, emesis, belching and diarrhoea.
Needling   : 0.5 to 1 t-sun, straight.

K-22 (355) Bulang (Pulang)
Location   : On the front of the chest in the 5th intercostal space, 2 t-sun lateral to the midline.
Indications   : Thickened pleura, pleuritis, pleurisy, intercostal neuralgia, herpes, bronchitis.
Needling   : 0.5 t-sun or less, slanting.

K-23 (356) Shenfeng
Location   : On the front of the chest in the 4th intercostal space, 2 t-sun lateral to Shanzhong (CV-17).
Indications   : Chronic mastitis, pleuritis, bronchitis, intercostal neuralgia.
Needling   : 0.5 t-sun or less, slanting.

K-24 (357) Lingxu (Linghsu)
Location   : 3rd intercostal space, 2 t-sun lateral to the midline.
Indications   : Chronic mastitis, thoracalgia, bronchitis, vomiting.
Needling   : 0.5 t-sun or less, slanting.

K-25 (358) Shencang (Shentsang)
Location   : 2nd intercostal space, 2 t-sun lateral to midline.
Indications   : Intercostal neuralgia, cough, bronchitis, emesis.
Needling   : 0.5 t-sun or less slanting.

K-26 (359) Yuzhong (Yuchung)
Location   : 1st intercostal space, 2 t-sun lateral to the midline, midway between the sternal and mammilary lines.

Indications   :   Thoracalgia, cough, bronchitis, vomiting.
Needling   :   0.5 t-sun or less, slanting.

K-27 (360) Shufu

Location   :   In the hollow between the lower border of the clavicle and the 1st rib,
                         2 t-sun lateral to the midline (Fig. 14.47).
Peculiarity   :   It is a dangerous point.
Indications   :   Thoracalgia, cough, bronchitis, asthma, emesis.
Needling   :   0.5 t-sun or less slanting.

9. THE PERICARDIUM MERIDIAN

According to the traditional Chinese description it is a Yin channel associated with the element fire and possesses interior and exterior relationship with the triple warmer meridian.
Total number of points: 9.

Starting point   :   1 t-sun lateral to the nipple.
Terminal point   :   Tip of the middle finger.
Pathway   :   It originates from the upper warmer and pericardium and has two bran-
                     ches: inner branch and superficial branch.
1. Inner branch :   This starts from the pericardium and descends to the area of abdomen
                     through the diaphragm to the middle and lower warmer.
2. Superficial :   This branch emerges at the upper outer quadrant of the breast, 3 t-sun
   branch   below the anterior axillary fold and ascends to the axilla and
                     anterior aspect of the shoulder joint. It then courses downwards along
                     the medial aspect of the upper arm between the lung and heart
                     meridians to the cubital fossa.
                     It enters the front of the arm medial to the tendon of biceps brachii
                     muscle, runs in the middle of the palm and ends at the tip of the
                     middle finger (Fig. 14.48).

Therapeutic Indications

1. Disorders along she pathway of the meridian, e.g. diseases of the wrist joint, enlarged
   lymph glands, infections of the hand.
2. Diseases of the heart, e.g. palpitation, tachycardia, bradycardia, angina pectoris.
3. Mental diseases, e.g. schizophrenia, epilepsy, insomnia, insanity, mania, anxiety.
4. Upper abdominal disorders, e.g. gastralgia, gastritis, peptic ulcer, hiccough.

DESCRIPTION OF THE POINTS

P-1 (63) Tianchi (Tienchih)

Location   :   On the front of the chest in the 4th intercostal space, 1 t-sun lateral to
                     the nipple.
Peculiarity   :   It is a dangerous point.
Indications   :   Intercostal neuralgia, herpes, fullness and heaviness in the chest, defi-
                     cient lactation, enlarged lymph glands.
Needling   :   0.5 t-sun, slanting outwards (away from the breast tissue).

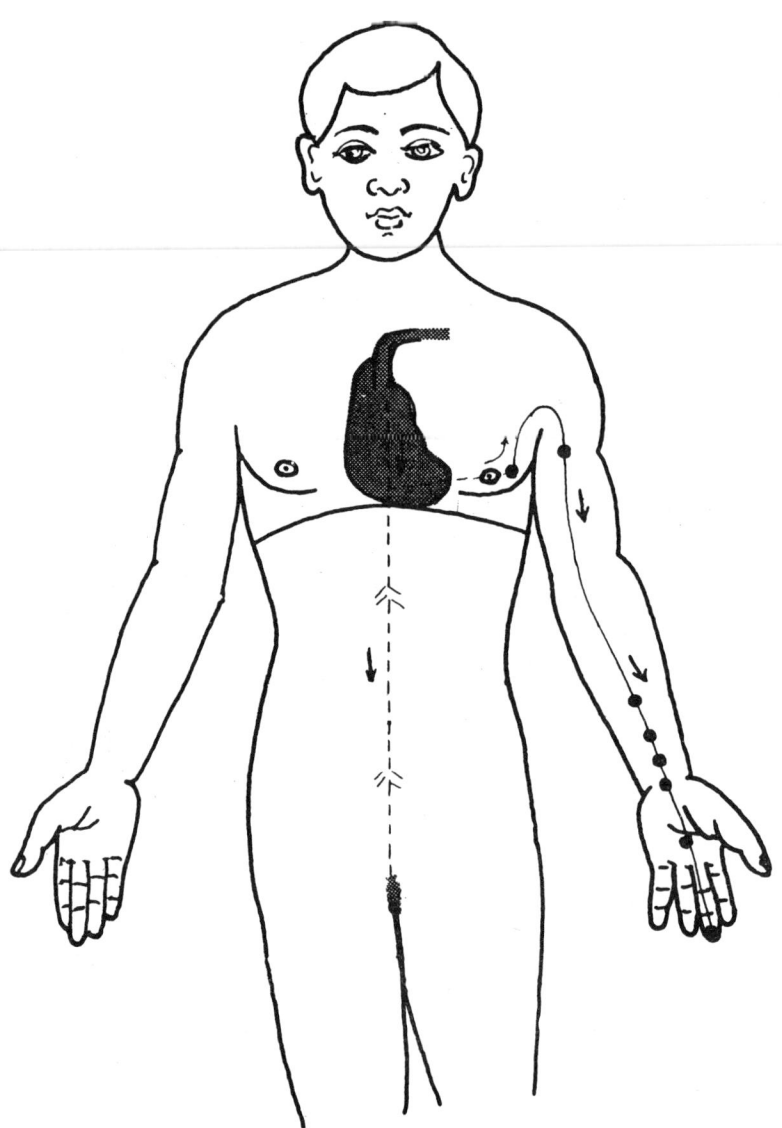

Fig. 14.48   The pericardium meridian.

P-2 (64) Tianquan (Tienchuan)

Location	:	Between the long and short heads of the biceps brachii muscle, 2 t-sun below the humeral end of the anterior axillary fold.
Indications	:	Thoracodyrnia and costalgia, cough, pain in the back and inner side of the upper arm.
Needling	:	1 to 2 t-sun deep, straight.

P-3 (65) Quze (Chutse)

Location	:	Medial to the tendon of the biceps brachi muscle on the transverse crease of the elbow (Fig. 14.49).
Indications	:	Palpitation, angina pectoris, contracture and arthritis of the elbow, tremors, pain in the arm and forearm, gastralgia, fever and psoriasis.
Needling	:	1 to 2 t-sun, straight. In case of skin disorders point can be made to bleed.

P-4 (66) Ximen (Hsimen)

Location	:	On the front of the forearm, 5 t-sun above the transverse crease of the wrist between the tendons of the muscle flexor carpi radialis and palmaris longus.

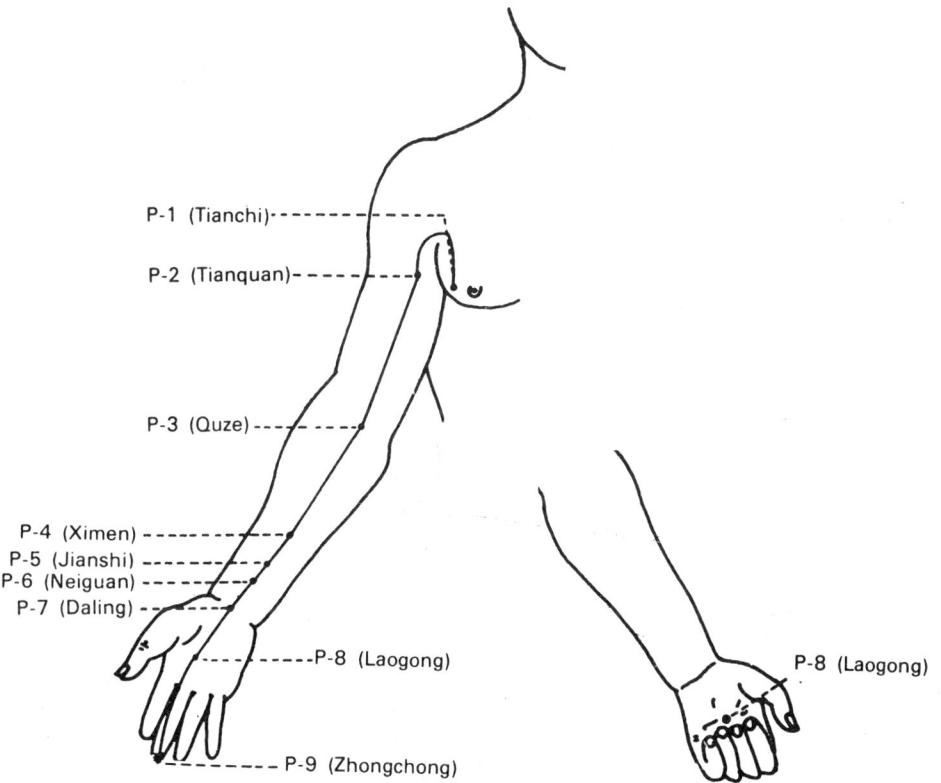

Fig. 14.49

Peculiarity   : It is the Xi-cleft point.
Indications   : Angina pectoris, tachycardia, palpitation, mastitis, pleuritis, acute psychosis and neurasthenia.
Needling   : 1 to 2 t-sun straight.

P-5 (67) Jianshi (Chienshih)

Location   : On the front of the forearm 3 t-sun above the distal transverse wrist crease, between the tendon of flexor carpi radialis and palmaris longus muscle.
Indications   : Tachycardia, palpitation, angina pectoris, schizophrenia, neurasthenia, psychosis, epilepsy and malaria.
Needling   : 1 to 1.5 t-sun deep, straight.

P-6 (68) Neiguan (Neikuan)

Location   : 2 t-sun above the distal transverse wrist crease between the tendons of the flexor carpi radialis and palmaris longus muscles.
Peculiarities   : 1. It is a distal point for abdominal and chest disorders.
                   2. It is a Luo-connecting point of the pericardium with the triple warmer meridian.
Indications   : 1. Thoracodynia and costalgia.
                   2. Paralysis, poliomyelitis, muscular wasting and myopathies.
                   3. Brachial neuralgia and carpal tunnel syndrome.
                   4. Gastralgia, gastritis, hiccough, hiatus hernia, anorexia, nausea, emesis.
                   5. Palpitation, angina pectoris.
                   6. Hysteria, epilepsy anxiety.
                   7. Asthma.
Needling   : 0.5 to 1 t-sun, straight.
Note   : Acupressure can be given for vomiting and travel sickness.

P-7 (69) Daling (Taling)

Location   : Midpoint of the distal transverse wrist crease, between the tendons of the flexor carpiradialis and palmaris longus muscles.
Peculiarity   : It is the Yuan (source) point.
Indications   : Myocarditis, intercostal neuralgia, tonsilitis, mental disorders, carpal tunnel syndrome, arthritis of the wrist joint, paralysis, epilepsy and insomnia.
Needling   : 0.5 to 1 t-sun, straight.

P-8 (70) Laogong (Laokung)

Location   : Middle of the palm. Flex the fingers at metacarpophalangeal and interphalangeal joints so that they touch the central part of the palm. The point between the tip of the middle and ring fingers is this point and it is close to the 3rd metacarpal bone.
Indications   : Polyneuropathy of the hand, paralysis, wasting, contracture of the fingers, carpal tunnal syndrome, stomatitis, chronic skin infections, epilepsy.

Needling : 0.3 to 0.5 t-sun deep, straight.

P-9 (71) Zhongchong (Chungchung)

Location : Midpoint of the tip of the middle finger.
Peculiarity : In is a Jing-well point.
Indications : 1. All acute emergencies.
2. Angina pectoris, shock, coma, hyperpyrexia.
Needling : 1. 0.1 t-sun, straight.
2. This point can be made to bleed by using three-edged needle.

10. THE TRIPLE WARMER MERIDIAN

According to the traditional Chinese description it is a Yang channel associated with the element fire and possesses interior and exterior relationship with the pericardium meridian.

The term triple warmer indicates three burning cavities of the body, namely, chest, abdomen and pelvis, controlling respiration, digestion and urogenital functions, respectively. Because of their location, chest is known as upper warmer, abdomen as middle warmer and pelvis as lower warmer. In the Chinese texts, triple warmer is termed as Sanjiao channel (Sanjiao means "three burning spaces") (Fig. 14.50).

Total number of points 23.

Starting point : Corner of the nail of ring finger on the ulnar side.
Terminal point : Lateral end of the eye brow.
Pathway : It originates from the medial corner of the nail of the ring finger, passes on the dorsum of the hand between fourth and fifth metacarpal bones and crosses the dorsum of the wrist and inferior radioulnar joints to take the position between radius and ulna on the dorsum of the forearm. It ascends to the olecranon and along the posterior aspect of the upper arm to the shoulder joint where it enters the neck to reach the supraclavicular fossa and divides into two branches: (i) cervical branch and (ii) inner branch.
1. Cervical branch : It runs superficially to the neck, along the posterior border of the ear, turns downwards to the cheek and terminates in the infraorbital region.
2. Inner branch : This branch descends through the diaphragm and goes to the abdomen and pelvis (Fig. 14.51).

Therapeutic indications

1. All disorders along the pathway of the meridian.
2. Diseases of the ear, i.e. tinnitus, vertigo, labyrinthitis, deafness (because one of its branch goes to the ear).
3. Gastrointestinal disorders like constipation and diarrhoea (due to its homeotatic effect).
4. Diseases of the eye (because the meridian passes close to the eye).
5. Painful shoulder and back.
6. Heart and mental disorders.

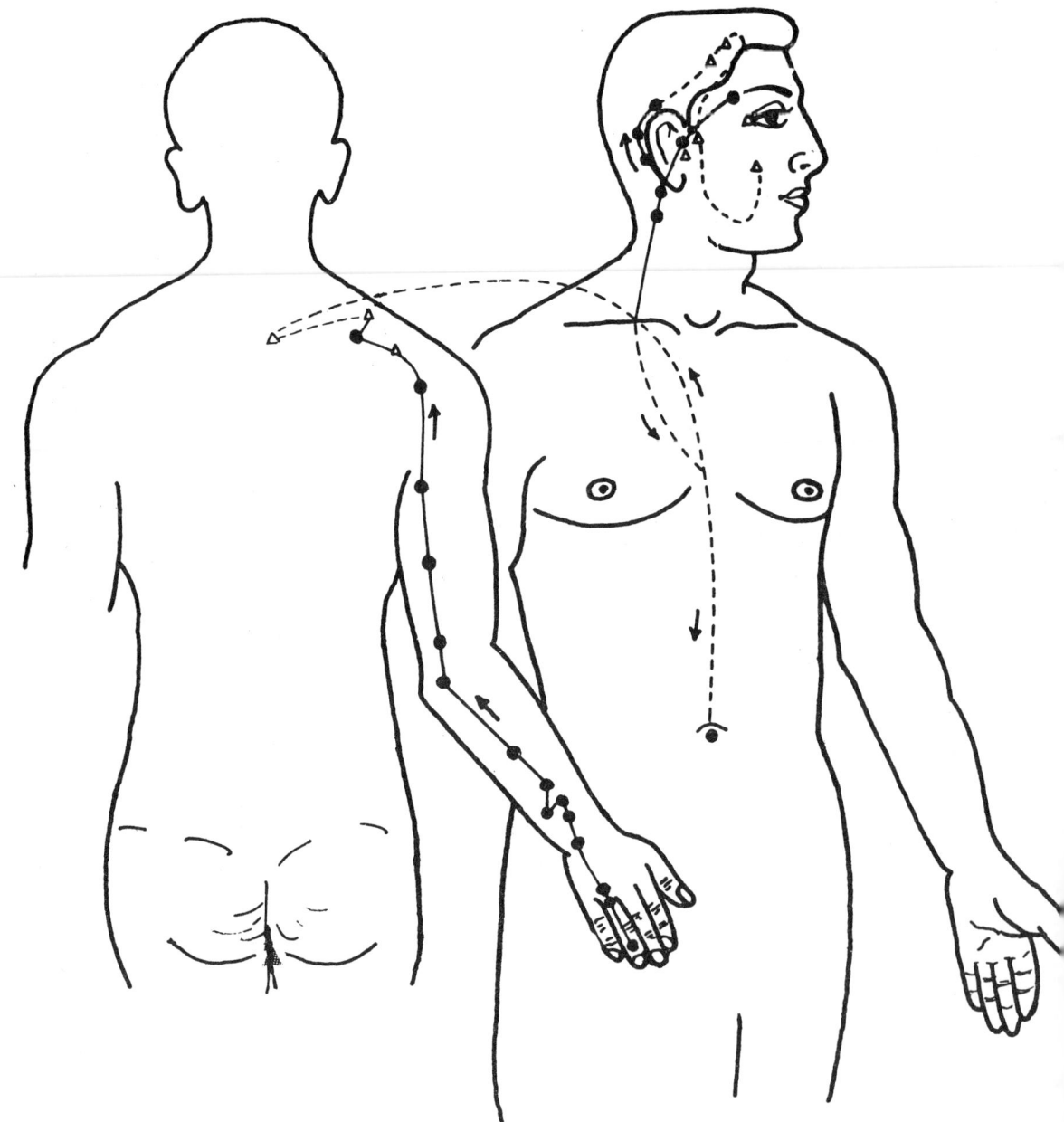

Fig. 14.50 The triple warmer meridian.

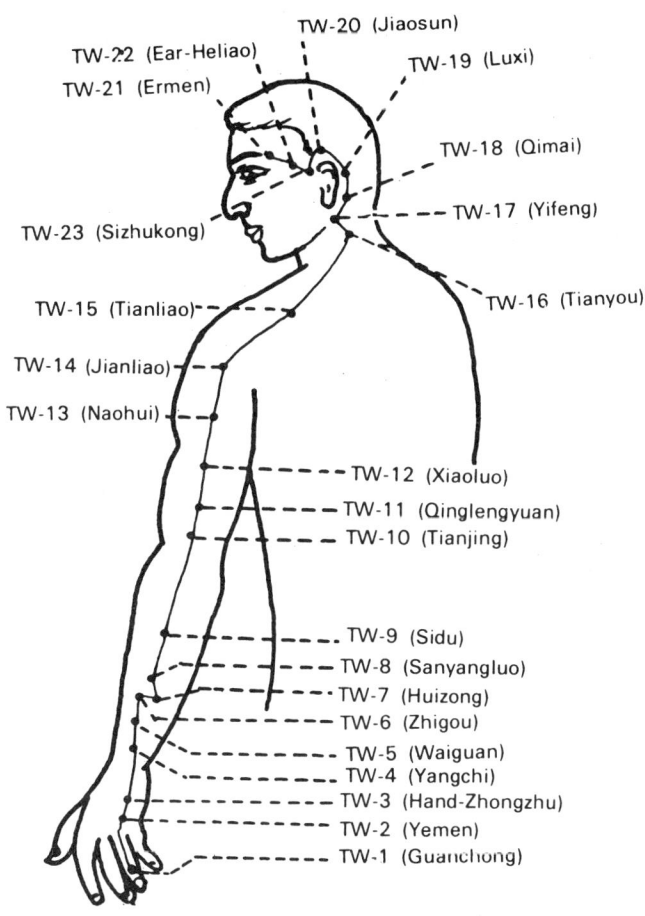

Fig. 14.51

DESCRIPTION OF THE POINTS

TW-1 (101) Guanchong (Kuangchung)

Location	: 0.1 t-sun proximal to the medial corner of the nail of the ring finger (Fig. 14.52).
Peculiarity	: It is a Jing-well point.
Indications	: All acute emergencies, pharyngitis, hyperpyrexia and acute headache.
Needling	: 0.1 to 0.3 t-sun, straight.

TW-2 (102) Yemen

Location	: 0.5 t-sun above the margin of the 4th web (between the little and ring fingers).
Indications	: Deafness, malaria, spastic fingers, pain in hand and arm, headache.
Needling	: 0.3 to 0.5 t-sun, straight.

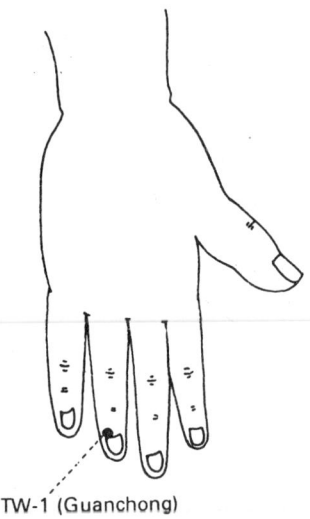

TW-1 (Guanchong)

Fig. 14.52

TW-3 (103) Zhongzhu (Chungchu)

Location	:	Dorsum of the hand in the 4th intermetacarpal space (between 4th and 5th metacarpal bones) in a hollow proximal to the metacarpophalangeal joints [1 t-sun proximal to Yenmen (TW-2)].
Indications	:	Deafness, tinnitus, labyrinthitis, vertigo, spastic hand, paralysis, polyneuropathy, painful shoulders.
Needling	:	0.5 t-sun, straight.

TW-4 (104) Yangchi (Yangchih)

Location	:	On the dorsal wrist crease medial to the tendon of the extensor digitorum communis muscle. This point is just distal to the extensor retinaculum.
Peculiarity	:	It is a Yuan (source) point.
Indications	:	Arthritis of the wrist, wrist drop, malaria.
Needling	:	0.3 to 0.5 t-sun, straight.

TW-5 (105) Waiguan (Waikuan)

Location	:	On the dorsal aspect of the forearm, 2 t-sun proximal to the dorsal transverse wrist crease between the two bones of the forearm.
Peculiarity	:	It is a Luo-connecting point.
Indications	:	Pain and paralysis of the upper extremity, arthritis of the small joints of hand and fingers, wrist drop, writer's cramps, neck pain, headache, deafness, fever, optic atrophy.
Needling	:	0.5 to 1.5 t-sun, straight [point to point with Neiguan (P-6)].

TW-6 (106) Zhigou (Chihkou)

Location	:	1 t-sun above Waiguan (TW-5).
Indications	:	Constipation, paralysis of the upper extremities.
Needling	:	1 to 1.5 t-sun, straight.

TW-7 (107) Huizhong (Huitsung)

Location	:	3/4 t-sun lateral to Zhigou (TW-6).
Peculiarity	:	It is a Xi-cleft point.
Indications	:	Epilepsy, deafness, pain and paralysis of the upper extremity.
Needling	:	1 to 1.5 t-sun, straight.

TW-8 (108) Sanyangluo (Sanyanglo)

Location	:	2 t-sun proximal to Waiguan (TW-5) midway between the radius and the ulna.
Peculiarity	:	Three Yang channels of the arm meet on this point.
Indications	:	Pain and paralysis of the upper extremities, deafness, aphasia, herpes zoster, intercostalneuralgia.
Needling	:	0.5 to 1 t-sun, straight.

TW-9 (109) Sidu (Szutu)

Location	:	5 t-sun below the tip of the olecranon, between the two bones of the forearm.
Indications	:	Pain and paralysis of the upper extremity, toothache and nephritis.
Needling	:	1 to 1.5 t-sun, straight.

TW-10 (110) Tianjing (Tienching)

Location	:	On the back of the elbow, 1 t-sun proximal to the tip of the olecranon [flex the elbow at right angle. Tianjing (TW-10) lies in the centre of the depression above the olecranon].
Indications	:	1. Diseases of the elbow joint and the soft tissue around it.
		2. Hemiplegia.
		3. Painful arm, shoulder and chest.
		4. Lymphadenitis.
Needling	:	0.5 to 1 t-sun, straight.

TW-11 (111) Qingleng Yuan (Chingleng Yuan)

Location	:	1 t-sun proximal to Tianjing (TW-10) on the back of the upper arm.
Indications	:	Periarthritis and other painful condition of the shoulder, pain in the arm.
Needling	:	0.5 to 0.8 t-sun, straight.

TW-12 (112) Xiaoluo (Hsiaolo)

Location	:	On the back of the arm, 6 t-sun above olecranon, midway between the Qingleng Yuan (TW-11) and Naohui (TW-13).
Indications	:	Pain in arm and vertex.
Needling	:	1 to 1.5 t-sun, straight.

TW-13 (113) Naohui

Location   : 3 t-sun below Jianliao (TW-14) on the back of the arm.
Indications   : Diseases of the eye, pain in the arm, shoulder and scapular joint.
Needling   : 1 to 1.5 t-sun, straight.

TW-14 (114) Jianliao (Chienliao)

Location   : 1. Between the acromion and greater tuberosity of the humerus, when the arm is kept by the side of the body.
                  2. When the arm is abducted two hollows appear on the shoulder. The posterior hollow is Jianliao (TW-14), while the anterior hollow is Jianyu (LI-15).
Indications   : 1. Periarthritis and other diseases of the shoulder joint and diseases of the soft tissue around the shoulder.
                  2. Pain and paralysis of the upper extremity.
Needling   : 1 to 1.5 t-sun, towards Jiquan (H-1) straight. Upper arm is kept horizontally in abduction while needling.

TW-15 (115) Tianliao (Tienliao)

Location   : Midway between the tip of the acromion and centre point of the intervertebral space between C-7 and T-1 (cervical-7 and thoracic-1 vertebrae), in suprascapular fossa, 1 t-sun below GB-21.
Indications   : Pain and paralysis of the upper extremities, painful shoulder and neck.
Needling   : 0.5 to 1 t-sun, straight.

TW-16 (116) Tianyou (Tienyu)

Location   : Behind and below the tip of the mastoid process, at the level of the angle of the mandible. This point lies on the posterior border of the sternocleido mastoideus muscle near the natural hair line.
Indications   : Deafness, stiffness of the neck.
Needling   : 1.5 to 2 t-sun, straight.

TW-17 (117) Yifeng

Location   : Behind the lobule of the ear in the depression between the mastoid process and the angle of the mandible.
Indications   : 1. All disorders of the ear like deafness, tinnitus aurium, otitis media.
                  2. Facial nerve paralysis.
                  3. Parotitis.
                  4. Trigeminal neuralgia.
Needling   : 1.5 to 2 t-sun, slanting.

TW-18 (118) Qimai (Chihmo)

Location   : Centre of the mastoid process.
Indications   : Facial nerve paralysis, deafness, tinnitus aurium.
Needling   : 0.1 to 0.3 t-sun, slanting.

TW-19 (119) Luxi (Luhsi)

Location   : 1 t-sun above Qimai (TW-18).

Indications   : Otitis media, mastoiditis, tinnitus aurium, emesis.
Needling   : 0.2 to 0.3 t-sun, slanting.

TW-20 (120) Jiaosun (Chuehsun)
Location   : On the natural hair line, above the apex auriculae.
Indications   : Toothache, infections of the external ear, corneal opacities.
Needling   : 0.2 to 0.3 t-sun, slanting.

TW-21 (121) Ermen (Erhmen)
Location   : In the depression in front of the superior notch of the tragus when the mouth is open.
Indications   : Deafness, tinnitus, labyrinthitis, vertigo, trismus, otitis media and otitis externa, arthritis of the temporomandibular joint.
Needling   : Mouth is kept open while needling.

TW-22 (122) Ear Heliao (Holiao)
Location   : At the level with the superior margin of the root of the auricle along superficial temporal artery.
Indications   : Facial nerve paralysis, tinnitus, headache.
Needling   : 0.2 to 0.3 t-sun, slanting.

TW-23 (123) Sizhukong (Ssuchukung)
Location   : Lateral end of the eyebrow.
Indications   : Frontal sinusitis, migraine, frontal and temporal headaches, diseases of the eye.
Needling   : 0.5 to 1 t-sun slanting posteriorly towards Shnaign (GB-8).

11. THE GALL BLADDER MERIDIAN

According to the traditional Chinese description it is a Yang channel associated with the element wood and possesses interior and exterior relationship with the liver meridian.

Total number of points : 44.
Starting point   : Lateral canthus of the eye.
Terminal point   : Tip of the fourth toe.
Pathway   : This channel originates at the lateral canthus and divided into two branches: (i) anterior branch, and (ii) posterior branch.
Anterior branch : It has no point in its course and not considered as a useful branch.
Posterior branch : It ascends to the corner of the forehead and then curves downwards to reach behind the ear.   It then runs along the lateral aspect of the neck and finally goes to the supraclavicular area where it divides into two branches—inner branch and superficial branch.
Inner branch   : This branch goes to the liver and gall bladder and emerges at the inguinal area.   It joins superficial branch at the hip joint.
Superficial branch   : From supraclavicular fossa, this branch courses downwards in front of the axilla and then along the lateral aspect of the chest, passes through the free ends of the 11th ribs to the hip region where it connects with the inner branch.

After union of the inner branch and the superficial branch, the main meridian descends along the lateral aspect of the thigh and knee antero-lateral aspect of the leg and dorsum of the foot and reaches the fourth toe where it terminates on the lateral side of its tip (Figs. 14.53 and 14.54).

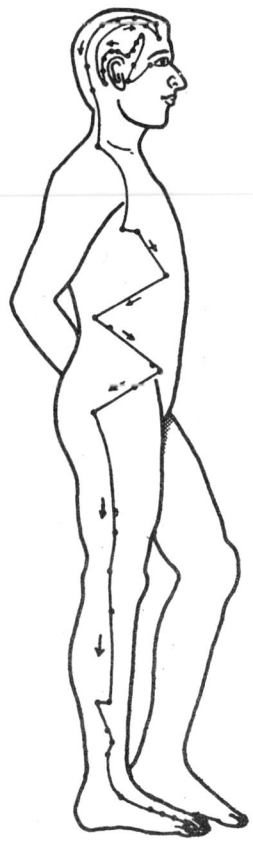

Fig. 14.53 Gall bladder meridian.

Therapeutic indications

1. All the disorders along the pathway of the channel.
2. Points on the face are used for eye and ear disorders, facial paralysis, trigeminal neuralgia and pain in the neck.
3. Points on the chest are used for lactation disorders.
4. Points on the abdomen are used for the liver and gall bladder disorders.
5. Points of the lower extremity are used for the treatment of sciatica, paralysis, poliomyelitis, and arthritis of the knee and ankle.
6. Points below knee are used as distal points for the treatment of proximal disorders.

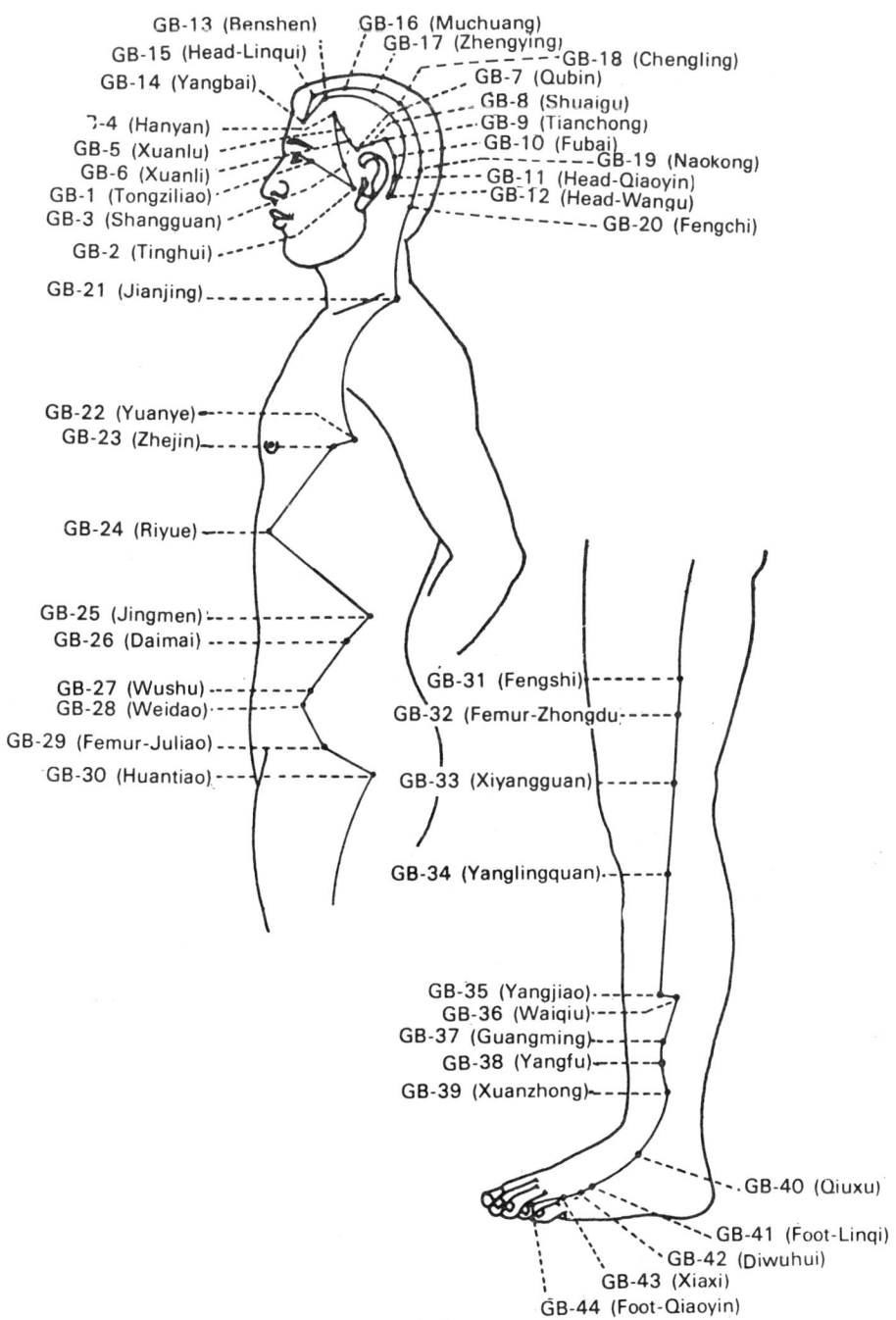

GB-13 (Benshen) GB-16 (Muchuang)
GB-15 (Head-Linqui) GB-17 (Zhengying)
GB-14 (Yangbai) GB-18 (Chengling)
GB-7 (Qubin)
GB-8 (Shuaigu)
GB-4 (Hanyan) GB-9 (Tianchong)
GB-5 (Xuanlu) GB-10 (Fubai)
GB-6 (Xuanli) GB-19 (Naokong)
GB-1 (Tongziliao) GB-11 (Head-Qiaoyin)
GB-3 (Shangguan) GB-12 (Head-Wangu)
GB-2 (Tinghui) GB-20 (Fengchi)

GB-21 (Jianjing)

GB-22 (Yuanye)
GB-23 (Zhejin)

GB-24 (Riyue)

GB-25 (Jingmen)
GB-26 (Daimai)

GB-27 (Wushu) GB-31 (Fengshi)
GB-28 (Weidao) GB-32 (Femur-Zhongdu)
GB-29 (Femur-Juliao) GB-33 (Xiyangguan)
GB-30 (Huantiao)

GB-34 (Yanglingquan)

GB-35 (Yangjiao)
GB-36 (Waiqiu)
GB-37 (Guangming)
GB-38 (Yangfu)
GB-39 (Xuanzhong)

GB-40 (Qiuxu)
GB-41 (Foot-Linqi)
GB-42 (Diwuhui)
GB-43 (Xiaxi)
GB-44 (Foot-Qiaoyin)

Fig. 14.54 Gall bladder meridian.

DESCRIPTION OF THE POINTS

GB-1 (188) Tongziliao (Tungtzuliao)

Location	:	0.5 t-sun lateral to the lateral canthus of the eye (Fig. 14.55).

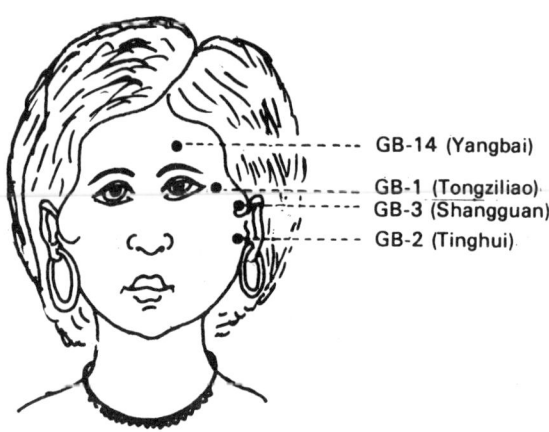

GB-14 (Yangbai)
GB-1 (Tongziliao)
GB-3 (Shangguan)
GB-2 (Tinghui)

Fig. 14.55

Indications	:	Keratitis, conjunctivitis, headache, facial paralysis, migraine (of the same side) trigeminal neuralgia.
Needling	:	0.2 to 0.5 t-sun, straight.
		Transverse 0.5 to 1 t-sun towards Taiyang (Ex.-2).

GB-2 (189) Tinghui (Tinghui)

Location	:	Depression in front of the inferior notch of the tragus or on the posterior margin of the condyloid process of the mandible (Fig. 14.55).
Indications	:	Deafness, tinnitus, otitis media, trigeminal neuralgia, upper toothache, arthritis of the tempromandibular joint, facial paralysis.
Needling	:	0.3 to 0.5 t-sun, straight or point to point with Ermen (TW-21).

GB-3 (190) Shangguan (Shangkuan)

Location	:	Anterior to the ear, the upper border of the zygomatic arch vertically above Xiaguan (St-7).
Indications	:	Tinnitus aurium, deafness, facial paralysis.
Needling	:	0.5 to 1 t-sun, straight.

GB-4 (191) Hanyan

Location	:	1 t-sun below Touwei (St-8) on the temple.
Indications	:	Migraine, tinnitus, facial paralysis.
Needling	:	0.3 to 0.5 t-sun, slanting.
Note	:	Xuanlu (GB-5), Xuanli (GB-6) and Qubin (GB-7) fall on a line drawn between the points Hanyan (GB-4) and the crossing point of the horizontal line of the auricle and verticle line in front of the anterior

auricle. The crossing point is Qubin (GB-7) while Xuanlu (GB 5) line at the junction of anterior and middle third and Xuanli (GB-6) at the junction of inferior and middle third of this line.

GB-5 (192) Xuanlu (Hsuanlu)
Location : As above on Hanyan (GB-4) to Qubin (GB-7) line.
Indications : Migraine, toothache, neurasthenia.
Needling : 0.2 to 0.3 t-sun, slanting.

GB-6 (193) Xuanli (Shuanli)
Location : As above on Hanyan (GB-4) to Qubin (GB-7) line.
Indications : Similar to Xuanlu (GB-5).
Needling : 0.3 to 0.5 t-sun, slanting.

GB-7 (194) Qubin (Chupin)
Location : Crossing point as described above.
Indications : Stiffness of the neck, trismus, headache, swollen and painful cheeks.
Needling : 0.3 to 0.5 t-sun, slanting.

GB-8 (198) Shuaigu (Shuaiku)
Location : Directly above the apex of the auricle, 1.5 t-sun above the natural hair line. To mark the apex auricle should be folded upon itself vertically.
Indications : Migraine, parietal headache, forgetfulness, vertigo, diziness, all ear disorders and psychosomatic disorders.
Needling : 0.3 to 0.5 t-sun, slanting anteriorly or posteriorly.

GB-9 (199) Tianchong (Tienchung))
Location : 0.5 t-sun behind Shuaigu (GB-8), 2 t-sun above the natural hair line.
Indications : Epilepsy, headache, gingivitis.
Needling : 0.5 to 0.8 t-sun, slanting.

GB-10 (197) Fubai (Fupai)
Location : Behind the ear, 1 t-sun below Tianchong (GB-9) on the postero-superior part of the mastoid process.
Indications : Tonsillitis, deafness, tinnitus aurium.
Needling : 0.5 to 0.8 t-sun, slanting.

GB-11 (198) Head-Qiaoyin (Chiaoyin)
Location : Midway between Fubai (GB-10 and Head Wangu (GB-12).
Indications : Pain in the eyes, headache (vertex pain).
Needling : 0.5 to 0.8 t-sun, slanting.

GB-12 (199) Head-Wangu (Wanku)
Location : In the hollow made my bending the neck behind and below the mastoid process.
Indications : Bell's palsy, toothache, tinnitus.
Needling : 0.5 to 0.8 t-sun, slanting.

GB-13 (200) Benshen (Penshen)
Location   : Vertically above the outer canthus of the eye, 0.5 t-sun above the natural hair line.
Indications   : Epilepsy, cervical spondylosis, stiff neck, eye diseases, facial paralysis.
Needling   : 0.5 to 0.8 t-sun, slanting.

GB-14 (201) Yangbai (Yangpai)
Location   : On the forehead 1 t-sun vertically above the midpoint of the eyebrow.
Indications   : Bell's palsy, headache (frontal), frontal sinusitis, trigeminal neuralgia, night blindness, glaucoma.
Needling   : 0.3 to 0.5 t-sun, horizontally directed inferiorly.

GB-15 (202) Head-Linqi (Linchi)
Location   : 0.5 t-sun inside the hair line vertically above the pupil. Patient is asked to look straight ahead while locating the point.
Indications   : Diseases of the eye, obstructed and stuffy nose, epilepsy.
Needling   : 0.5 to 0.8 t-sun, slanting.

GB-16 (203) Muchuang
Location   : 1 t-sun above Head-Linqi (GB-15).
Indications   : Diseases of the eye, oedema and cellulitis of the face.
Needling   : 0.5 to 0.8 t-sun, slanting.

GB-17 (204) Zhengying (Chengying)
Location   : 1 t-sun behind and 1 t-sun above Head-Linqi (GB-15).
Indications   : Epoplexy, toothache, headache.
Needling   : 0.5 to 0.8 t-sun, slanting.

GB-18 (205) Chengling
Location   : 1 t-sun above 1.5 t-sun behind Head-Linqi (GB-15).
Indications   : Epistaxis, headache, stuffy nose, rhinitis.
Needling   : 0.5 to 0.7 t-sun, slanting.

GB-19 (206) Naokong (Naokung)
Location   : 1.5 t-sun above Fengchi (GB-20) lateral to the external occipital protuberance.
Indications   : Bronchial asthama, headache, cervical spondylosis, stiffness of the neck.
Needling   : 0.5 to 0.7 t-sun, slanting.

GB-20 (207) Fengchi (Fengchih)
Location   : At the apex of the posterior triangle of the neck, in the hollow directly below and between the external occipital protuberance and the mastoid process. It lies between the insertions of the trapezius and sterno cliedo mastoid muscles (Fig. 14.56).
Indications   : 1. Stiff neck, cervical spondylosis and all other painful disorders of the occipital region.

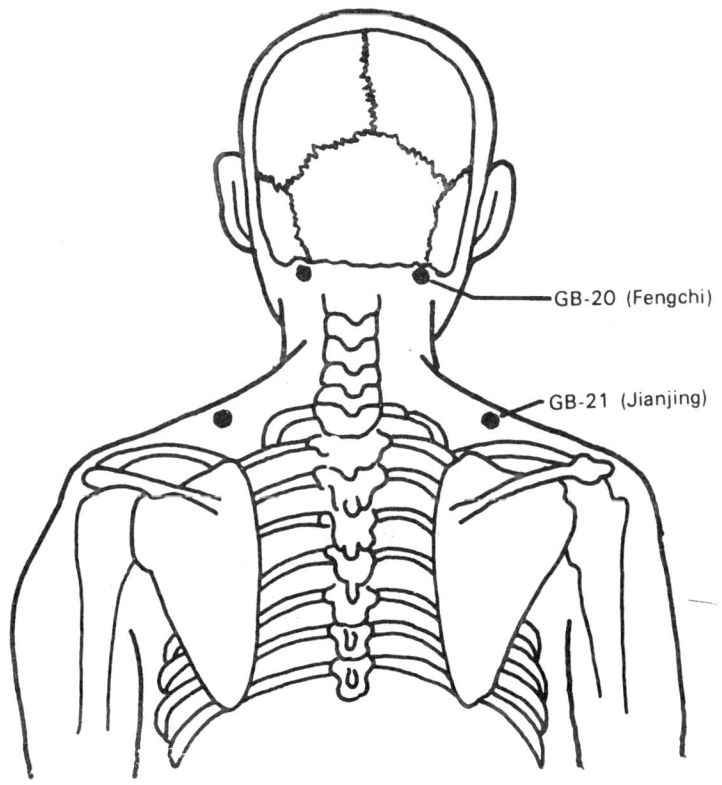

GB-20 (Fengchi)

GB-21 (Jianjing)

Fig. 14.56

2. Headache, common cold, vertigo, tinnitus, influenza.
3. Hypertension.
4. Meningitis.

Needling : 0.5 to 0.8 t-sun, slanting.
Directed towards the opposite eye.

GB-21 (208) Jianjing (Chien Ching)

Location : Highest point of the shoulder [it is located midway between Dazhui (GV-14) and acromion].

Peculiarity : It is a dangerous point.

Indications : Frozen shoulder, backache, stiffness of the neck, cervical spondylosis, motor disorders of the upper extremity, menstrual disorders of the endocrine origin, functional uterine bleeding, hyperthyroidism, mastitis.

Needling : 0.5 to 1 t-sun, straight (deep insertion is prohibited).

GB-22 (209) Yuanye (Yuanyeh)

Location   : 3 t-sun below the mid-axilliary fold.   To locate the point with accuracy ask the patient to abduct the arm.   The point lies in the anterior axillary line in the fourth intercostal space.

Indications   : Intercostal neuralgia, herpes zoster, pleuritis, thickened pleura, axillary lymphadenitis.

Needling   : 0.5 to 1 t-sun, oblique.

GB-23 (210) Zhejin (Chechin)

Location   : On the chest in the fourth intercostal space 1 t-sun anterior to Yuanye (GB-22).

Indications   : Hyperacidity, excessive salivation, water brash, heart burn, emesis, bronchial asthma.

Needling   : 0.5 to 1 t-sun slanting.

GB-24 (211) Riyue (Jihyueh)

Location   : In the 7th intercostal space directly below the nipple.

Indications   : Epigastric pain, herpes zoster, hepatitis, cholecystitis, hiccough, myalgia chest, lactational defects.

Needling   : 0.5 to 1 t-sun, slanting outwards.

GB-25 (212) Jingmen (Chingmen)

Location   : On the abdominal wall at the lower border of the free end of the 12th rib.

Indications   : Intercostal neuralgia, fever, gall bladder disorders, fibrositis chest, hepatic disorders.

Needling   : 0.3 to 0.5 t-sun, slanting.

GB-26 (213) Daimai (Taimo)

Location   : On the abdominal wall, midway between the free ends of the 11th and 12th rib at level of umbilicus.

Indications   : Menstrual disorders like dysmenorrhoea, menorrhagia and metorrhagia, endometritis, cystitis, lumbago, cholecystitis, hepatitis and intercostal neuralgia.

Needling   : 1 to 1.5 t-sun, slanting.

GB-27 (214) Wushu

Location   : In front of the anterior superior iliac spine at the level with Guan Yuan (CV-4).

Indications   : Lower abdominal pain, endometritis, orchitis and impotence.

Needling   : 1 to 1.5 t-sun, straight.

GB-28 (215) Weidao (Weitao)

Location   : 0.5 t-sun below the anterior to Wushu (GB-27).

Indications   : Lower abdominal pain, pelvic cellulitis dysmenorrhoea, habitual constipation.

Needling   : 1 to 1.5 t-sun straight.

GB-29 (216) Femur-Juliao (Chuliao)

Location	:	Midway between the highest point of the greater trochanter of the femur and the anterior superior iliac spine.
Indications	:	Lumbago, lower abdominal pain, orchitis, endometritis, diseases of the hip joint.
Needling	:	1 to 2 t-sun, straight.

GB-30 (217) Huantiao

Location	:	At the junction of the outer one third and the middle two-thirds of a line drawn between the highest point of the greater trochanter and sacral hiatus (Fig. 14.57).

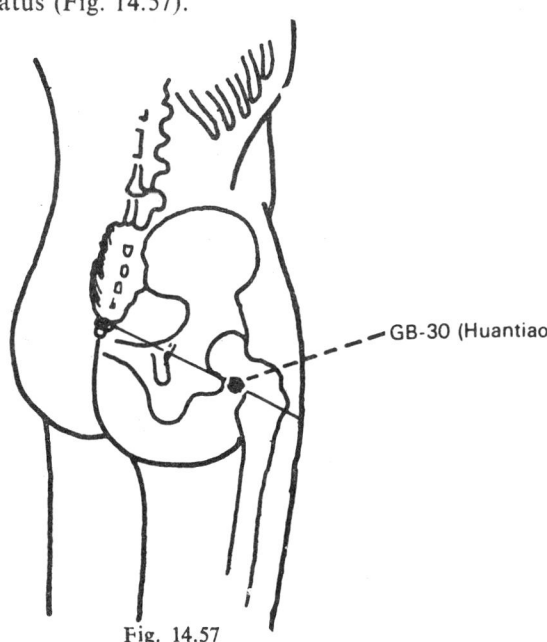

GB-30 (Huantiao)

Fig. 14.57

Indications	:	Prolapsed intervertebral disc, acute sciatica, paralysis of the lower extremities, poliomyelitis, arthritis of the hip joint.
Needling	:	2.5 to 5 t-sun, straight.

GB-31 (218) Fengshi (Fengshih)

Location	:	7 t-sun above the outer end of the transverse popliteal crease on the lateral aspect of the thigh.
	:	An easy way of locating the point is to ask the patient to extend arm and forearm while standing or lying down, by the side of the body so that the palm touches the thigh. The tip of the middle finger indicates the point.
Indications	:	Poliomyelitis, paralysis of the lower extremities, lumbago, sciatica, neurodermatitis of the outer aspect of the thigh.
Needling	:	1.5 to 3 t-sun, straight.

GB-32 (219) Femur Zhongdu (Chungtu)

Location	:	2 t-sun below the Fengshi (GB-31).
Indications	:	Slipped disc syndrome, sciatica, hemiplegia.
Needling	:	1 to 3 t-sun, straight.

GB-33 (220) Xiyangguan (Hsiyangkuan)

Location	:	3 t-sun vertically above Yanglingquan (GB-34) on the outer aspect of the knee.
Indications	:	Painful disorders of the knee joint, paralysis of the lower limb.
Needling	:	1 to 2 t-sun, straight.

GB-34 (221) Yanglingquan (Yanglingchuan)

Location	:	On the antero-lateral aspect of the leg in the depression in front and below the head of the fibula (Fig. 14.58).

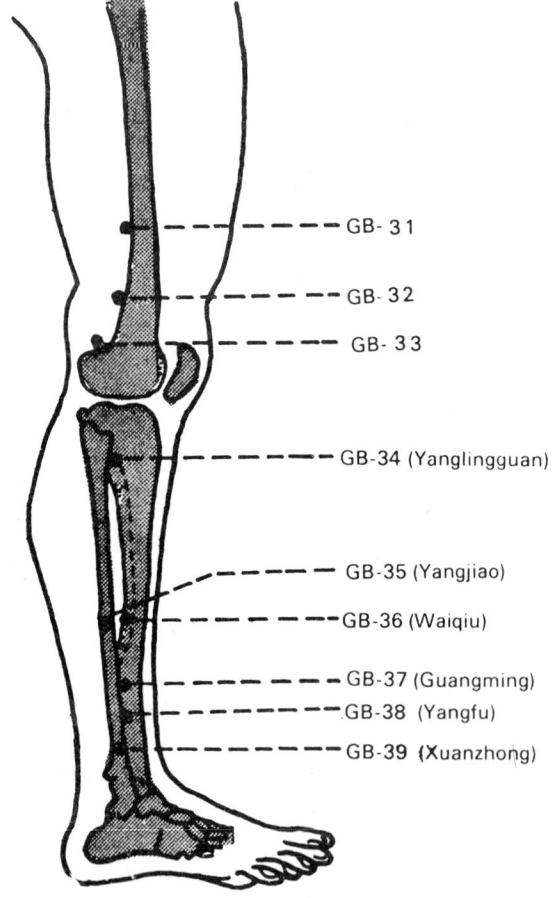

Fig. 14.58

Peculiarities	:	It is the influential point for the tendon and muscle.
Indications	:	Hemiplegia, poliomyelitis, tenosynovitis, myopathies and muscular dystrophies, mental disorders, diseases of the knee joint, foot drop, diseases of gall bladder, lumbago, hyperacidity, vertigo, labyrinthitis, and dizziness.
Needling	:	1 to 1.5 t-sun, straight.

GB-35 (222) Yangjiao (Yangchiao)

Location	:	On the anterior border of the fibula, 7 t-sun above the tip of the lateral malleolus.
Indications	:	Sciatica, asthma.
Needling	:	1 to 1.5 t-sun, straight.

GB-36 (223) Waiqiu (Waichiu)

Location	:	1 t-sun bihind Yangjiao (GB-35).
Indications	:	Sciatica, leg cramps, myoclonus, stiff neck.
Needling	:	1 to 1.5 t-sun, straight.

GB-37 (224) Guangming (Kuangming)

Location	:	2 t-sun below Yangjiao (GB-35) in front of the fibula.
Peculiarities	:	It is the Luo-connecting point of the gall bladder channel. It is a distal point for eye diseases.
Indications	:	Eye diseases, sciatica and pain of the lateral side of the leg, migraine, headache.
Needling	:	1 to 1.5 t-sun, straight.

GB-38 (225) Yangfu

Location	:	3 t-sun below Yangjiao (GB-35) in front of the fibula.
Indications	:	Diseases of the knee joint like arthritis and synovitis, lumbago.
Needling	:	1 to 1.5 t-sun, straight.

GB-39 (226) Xuanzhong (Hsuanchung)

Location	:	3 t-sun above the lateral malleolus.
Peculiarity	:	It is an influential point for bone marrow and a distal point for the neck.
Indications	:	Poliomyelitis, paralysis, anaemia, cervical spondylosis.
Needling	:	0.5 to 1 t-sun straight.

GB-40 (227) Qiuxu (Chiuhsu)

Location	:	In the depression anterior and inferior to the lateral malleolus.
Peculiarity	:	It is a distal point for the chest and buttock.
Indications	:	Axillary lymphadenitis, costalgia, cholecystitis, sciatica, arthritis of the ankle joint, foot drop, véricose and other chronic ulcers of the ankle, pain in the chest, painful conditions of the hip.
Needling	:	0.5 to 1 t-sun, slanting.

GB-41 (228) Foot Linqi (Tsulingchi)

Location	:	In the depression anterior to the 4th intermetatarsal joint (junction of the 4th and 5th matatarsal bones of the foot).

Peculiarities   :   It is one of the best distal points for ear and breast, and one of the confluent points of the eight extra channels.

Indications   :   Conjunctivitis, metatarsalgia, costalgia, mastitis, lymphadenitis, to stop the milk secretion, deafness and tinnitus.

Needling   :   0.3 to 0.5 t-sun, straight.

GB-42 (229) Diwuhui (Tiwuhui)

Location   :   4th intermetatarsal space (between 4th and 5th metatarsal bones) 0.5 t-sun distal to Foot Linqi (GB-41).

Indications   :   Axillary lymphadenitis, painful axilla, tinnitus aurium.

Needling   :   0.3 to 0.5 t-sun, straight.

GB-43 (230) Xiaxi (Hsiahsi)

Location   :   0.5 t-sun proximal to the margin of the 4th web (between 4th toe and the little toe).

Indications   :   Deafness, dizziness intercostal neuralgia.

Needling   :   0.4 to 0.5 t-sun, straight.

GB-44 (231) Foot Qiaoyin (Tsuchiaoyin)

Location   :   On the lateral side of the tip of the 4th toe, 0.1 t-sun proximal to the corner of the nail.

Peculiarity   :   It is a Jing-well point.

Indications   :   Asthma, pleuritis, acute emergencies.

Needling   :   0.1 to 0.2 t-sun, straight or until bleeding.

12. THE LIVER MERIDIAN

According to the traditional Chinese description it is a Yin channel associated with the element wood and possesses interior and exterior relationship with the gall bladder meridian (Fig. 14.59).

Total number of points : 14.

Starting point   :   Dorsum of the big toe.

Terminal point   :   6th intercostal space, below the nipple.

Pathway   This channel originates from the lateral side of the great toe, ascends over the dorsum of the foot and reaches in front of the medial malleolus. In its course on the medial side of the leg it meets the spleen and kidney meridian at the point Sanyinjiao (Sp-6) and then ascends upwards along the medial side of the knee and thigh, curves around external genitalia in the pubic region and reaches the lower abdomen, where it divides into two branches : (i) superficial branch, and (ii) inner branch.

1. Superficial :   From the level of the symphysis pubis, this branch turns upwards,
branch   reaches the free end of the 11th rib and ends in the 6th intercostal space where it meets the inner branch.

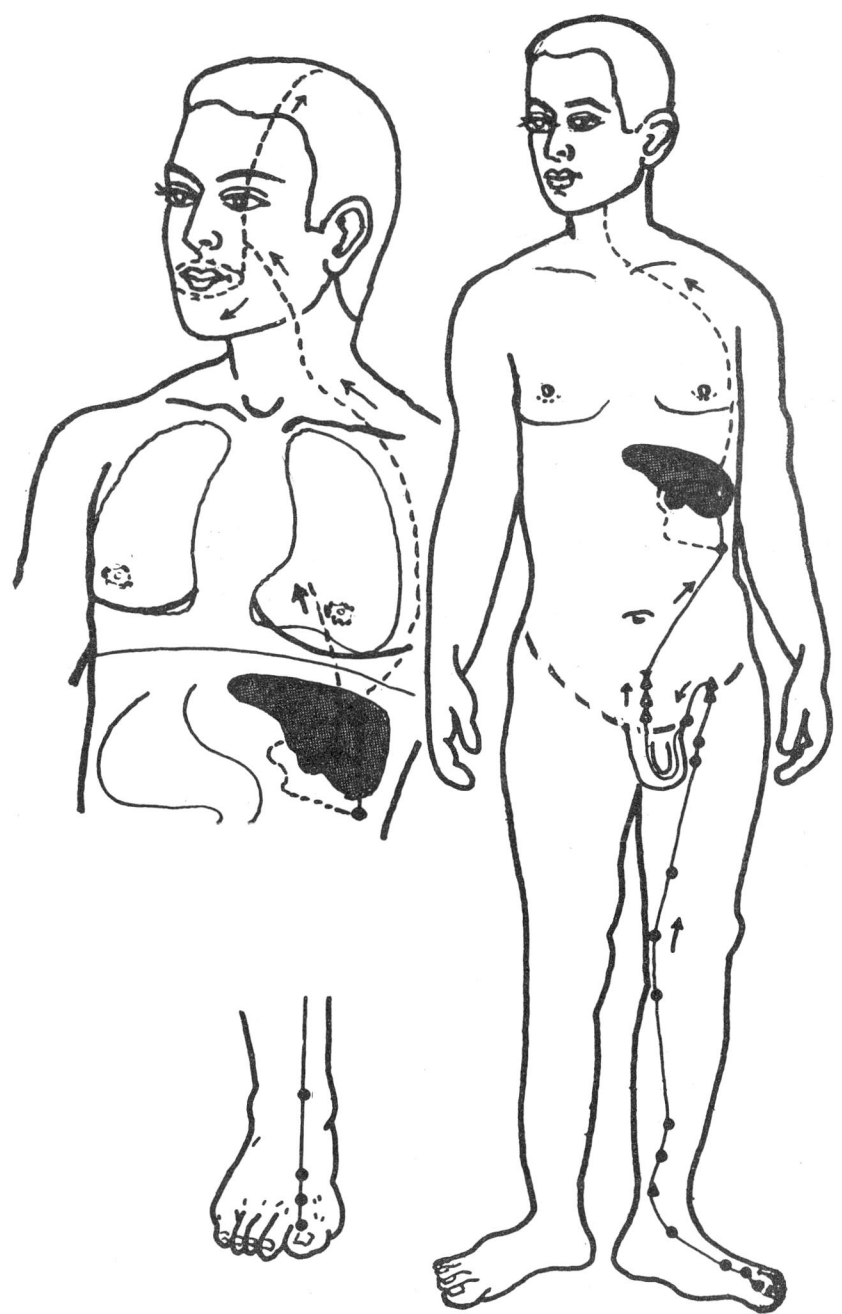

Fig. 14.59 Liver meridian.

2. Inner branch : It goes to the abdomen, encircles the stomach and then enters the pertaining organ, liver. Here it communicates with the gall bladder and then passes further upwards to the diaphragm and ascends along the posterior aspect of the throat to the nasopharynx and connects with the eye and brain. It then again becomes superficial in its course, leads to the forehead and meets the governing vessel meridian. A small branch goes to the mouth but it has no point.

Therapeutic Indications

1. All the disorders along the pathway of the channel.
2. Diseases of the liver and gall bladder.
3. Eye disorders.
4. Disorders of the spleen.
5. Convulsion and headache.

DESCRIPTION OF THE POINTS

Liv-1 (320) Dadun (Tatun)

Location : On the outer side of the dorsum of the terminal phalanx of the big toe, midway between the interphalangeal joint and the lateral corner of the nail (Fig. 14.60).

Peculiarities : It is a Jing-well point. It is a specific point for pruritis of the genital organs.

Indications : Pruritis of the genital organs, menorrhagia, prolapse of the uterus, enuresis, hernia, colic and all acute emergencies.

Needling : 0.3 to 0.5 t-sun, slanting.

Liv-2 (321) Xingjian (Hsingchien)

Location : On the dorsum of the foot 0.5 t-sun proximal to the margin of the web between the big toe and the second toe.

Indications : Headache, fainting, infantile convulsions, insomnia, epilepsy, intercostal neuralgia, hypertension, night sweating, urethritis, enuresis.

Needling : 0.3 to 0.5 t-sun, straight.

Liv-3 (322) Taichong (Taichung)

Location : On the dorsum of the foot, in the first intermetatarsal space, 2 t-sun proximal to the margin of the web (Fig. 14.60).

Peculiarity : It is physiological danger point as it lowers the blood pressure very suddenly.

Indications : Headache, fainting, uterine bleeding, disorders of the eye, hypertension, epilepsy.

Needling : 0.3 to 0.5 t-sun, straight, or 0.3 to 0.5 t-sun obliquely upwards.

Liv-4 (323) Zhongfeng (Chungfeng)

Location : On the ankle 1 t-sun anterior to the medial malleolus, in between the tendons of the extensor hallusis longus muscle and the tibialis anterior muscle.

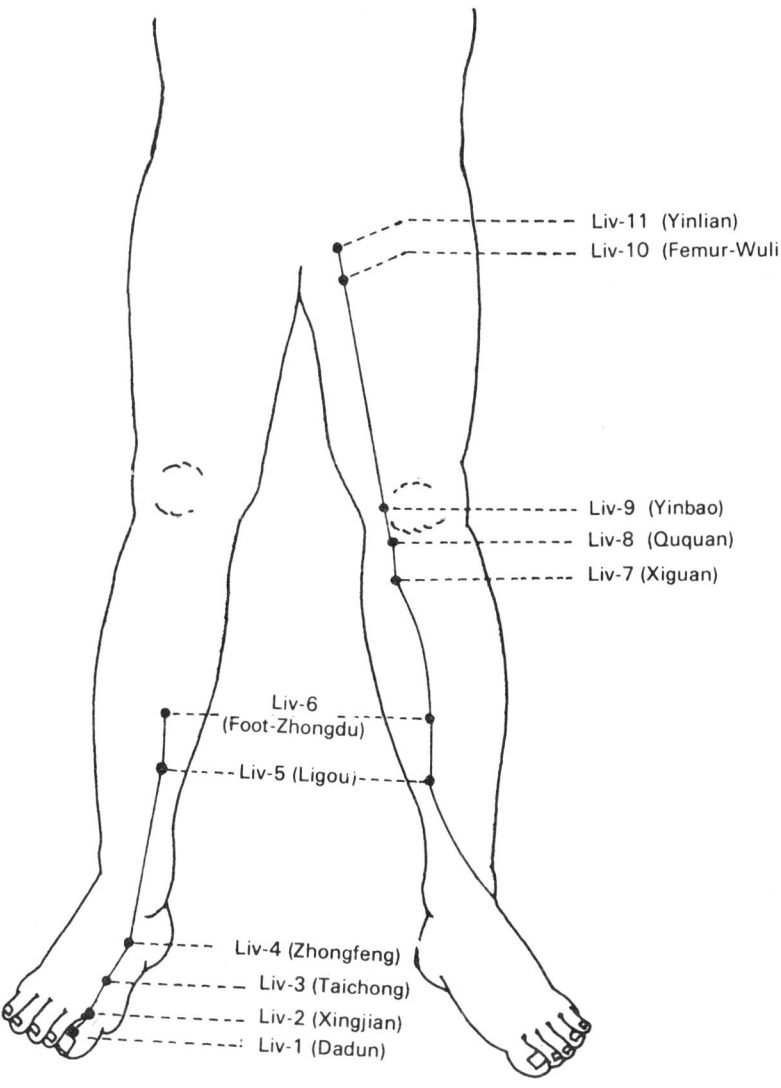

Liv-11 (Yinlian)
Liv-10 (Femur-Wuli)

Liv-9 (Yinbao)
Liv-8 (Ququan)
Liv-7 (Xiguan)

Liv-6
(Foot-Zhongdu)
Liv-5 (Ligou)

Liv-4 (Zhongfeng)
Liv-3 (Taichong)
Liv-2 (Xingjian)
Liv-1 (Dadun)

Fig. 14.60

Indications   : Lower abdominal pain, pelvic cellulitis, nocturnal pollution, pain in
                  the penis, urinary retention, phosphaturea, spermatorrhoea.
Needling   : 0.3 to 0.5 t-sun, straight.

Liv-5 (324) Ligou (Likou)

Location   : On the medial aspect of the leg, along the posterior border of the
                  tibia, 5 t-sun above the tip of the medial malleolus.
Peculiarity   : It is a Luo-connecting point.

Indications	:	Impotence, spermatorrhoea, schizophrermia, pelvic cellulitis, urinary retention, pain in the legs.
Needling	:	0.5 to 1 t-sun, straight.

Liv-6 (325) Foot Zhongdu (Chungtu)

Location	:	2 t-sun above Ligou (Liv-5) on the posterior border of the tibia.
Peculiarity	:	It is a Xi-cleft point and the alarm point for the liver.
Indications	:	Diseases of the liver and of gall bladder, pain in the joints of the lower limbs, menorrhagia, colic.
Needling	:	0.5 to 1 t-sun, straight.

Liv-7 (326) Xiguan (Hsikuan)

Location	:	1 t-sun behind Yinlingquan (Sp-9) on the postero-inferior aspect of the medial condyle of the tibia.
Indications	:	Painful disorders of the knee joint.
Needling	:	1 to 2 t-sun, straight.

Liv-8 (327) Ququan (Chuchuan)

Location	:	On the medial end of the transverse popliteal crease, in front of the semimemberanous muscle behind the lower end of the femur.
Peculiarity	:	It is a specific distal point for impotence.
Indications	:	Impotence, spermatorrhoea, poliomyelitis, prolapse of uterus, urethritis cystitis, endometritis.
Needling	:	1 to 2 t-sun, straight.

Liv-9 (328) Yinbao (Yinpao)

Location	:	On the medial aspect of the thigh, 4 t-sun above the medial epicondyle of the femur in between the sartorius muscle and vastus medialis muscle.
Indications	:	Lower abdominal pain, pelvic cellulitis, lumbago, urinary incontinence, irregular menstruation.
Needling	:	1 to 2 t-sun, straight.

Liv-10 (329) Femur-Wuli (Wuli)

Location	:	On the medial aspect of the thigh, 1 t-sun distal to Yinlian (Liv-11).
Indications	:	Distension of the abdomen, enuresis, urinary retention, eczema of the scrotum.
Needling	:	1 to 2 t-sun, straight.

Liv-11 (330) Yinlian (Yinlien)

Location	:	On the front of the thigh below inguinal ligament, 1 t-sun distal to the lateral wall of the femoral artery (palpate the artery to locate the point).
Indications	:	Neuralgia of the femoral nerve, lumbago, paraplegia, hemiplegia, pain in legs, irregular menstruation.
Needling	:	1 to 2 t-sun, straight.

Liv-12 (331) Jimai (Chimo)

Location	:	2.5 t-sun lateral from the centre of the symphysis pubic, in the inferio-lateral part of the pubic tubercle.
Indications	:	Pain in the penis, prolapse of uterus, lower abdominal pain, pelvic cellulitis, pain in the lateral side of the thigh fibrositis.
Neelding	:	0.5 to 1 t-sun, straight.

Liv-13 (332) Zhangmen (Changmen)

Location	:	On the tip of the free end of the 11th rib (Fig. 14.61).
Peculiarity	:	It is the influential point for the solid organs.
Indications	:	Subcostal pain, emesis, di. hoea, flatulence, abdominal distension, diseases of the liver and spl.

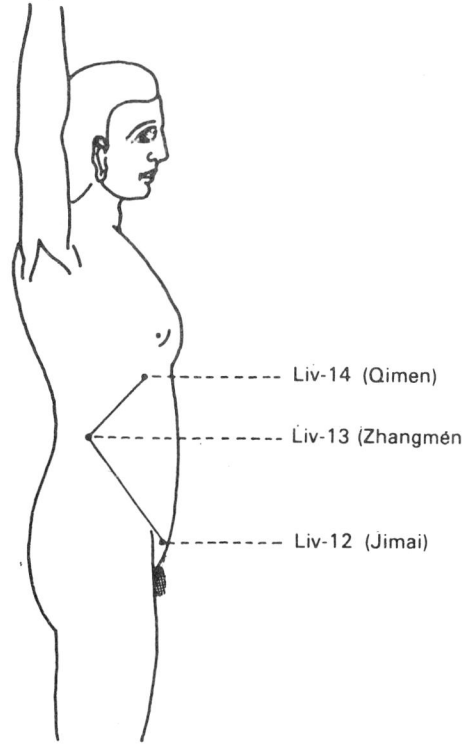

Liv-14 (Qimen)

Liv-13 (Zhangmén)

Liv-12 (Jimai)

Fig. 14.61

Liv-14 (333) Qimen (Chimen)

Location	:	On the front of the chest directly below the nipple, on the 6th inter-costal space.
Peculiarity	:	It is a dangerous point.
Indications	:	Neuralgia, indigestion, pleurisy, hepatitis, chest pain, heart diseases, lactational disorders, bronchial as thma.
Needling	:	0.5 t-sun slanting.

13. THE GOVERNING VESSELS MERIDIAN (The Du Channel)

This meridian is not linked to any organ but it possesses a governing influence on all the Yang channels of the body. The word 'Du' means 'Governor' (Fig. 14.62).

Total number of points: 28.

Starting point	:	In the perineum in between the coccyx and the anus.
Terminal point	:	Junction of the upper lip and gum.
Pathway	:	This meridian originates in the pelvic cavity, runs downwards and emerges externally in between the tip of the coccyx and anus. It then runs exactly in the posterior midline along the spinous processes of the vertebral column, and then in the midline of the skull to reach vertex. It winds round the scalp and forehead to reach the columella of the nose, descends to frenulum of the upper lip and ends in between the junction of the upper lip and gum. In its course it communicates with the kidney in the lumbar region and brain near vertex.

Therapeutic Indications

1. All the disorders along the pathway of channel.
2. Mental and neurological disorders.
3. Deaf mutism.
4. Anorectal and oral disorders.
5. Backache, spondylosis, ankylosing-spondylitis.
6. Febrile conditions.
7. Debility and other disorders associated with low body resistance.

DESCRIPTION OF THE POINTS

GV-1 (27) Changqiang (Chang Chiang)

Location	:	In between the tip of the coccyx and the anus (best located in the knee-chest position) (Fig. 14.63).
Indications	:	Anal fissure, haemorrhoids, prolapse of rectum, diarrhoea, pruritis of the anal region, coccydynia.
Needling	:	0.5 to 1.0 t-sun, slanting upwards.

GV-2 (26) Yaoshu

Location	:	Centre of the sacro-coccygeal junction (in the sacral hiatus).
Indications	:	Coccydynia, pain in the lumbosacral region, haemorrhoids, prolapse of the anus, paralysis of the lower limbs, cauda-equina syndrome, irregular menstruation, spermatorrhoea, impotence, enteritis, diarrhoea.
Needling	:	0.5 to 1 t-sun, slanting.

GV-3 (25) Yaoyangguan (Yangkuan)

Location	:	In the centre of the interspace between the dorsal spinous processes of the 4th and 5th lumbar vertebrae.
Indications	:	Pain in the lumbosacral region, sciatica, paralysis of the lower limbs, irregular menstruation, impotence, nocturnal emissions, enteritis, diarrhoea.

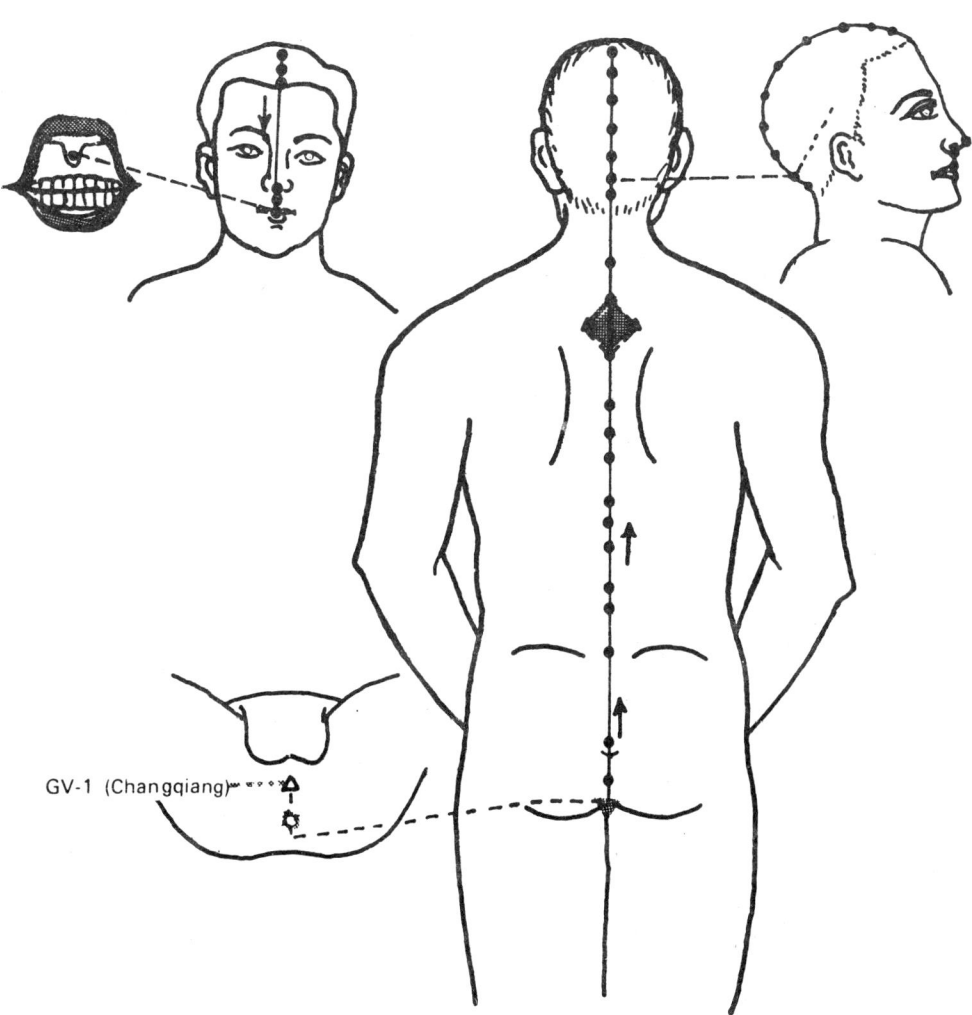

GV-1 (Changqiang)

Fig. 14.62 The governing vessels meridian.

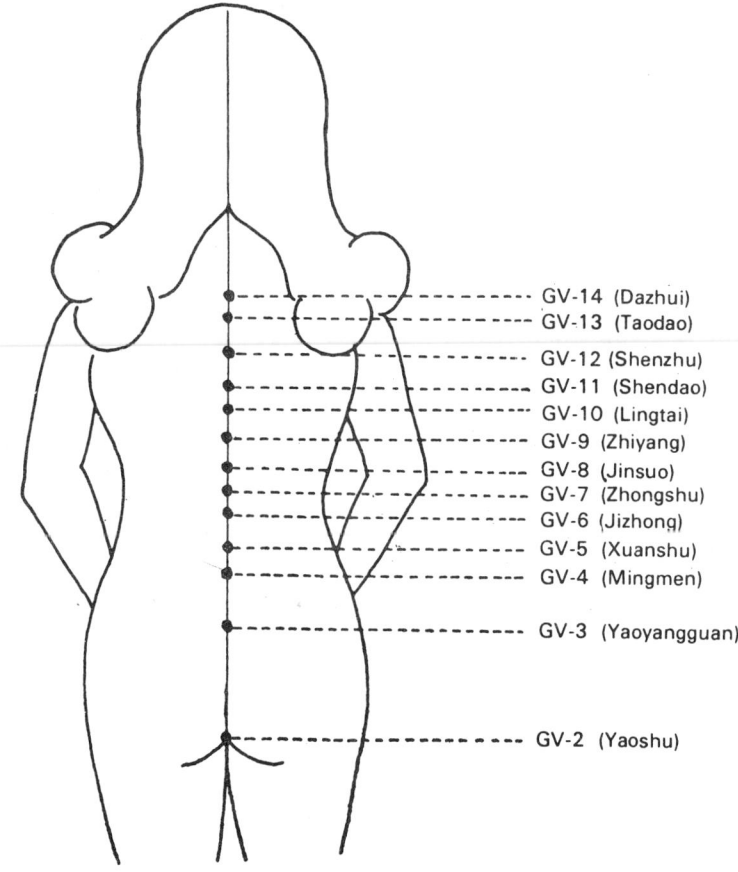

GV-14 (Dazhui)
GV-13 (Taodao)
GV-12 (Shenzhu)
GV-11 (Shendao)
GV-10 (Lingtai)
GV-9 (Zhiyang)
GV-8 (Jinsuo)
GV-7 (Zhongshu)
GV-6 (Jizhong)
GV-5 (Xuanshu)
GV-4 (Mingmen)
GV-3 (Yaoyangguan)
GV-2 (Yaoshu)

Fig. 14.63

| Needling | : | 0.5 to 1 t-sun, slanting upwards. |

GV-4 (24) Mingmen

Location	:	In the centre of the interspace between the dorsal spines of 2nd and 3rd lumbar vertebrae.
Indications	:	Nephritis, pyelitis, renal colic, enuresis, impotence, spermatorrhoea, sciatica, lumbago.
Note	:	It is also used in acupuncture anaesthesia for caessarian section and urogenital operations.
Needling	:	0.5 to 1 t-sun, slanting upwards.

GV-5 (23) Xuanshu (Hsuanshu)

Location	:	In the centre of the interspace between the spinous process of 1st and 2nd lumbar vertebrae.
Indications	:	Backache, dyspepsia, diarrhoea.
Needling	:	0.5 to 1 t-sun, slanting upwards.

GV-6 (22) Jizhong (Chichung)

Location   : In the centre of the interspace between the 11th and 12th dorsal sspines.
Indications   : Epilepsy, jaundice, diarrhoea, prolapse of the anus in children, piles.
Note   : This is a specific point for relaxation of muscle spasm together with Yaogi (Extra-20)
Needling   : 0.5 to 1 t-sun, slanting upwards.

GV-7 (21) Zhongshu (Chungshu)

Location   : In the centre of the interspace between 10th and 11th dorsal spines.
Indications   : Diminished vision, gastralgia, backache.
Needling   : 0.5 to 1 t-sun, slanting upward.

GV-8 (20) Jinsuo (Chinso)

Location   : In the centre of the interspace between the 9th and 10th dorsal spines.
Indications   : Gastralgia, backache, hysteria, epilepsy, neurasthenia.
Needling   : 0.5 to 1 t-sun, slanting upwards.

GV-9 (19) Zhiyang (Chihyang)

Location   : In the centre of the interspace between the 7th and 8th dorsal spines.
Indications   : Pneumonitis, cholecystitis, gastralgia, backache.
Needling   : 0.5 to 1 t-sun, slanting upwards.

GV-10 (18) Lingtai

Location   : In the centre of the interspace between the 6th and 7th dorsal spine.
Indications   : Gastralgia, backache, asthma bronchitis.
Needling   : 0.5 to 1 t-sun, slanting upwards.

GV-11 (17) Shendao (Shentao)

Location   : In the centre of the interspace between 5th and 6th dorsal spine.
Indications   : Neurasthenia, cough, backache, malaria, asthma, infantile convulsions.
Note   : It is a specific point for loss of memory.
Needling   : 0.5 to 1 t-sun, slanting upwards.

GV-12 (16) Shenzhu (Shenchu)

Location   : In the centre of the interspace between 3rd and 4th dorsal spine.
Indications   : Bronchitis pneumonitis, fibrositis-chest, backache, insanity, epilepsy, poor memory.
Needling   : 0.5 to 1 t-sun, slanting upwards.

GV-13 (15) Taodao (Taotao)

Location   : In the centre of the interspace between 1st and 2nd dorsal spine.
Peculiarity   : It is an immunity improving point.
Indications   : Malaria, headache, stiff and painful spine, epilepsy, insanity, febrile conditions, skin diseases.
Needling   : 0.5 to 1 t-sun, slanting upwards.

GV-14 (14) Dazhui (Tachui)

Location   : Midway between the spinous process of the 7th cervical and 1st thoracic vertebrae.

Peculiarities : It is an immunity enhancement (most potent) point with homeostatic effects; also a potent sedative point.

Indications : Infections, fever, heat stroke, bronchitis, asthma, frozen shoulder, severe backache, cervical spondylosis, torticollis, stiff neck, ankylosing spondylitis, epilepsy, headache, migraine, anxiety states.
Many times it is used in place of Baihui (GV-20) for sedation (when the patient is sensitive to Baihui).

Needling   : 0.5 to 1 t-sun, slanting upwards.

GV-15 (13) Yamen

Location   : Between the spinous processes of the atlas and axis cervical vertebrae (1st and 2nd cervical) on the nape of the neck, 3.5 t-sun above the prominence of the 7th cervical vertebra when the head is erect (Fig. 14.64).

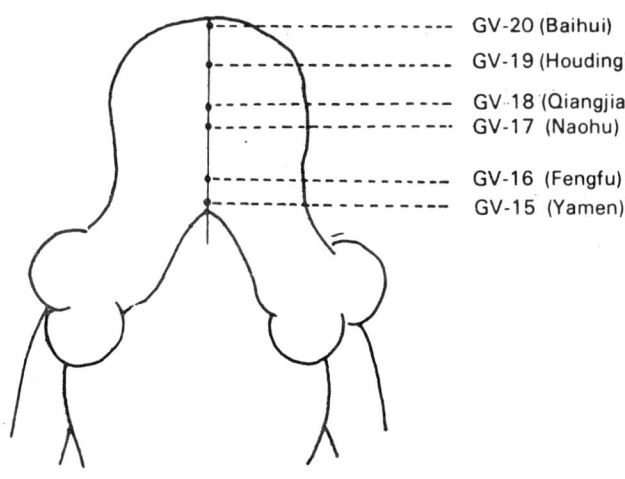

GV-20 (Baihui)
GV-19 (Houding)
GV-18 (Qiangjian)
GV-17 (Naohu)
GV-16 (Fengfu)
GV-15 (Yamen)

Fig. 14.64

Peculiarity : It is a dangerous point.

Indications : Deaf mutism (specific point), epilepsy, paralysis, headache, aphasia, aphonia, stiff neck.

Needling   : 0.5 t-sun or less, towards the chin when the neck is bent slightly forward. There should be no stimulation and no manipulation.

GV-16 (12) Fengfu

Location   : In the depression directly below the external occipital protuberance, in the midline.

Peculiarity	:	It is a very dangerous point therefore only very experienced acupuncturist should use it. As its indications are few and there are many other effective points available we consider this to be a forbidden point.
Indications	:	Cold, insanity, headache, epilepsy, apoplexy.
Needling	:	0.5 to 0.8 t-sun, slanting.

GV-17 (11) Naohu

Location	:	Superior to external occipital protuberance, 1.5 t-sun above Fengfu (GV-16).
Indications	:	Occipital headache, stiffness and pain in the neck, vertigo, unsteadyness, epilepsy.
Needling	:	0.5 to 0.8 t-sun, slanting.

GV-18 (10) Qiangjian (Chiang Chien)

Location	:	3 t-sun behind Baihui (GV-20).
Indications	:	Unsteadyness, headache, emesis.
Needling	:	0.5 to 0.8 t-sun, slanting.

GV-19 (9) Houding (Houting)

Location	:	1.5 t-sun behind Baihui (GV-20).
Indications	:	Vertigo, dizziness, headache, stiff neck, mental disorders.
Needling	:	0.5 to 0.8 t-sun, slanting.

GV-20 (8) Baihui (Paihui)

Location	:	On the scalp in the midline, 7 t-sun above the posterior hair line, 5 t-sun behind the anterior hair line, midway on a line connecting the apex of both the auricles.
Peculiarities	:	It governs all the Yang channels (in Sri Lanka it is known as *Adhipathi*—Governor); it possesses powerful sedative and tranquilising effect; acts as distal point for ano-rectal disorders. It brings about co-ordination amongst the channels. (In Chinese Baihui means the meeting point of a hundred points.)
Indications	:	Epilepsy, schizophrenia, headache, vertigo, apoplexy, insomnia, nuresthenia anxiety, parkinsonism, bronchial asthma, psoriasis, impotence, premature ejaculations, cerebro-vascular accidents, loss of memory, alopecia, pruritis ani.
Note	:	Is a governing and co-ordination point in the treatment along with all other points.
Needling	:	0.3 t-sun, slanting posteriorly.

GV-21 (7) Qianding (Chienting)

Location	:	1.5 t-sun in front of Baihui (GV-20) in the midline.
Indications	:	Infantile convulsion, cellulitis and oedema of the face, vertical headache, vertigo, dizziness, insomnia.
Needling	:	0.5 fo 0.8 t-sun, slanting.

GV-22 (6) Xinhui (Hsinhui)

Location	:	1.5 t-sun anterior to Qianding (GV-21).
Indications	:	Headache, pain in the eye, rhinitis, occlusion of the nose, epistaxis, convulsive states of children.
Needling	:	0.5 to 0.8 t-sun, slanting.

GV-23 (5) Shang Xing (Shanghsing)

Location	:	4 t-sun anterior to Baihui (GV-20) in the midline.
Indications	:	Epistaxis, rhinitis, frontal sinusitis, frontal headache, stuffy nose, eye diseases, insomnia.
Needling	:	0.5 to 0.8 t-sun, slanting downwards.

GV-24 (4) Shenting

Location	:	0.5 t-sun inside the anterior natural hair line in the midline.
Indications	:	Headache, frontal sinusitis, epilepsy, anxiety, insomnia, rhinitis, vertigo.
Needling	:	0.5 to 0.8 t-sun, slanting downwards.

GV-25 (3) Suliao

Location	:	At the tip of the nose.
Indications	:	Epistaxis, rhinitis, abscess of the nose, respiratory failure, shock, carbon monooxide poisoning, nasal obstruction.
Needling	:	0.2 to 0.3 t-sun, straight.

GV-26 (2) Renzhong (Jenchung)

Location	':	At the centre of the junction of the upper one-third and lower two-thirds of the philtrum of the upper lip (Fig. 14.65).
Peculiarity	:	It is a Jing-well point.
Indications	:	All the indications of a Jing-well point. Shock, heat stroke, facial paralysis, epilepsy.
Needling	:	0.3 to 0.5 t-sun, slanting upwards.

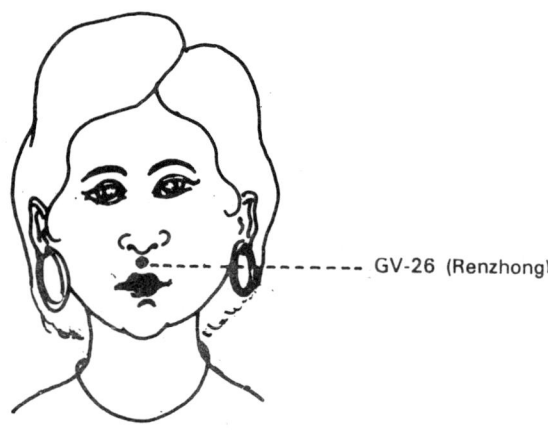

GV-26 (Renzhong)

Fig. 14.65

GV-27 (1) Duiduan (Tuituan)

Location   : Median tubercle of the upper lip.

Indications   : Stomatitis, thrust, foul breath, toothache.

Needling   : 0.2 to 0.3 t-sun, slanting.

GV-28 Mouth-Yinjiao (Yinchiao)

Location   : Midpoint between the inner surface of the superior lip and the root of the upper gum, in the frenulum of the upper lip (Fig. 14.66).

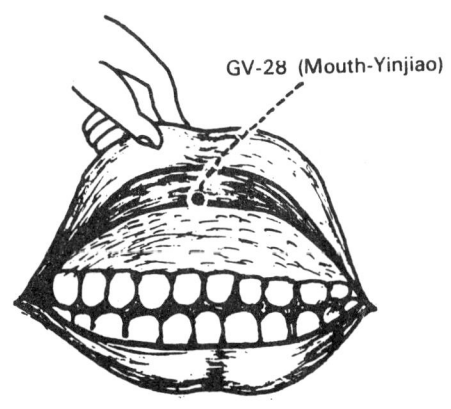

GV-28 (Mouth-Yinjiao)

Fig. 14.66

Indications   : Stomatitis, gingivitis, rhinitis, haemorrhoids.

Needling   : 0.2 to 0.3 t-sun, slanting upwards, or until bleeding (three edged needle can be used for bleeding).

14. THE CONCEPTIONAL VESSELS MERIDIANS (The Ren Meridian)

This meridian is not associated with any organ but it possesses Yin character and is endowed with a controlling influence over all the Yin meridians of the body. It is described as a conceptional vessel because of its special control over the reproductive functions and as 'Ren channel' because of anterior midline position in the body (*Ren* means front in Chinese record).

Total number of points : 24 (Fig. 14.67).

Starting point   : In the centre of the perineum in front of the anus.

Terminal point   : Middle of the mentolabial sulcus.

Pathway   : This meridian originates in the pelvic cavity and emerges at the perimeum between the anus and the external genitalia. It runs upwards in front of the pubic symphysis and then ascends along the anterior midline of the abdomen, chest and neck. It winds around the inferior surface of the lower jaw and ends at the mentolabial sulcus by dividing in two inner branches which go to both eyes and brain.

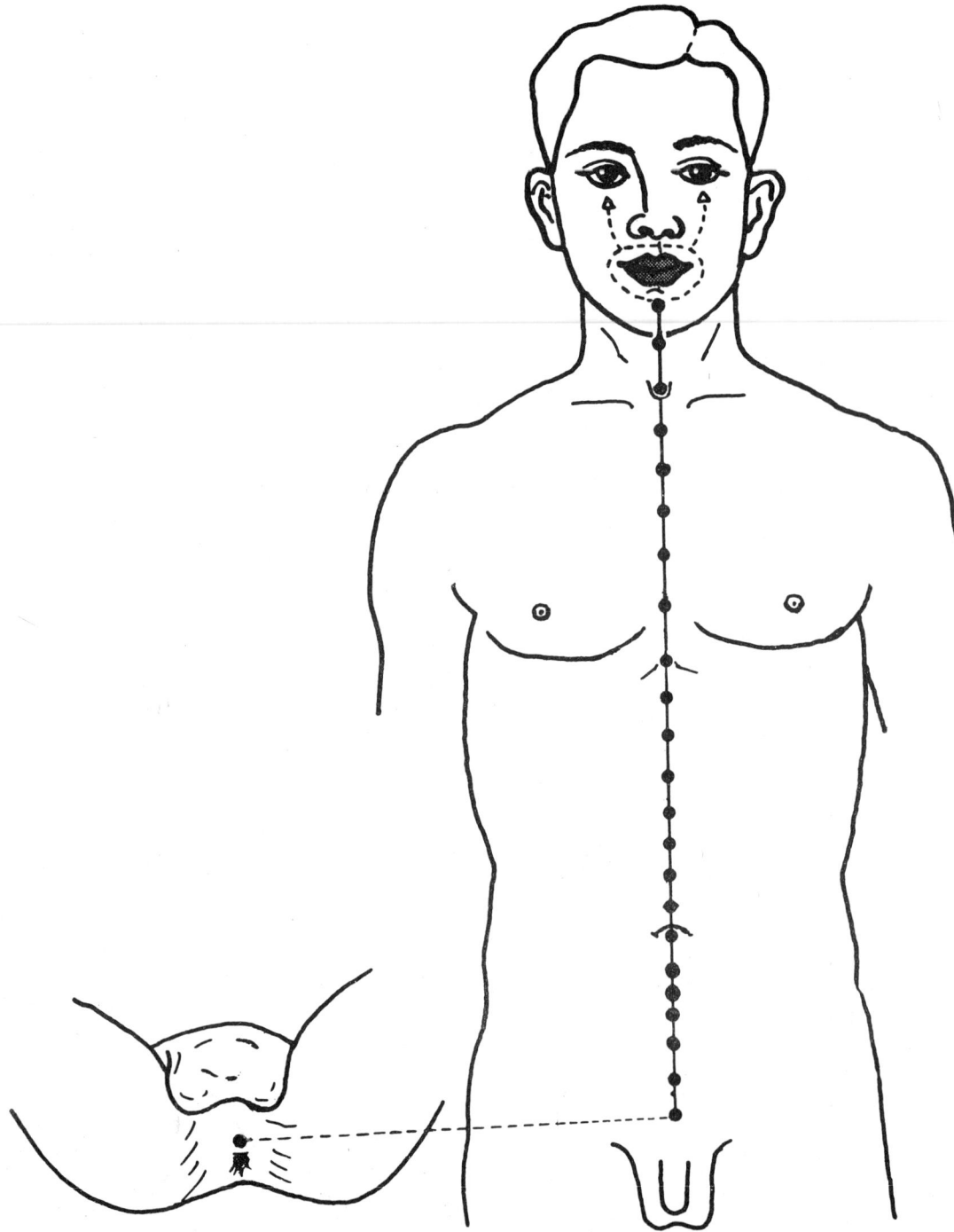

Fig. 14.67   The conceptional vessels meridian.

Therapeutic Indications
1. All the disorders along the pathway of the channel.
2. Genito-urinary disorders.
3. Abdominal disorders.
4. Heart and lung disorders.
5. Diseases of the breast.
6. Speech disorders.
7. Disorders of the mouth and face like Bell's palsy, trigeminal neuralgia, toothache, excessive salivation.
8. Painless child birth.
9. Oedema and ascites.

DESCRIPTION OF THE POINTS

CV·1 (51) Huiyin
Location   : Centre of the perineum in front of the anus.
Indications   : Haemorrhoids, prolapse of uterus, irregular menstruation, vaginitis.
Needling   : 0.5 to 1 t-sun, slanting upwards.

CV-2 (50) Qugu (Chuku)
Location   : Just above the superior border of the pubic symphysis in midline.
Indications   : Urinary incontinence, frequency of micturition, retention of urine, cystitis, pelvic cellutitis, spermatorrhoea, impotence, nocturnal emissions, premature ejaculations, irregular menstruation, dysmenorrhoea, functional uterine bleeding, leucorrhoea, retained placenta, postpartum haemorrhage, prolapse of uterus.
Needling   : 0.5 to 1 t-sun, straight.

CV-3 (49) Zhongji (Chung Chi)
Location   : On the anterior abdominal wall, 4 t-sun below the umbilicus in the anterior midline.
Indications   : Same as Qugu (CV-2).
Needling   : 0.5 to 1 t-sun, straight.

CV-4 (48) Guanyuan (Kuanyuan)
Location   : In the midline of the anterior abdominal wall, 3 t-sun below the umbilicus.
Indications   : Same as Qugu (CV-2).
Needling   : 0.5 to 1 t-sun, straight.

CV-5 (47) Shimen (Shihmen)
Location   : In the midline of the anterior abdominal wall, 2 t-sun below the umbilicus.
Indications   : Painless child birth, specific point for oedema, abdominal distension, irregular menstruation.
Caution   : In early pregnancy, this point may lead to abortion.
Needling   : 0.5 to 1 t-sun, straight.

CV-6 (46) Qihai (Chihai)

Location	:	In the midline of the anterior abdominal wall, 1.5 t-sun below the umbilicus.
Indications	:	Neurasthenia, abdominal pain, distended abdomen, menstrual disorders, enuresis, spermatorrhoea.
Needling	:	0.5 to 1 t-sun, straight.

CV-7 (45) Abdomen Yinjiao (Yinchiao)

Location	:	1 t-sun below umbilicus, in midline.
Indications	:	Endometritis, post partum pain, hernia.
Needling	:	0.5 to 1 t-sun, straight.

CV-8 (44) Shenjue (Shenchueh)

Location	:	In the centre of the umbilicus.
Peculiarity	:	It is a forbidden point.
Indications	:	It is an anatomical land mark; apoplexy.
Needling	:	No needling, indirect moxibustion with ginger or salt, moxa stick for 10 minutes.

CV-9 (43) Shuifen

Location	:	1 t-sun above umbilicus in the front of midline.
Indications	:	Oedema (specific point), hyperperistalsis, varicose veins, dysurea, diarrhoea.
Needling	:	1 to 1.5 t-sun, straight.

CV-10 (42) Xiawan (Hsiawan)

Location	:	2 t-sun above the umbilicus in the front midline.
Indications	:	Epigastric pain, gastralgia, gastroptosis, enteritis.
Needling	:	1 to 1.5 t-sun, straight.
Caution	:	Not to be used within two hours of the meals. It may induce vomiting.

CV-11 (41) Jianli (Chienli)

Location	:	3 t-sun above the umbilicus in the front midline.
Indications	:	Epigastric pain, gastralgia, emesis, oedema.
Needling	:	1 to 1.5 t-sun, straight.
Caution	:	Not to be used within two hours of the meals.

CV-12 (40) Zhongwan (Chungwan)

Location	:	Midway between the umbilicus and the tip of the xiphoid process in the front midline, 4 t-sun above the umbilicus (Fig. 14.68).
Peculiarity	:	It is the influential point for the hollow organ.
Indications	:	Gastralgia, epigastric pain, gastric ulcer, reflex oesophagitis, hiatus hernia, gastroptosis, heart burn, hiccough, dyspepsia, nausea and vomiting, retrosternal pain, pain in cardiac region.
Needling	:	1 to 1.5 t-sun, straight.
Caution	:	Not to be used within two hours of the meals.

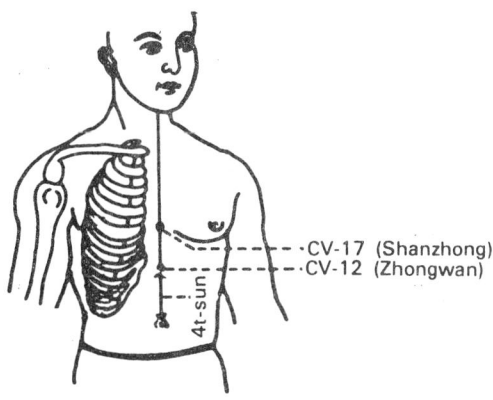

CV-17 (Shanzhong)
CV-12 (Zhongwan)
4t-sun

Fig. 14.68

CV-13 (39) Shangwan

Location	:	6 t-sun above the umbilicus in the front midline.
Indications	:	Same as Zhongwan (CV-12).
Needling	:	Same as Zhongwan (CV-12).

CV-14 (38) Jujue (Chuchueh)

Location	:	1 t-sun below the xiphoid process (7 t-sun above the umbilicus.)
Indications	:	Palpitation, anxiety, gastralgia.
Needling	:	1 t-sun or less, slanting downwards.

CV-15 (37) Jiuwei (Chiuwei)

Location	:	Below the xiphoid process in the front midline. (8 t-sun above the umbilicus).
Indications	:	Gastralgia, mental disorders, epilepsy, retrosternal pain, pain in cardiac region, emesis, hiccough, hiatus hernia.
Needling	:	0.5 to 1 t-sun, slanting upwards.

CV-16 (36) Zhongting (Chungting)

Location	:	On the sternum in the front midline, 1.5 t-sun below Shanzhong (CV-17), at the level of the 5th intercostal space.
Indications	:	Bronchitis, asthma, cough, vomiting, milk intolerance in infants.
Needling	:	0.5 to 1 t-sun, slanting upwards.

CV-17 (35) Shanzhong (Shanchung)

Location	:	On the midline of the sternum midway between the two nipples at the level of the 4th intercostal space.
Peculiarity	:	It is the specific point for the lung tissue.
Indications	:	Asthma, bronchitis, cough, pain in the chest, intercostal neuralgia, lactational deficiency, hiccough, heart diseases, acne vulgaris.
Needling	:	0.5 to 1 t-sun, slanting upwards.

CV-18 (34) Yutang

Location	:	On the midline, at the level of the 3rd intercostal space, 1.5 t-sun above Shanzhong (CV-17).
Indications	:	Asthma, cough, bronchitis, pleuritis.
Needling	:	0.5 to 1 t-sun, slanting.

CV-19 (33) Chest Zigong (Tzukung)

Location	:	In the front midline at the level of the 2nd intercostal space.
Indications	:	Asthma, bronchitis, pleurisy.
Needling	:	0.5 to 1 t-sun, slanting upwards.

CV-20 (32) Huagai (Huakai)

Location	:	In the centre of the manubrium and sternal junction.
Indications	:	Asthma, chest pain.
Needling	:	0.5 to 1 t-sun, slanting.

CV-21 (31) Xuanji (Hsuanchi)

Location	:	1 t-sun below Tiantu (CV-22) in midline.
Indications	:	Cough, asthma, chest pain, pharyngitis.
Needling	:	0.5 to 1 t-sun, slanting upwards.

CV-22 (30) Tiantu (Tientu)

Location	:	At the centre of the suprasternal fossa, 0.5 t-sun above the sternal notch.
Paculiarity	:	It is a dangerous point.
Indications	:	Acute attack of bronchial asthma, status asthmaticus, bronchitis globus hysterious, hiccough, dysphagia, pharyngitis.
Needling	:	Slanting downwards along the posterior border of the sternum 1 to 1.5 t-sun deep, only an experienced acupuncturist should use it. It should not be needled in the children and infants.

CV-23 (29) Lianquan (Lienchuan)

Location	:	Midway between the lower border of the mandible and the tip of the cricoid cartilage, in the front midline of the neck (Fig. 14.69).
Peculiarity	:	It is the specific point for aphasia.
Indications	:	Mutism, aphasia, hoarseness of voice, pharyngitis, laryngitis, excessive salivation, tonsillitis.
Needling	:	0.3 to 0.5 t-sun towards the root of the tongue, slanting upwards.

CV-24 (28) Chengjiang (Chengchiang)

Location	:	Centre of the mentolabial sulcus.
Indications	:	Facial paralysis, gingivitis, toothache, excessive salivation.
Needling	:	0.3 to 0.5 t-sun, straight.

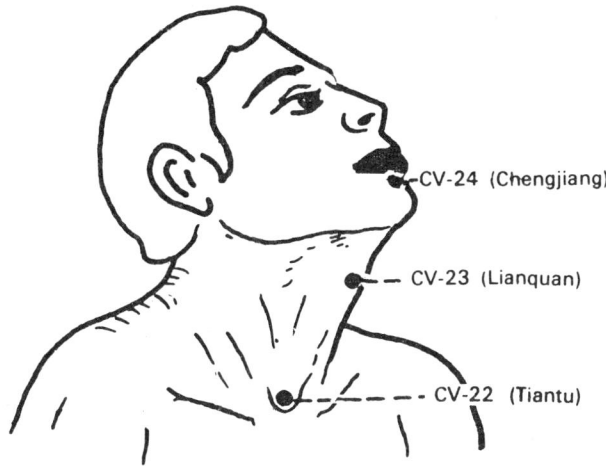

CV-24 (Chengjiang)

CV-23 (Lianquan)

CV-22 (Tiantu)

Fig. 14.69

15. THE EIGHT EXTRA MERIDIANS

The eight extra meridians are different from the main twelve meridians as they do not pertain to any of the internal organs. They act as reservoirs to unite, store and control the Chi.

The eight meridians are listed below:

1. The governing vessel (Du Mai).
2. The conceptional vessel (Ren Mai)
3. The belt vessel (Dai Mai)
4. The vital vessel (Chong Mai)
5. The yang ankle vessel (Yang Chiao Mai)
6. The yin ankle vessel (Yin Chiao Mai)
7. The yang regulating vessel (Yang Wei Mai)
8. The yin regulating vessel (Yin Wei Mai)

Out of these eight extra ordinary meridians, the governing vessel and the conceptional vessel meridians possess points of their own, but the remaining six have no acupuncture points of their own. Thes are the reservoir channels connecting main meridians.

BELT VESSEL MERIDIAN (DAI MAI)

Dai Mai means belt and this meridian is seen as a belt around the waist, binding up the Yin and Yang meridians (Fig. 14.70).

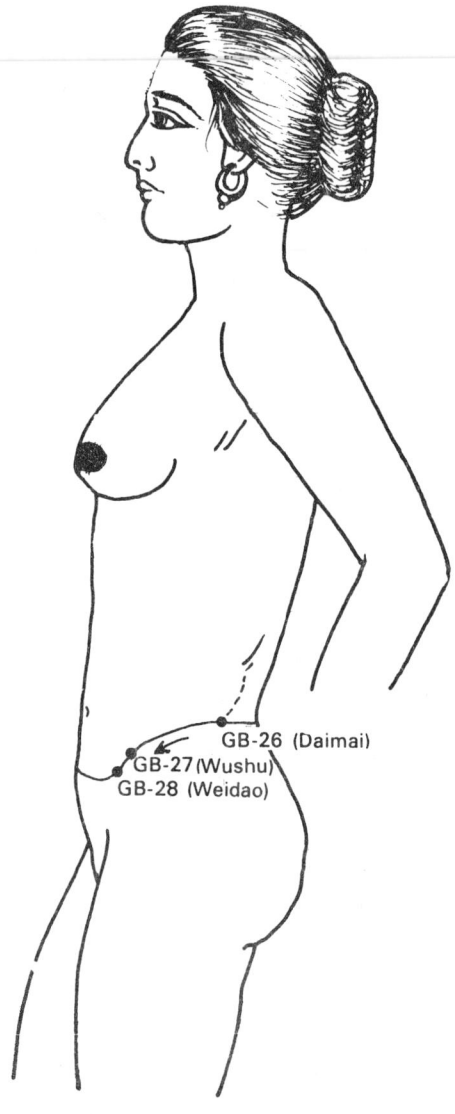

Fig. 14.70   Belt vessel meridian (Dai Mai).

Pathway   : It starts below the hypochondrium and runs obliquely through three points of the gall bladder meridian : Daimai (GB-26), Wushu (GB-27), Weidao (GB-28). Then it runs around the waist like a belt.

Therapeutic indications   : Fullness of abdomen, weakness or motor impairment of the lumbar region, articular rheumatism, general arthritis, anaemia, amenorrhoea, dysmenorrhoea, general fatigue, pruritis.

VITAL VESSEL MERIDIAN (CHONG MAI)

This vessel is supposed to control the T-chi (Qi) and blood of the whole body (Fig. 14.71).

Pathway   : It originates in the pelvic cavity and comes out on the body surface at the perineum. It splits into two and coincides with the kidney channel running upwards along both sides of the abdomen. Both branches encircle the lips and end over there.

Points   : Henggu (K-11), Dahe (K-12), Qixue (K-13), Siman (K-14), Abdomen Zhongzhu (K-15), Huangshu (K-16), Shangqu (K-17), Shiguan (K-18), Yindu (K-19), Abdomen Tonggu (K-20), Youmen (K-21).

Therapeutic indications   : Colic and abdominal pain, gynaecological disorders, gastric ulcer, vomiting, jaundice, endocarditis, bradycardia, myocarditis, palpitation. This vessel regulates menstruation.

YANG ANKLE VESSEL MERIDIAN (YANCHIAO MAI)

Pathway   : It starts from the lateral side of the heel, near Shenmai (UB-62), and ascends along the lateral aspect of the leg, thigh, posterolateral aspect of trunk and reaches the shoulder. It then penetrates the posterior axillary fold and ascends along the neck to reach the corner of the mouth. It further ascends on the face and reaches the inner canthus of the eye. Then it winds around the scalp to reach Fengchi (GB-20) (Fig. 14.72).

Points   : Shenmai (UB-62), Pushen (UB-61), Fuyang (UB-59), Femur Juliao (GB-29), Naoshu (SI-10), Jianyu (LI-15), Jugu (LI-16), Dicang (ST-4), Juliao (ST-3), Chengqi (ST-1), Jingming (UB-1), Fengchi (GB-20).

Therapeutic indications   : Insomnia, numbness, muscular atrophy of the lower extremities, hemiplegia, paraplegia, fecial paralysis, sciatica, lumbago.

YIN ANKLE VESSEL MERIDIAN (YINCHIAO MAI)

Pathway   : This meridian originates from the posterior aspect of the navicular bone and runs upwards along the medial malleolus, inner aspect of the leg, ascends along the posteromedial aspect of the thigh to the external genital organs. From here it reaches directly to the supraclavicular fossa, then runs further upwards along the front of the neck. It ends at the inner canthus of the eye (Fig. 14.73).

Points   : Coalescent points : Zhaohai (K-6), Jiaoxin (K-8), Jingming (UB-1).

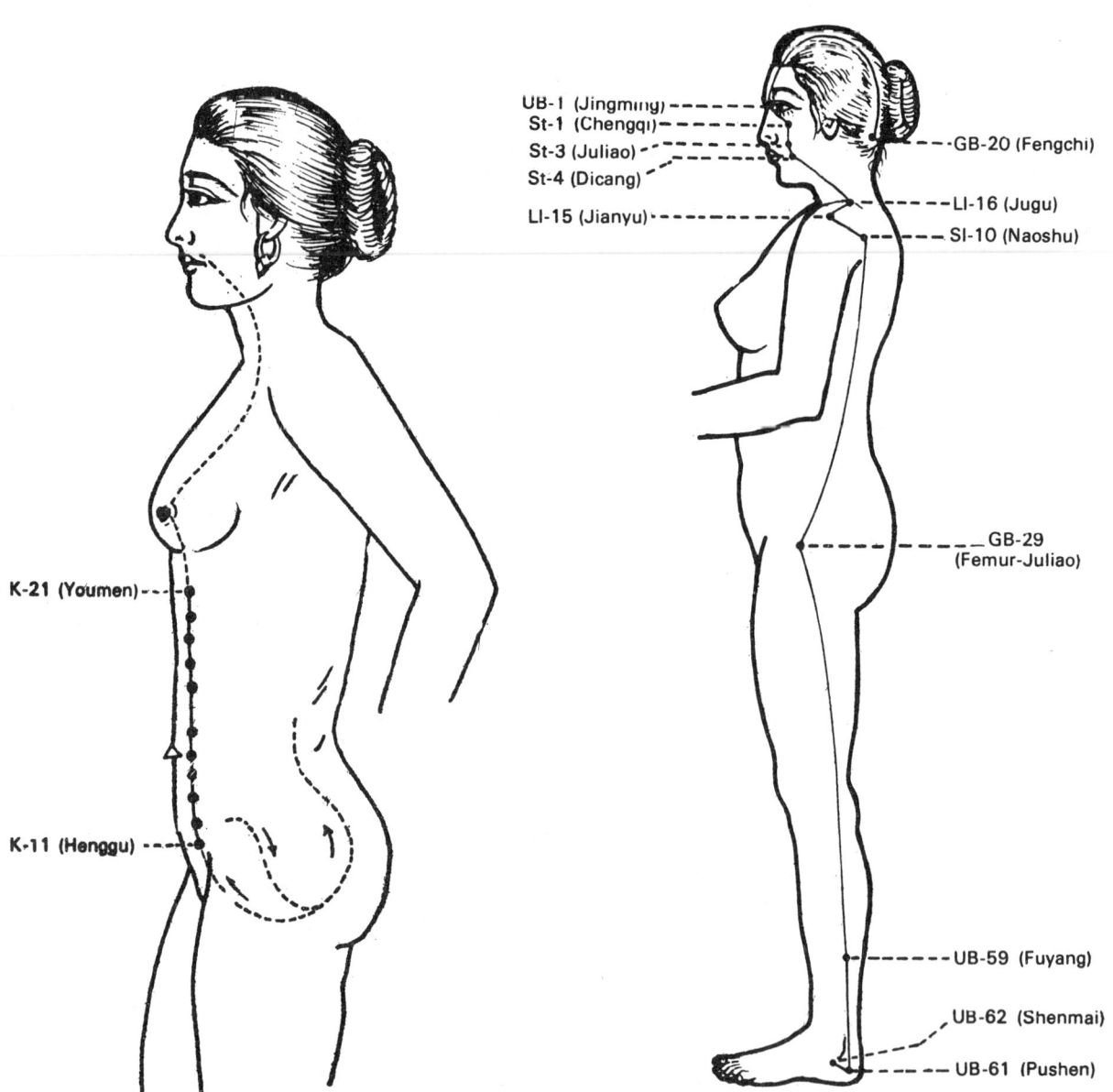

Fig. 14.71 Vital vessel meridian (Chong Mai).

Fig. 14.72 Yang ankle vessel meridian (Yangchiao Mai).

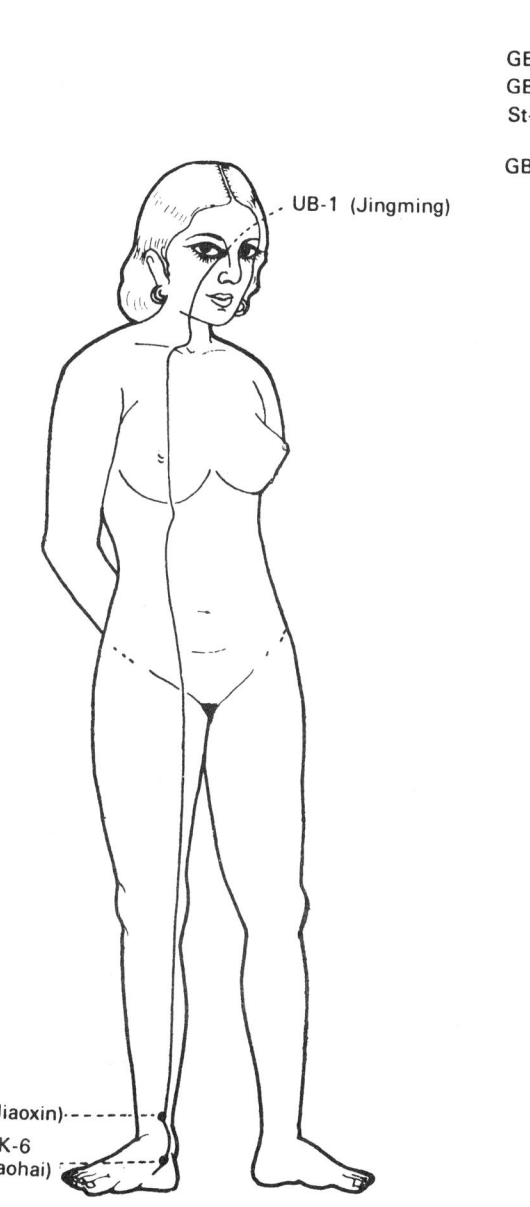

Fig. 14.73 Yin ankle vessel meridian (Yinchiao Mai).

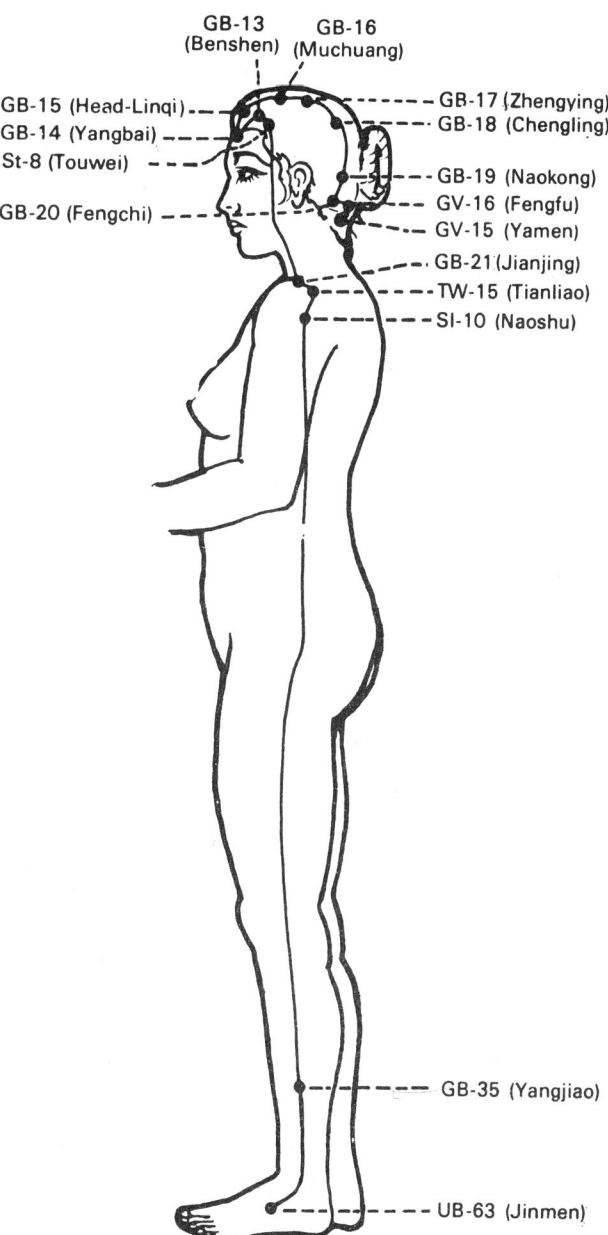

Fig. 14.74 Yang regulating vessel meridian (Yangwei Mai).

Therapeutic   : Impotence, frigidity, sterility, habitual abortions, difficult labour, post-
indications   partum haemorrhage, dysmenorrhoea in virgins, orchitis, anuria,
                  urinary retention, motor impairment, numbness, muscular atrophy of
                  lower extremities.

YANG REGULATING VESSEL MERIDIAN (YANGWEI MAI)

This is a Yang regulating meridian which connects the urinary bladder and the gall bladder
meridian.

Pathway   : It starts at the heel near Jinmen (UB-63) and ascends along the outer
                aspect of the leg along the gall bladder meridian. It runs along the

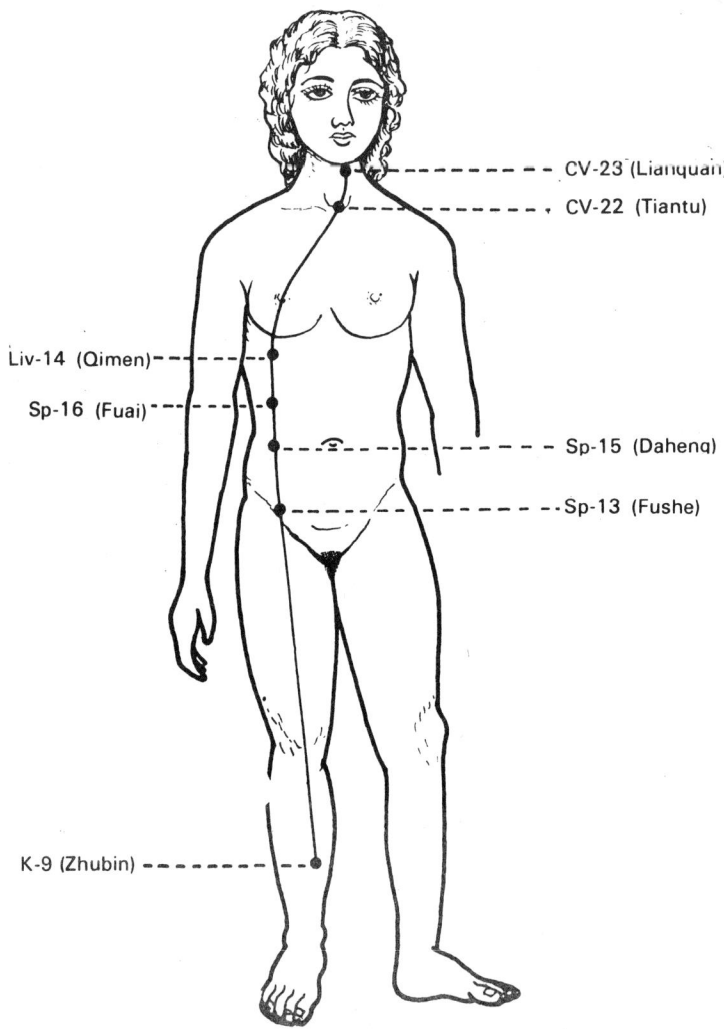

CV-23 (Lianquan)
CV-22 (Tiantu)

Liv-14 (Qimen)
Sp-16 (Fuai)
Sp-15 (Daheng)
Sp-13 (Fushe)

K-9 (Zhubin)

Fig. 14.75   Yin regulating vessels meridian (Yinwei Mai).

posterior aspect of the trunk and reaches the shoulder. It then runs along the neck, reaches forehead, winds around the head and turns backwards to the nape of the neck and communicates with the governing vessel meridian (Fig. 14.74).

Points : Coalesent points: Jinmen (UB-63), Yangjiao (GB-35), Naoshu (SI-10), Tianliao (TW-15), Jianjing (GB-21), Touwei (ST-8), Benshen (GB-13), Yangbai (GB-14), Head Linqi (GB-15), Muchuang (GB-16), Zhengying (GB-17), Chengling (GB-18), Naokong (GB-19), Fengchi (GB-20), Fengfu (GV-16), Yamen (GV-15).

Therapeutic indications : Chills and fever, headache, toothache, earache, neuralgia, rheumatoid arthritis, painful heel epistaxis, debility.

YIN REGULATING VESSEL MERIDIAN (YINWEI MAI)

This meridian connects the Yin meridians of the conception vessel, heart and lung.

Pathwav : It originates on the medial aspect of the lower part of the leg near Zhubin (K-9), runs along the medial aspect of the thigh, abdomen, chest and the neck. It communicates with the spleen meridian in the abdomen and conceptional vessel meridian on the chest and neck (Fig. 14.75).

Points : Coalescent points: Zhubin (K-9), Fushe (Sp-13), Daheng (Sp-15), Fuai (Sp-16), Qimen (Liv-14), Tiantu (CV-22), Lianquan (CV-23).

Therapeutic indications : Gastralgia, epigastric pain, chest pain, apprehension, delirium, agitation, epilepsy, indigestion, varicose veins.

15

THE EXTRA-ORDINARY POINTS

In this chapter we have described the extra points which do not belong to any of the meridians. Most of them lie outside the path of the traditionally described channels but a few of them like Yintang (Ex.-1) and Lanwei (Ex.-33) lie on the channel.

EXTRA-ORDINARY POINT ON THE HEAD AND NECK

Ex.-1 Yintang

Location : On the centre of the glabella, midway between the medial ends of the two eyebrows. It falls on the governing vessels meridian (Fig. 15.1).

Indications : Frontal sinusitis, frontal headache, migraine, stuffy nose, rhinitis, epistaxis, epilepsy, diseases of the eye, mental disorders, vertigo, labyrinthitis.

Needling : 0.5 to 0.7 t-sun, horizontally downward.

Ex.-2 Taiyang

Location : In the depression about 1 t-sun eral to the midpoint between the outer canthus of the eye and lateral end of the eyebrow (Fig. 15.2). To locate the point nicely, one imaginary line is extended from the lateral end of the eyebrow and another along the margin of the lower lid. The spot where these two lines meet is Taiyang.

Indication : Temporal headache, trigeminal neuralgia, migrane, facial paralysis, toothache, acupuncture anaesthesia.

Needling : 0.5 t-sun, slanting towards eye ball.

Ex.-3 Yuyao

Location : Midpoint of the eyebrow, in the line of the pupil.

Indications : Eye diseases, facial paralysis, frontal headache, frontal sinusitis, ptosis.

Needling : 0.3 to 0.5 t-sun, horizontally along the skin.

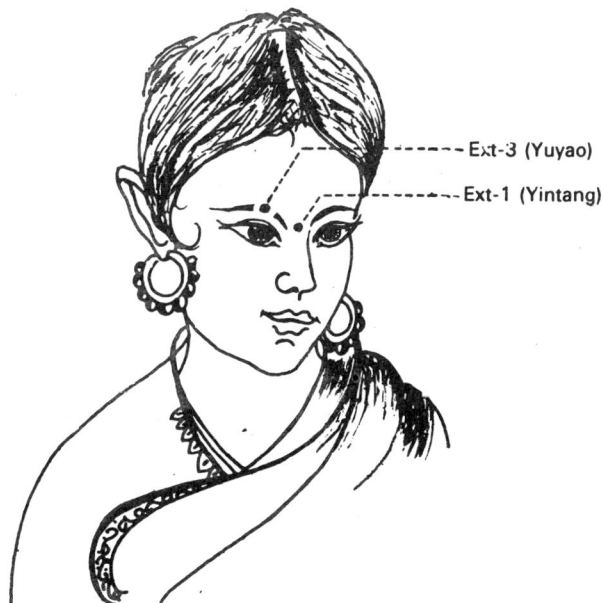

Ext-3 (Yuyao)
Ext-1 (Yintang)

Fig. 15.1

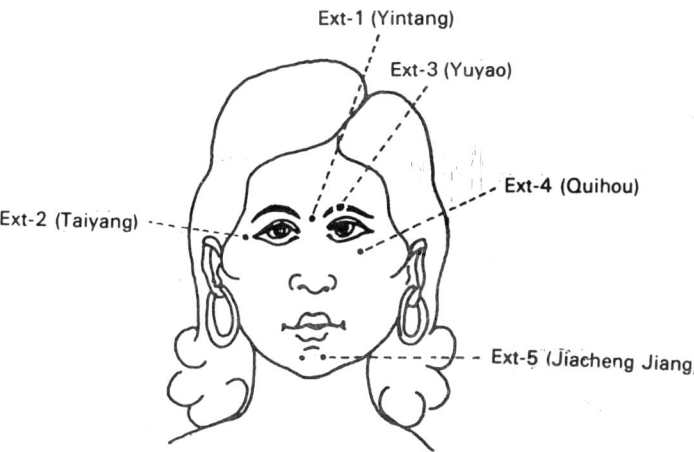

Ext-1 (Yintang)
Ext-3 (Yuyao)
Ext-4 (Quihou)
Ext-2 (Taiyang)
Ext-5 (Jiacheng Jiang)

Fig. 15.2

Ex.-4 Qiuhou

Location : At the junction of the lateral one-fourth and medial three-fourth of the infraorbital border.

Indications : Optic neuritis, optic nerve atrophy, myopia, glaucoma, keratitis and all other diseases of the eye.

Needling : 0.3 to 0.5 t-sun, towards the floor of the orbital cavity when the patient is asked to look upwards (only experienced acupuncturists should use this point).

Ex.-5 Jiacheng Jiang

Location : 1 t-sun lateral to Cheng Jiang (CV-24) it lies over the mental foramen (Fig. 15.2).

Indications . Trigeminal neuralgia, facial paralysis, lower toothache, excessive salivation.

Needling : 0.3 to 0.5 t-sun, straight.

Ex.-6 Sishencong

(Sishencong means four mental wisdoms in the Chinese description)

Location : These are a group of four points situated 1 t-sun anterior, posterior, right lateral and left lateral of Baihui (GV-20) on the scalp.

Indications : All types of the mental disorders: Cerebral palsy, forgetfulness, parkinsonism, epilepsy, schizophrenia, vertigo, addiction, anxiety. Indications of Baihui (GV-20) are also allotted to it.

Needling : 0.3 to 0.5 t-sun, horizontally slanting towards Baihui (GV-20).

Ex.-7 Yiming

Location : 1 t-sun posterior to Yifeng (TW-17), lies behind the lobule of the ear in the depression between the mastoid process and the mandible (Fig. 15.3).

Indications : Insomnia, myopia, optic atrophy, hypermetropia, night blindness, cataract, tinnitus, deafness, vertigo, otitis media, schizophrenia, occipital headache.

Needling : 1 to 1.5 t-sun, straight.

Ex.-8 Anmian-I

(In Chinese Anmian means "have good sleep")

Location : Midway between Yifeng (TW-17) and Yiming (Ex.-7)

Indications : Schizophrenia, insomnia.

Needling : 1 to 1.5 t-sun, straight.

Ex.-9 Anmian-II

Location : Midway between Yiming (Ex.-7) and Fengchi (GB-20).

Indications : Schizophrenia, insomnia.

Needling : 1 to 1.5 t-sun, straight.

Ex.-10 Jinjin Yuye

Location : On either side of the sublingual veins of the frenulum, the left one is Jinjin and the right one is Yuye.

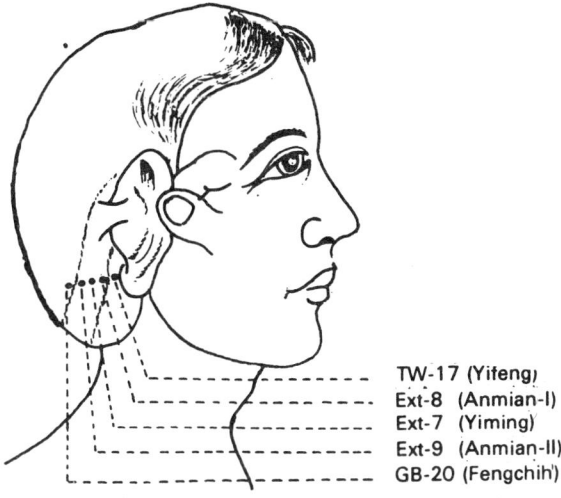

TW-17 (Yiteng)
Ext-8 (Anmian-I)
Ext-7 (Yiming)
Ext-9 (Anmian-II)
GB-20 (Fengchih)

Fig. 15.3

Indications	:	Stomatitis, glossitis, excessive thirst, excessive salivation, disorders of the taste, dryness of the mouth, infection of the salivery glands, mutism.
Needling	:	Needling with the three edged needles until bleeding.

Ex.-11 Zengyin

Location	:	On either side of the thyroid cartilage.
Indications	:	Muteness.
Needling	:	1 t-sun, slanting upwards towards the opposite side.

Ex.-12 Shanglianquan

Location	:	1 t-sun, below the middle of the mandible.
Indications	:	Mutism.
Needling	:	1.5 to 2 t-sun, slanting upwards, towards the root of the tongue.

Ex.-13 Jingbi

Location	:	At the junction of the lateral two-thirds and medial one-third of the clavicle on its upper border.
Indications	:	Pain, numbness and paralysis of the upper extremity.
Needling	:	0.5 to 0.8 t-sun, straight.
Caution	:	It is a dangerous point and deep insertion is not advisable.

EXTRA-ORDINARY POINTS ON THE TRUNK

Ex.-14 Weishang

Location	:	2 t-sun above and 4 t-sun lateral to Shenjue (CV-8) (Fig. 15.4).
Indications	:	Gastroptosis.
Needling	:	1.5 t-sun, slanting towards umblicus.

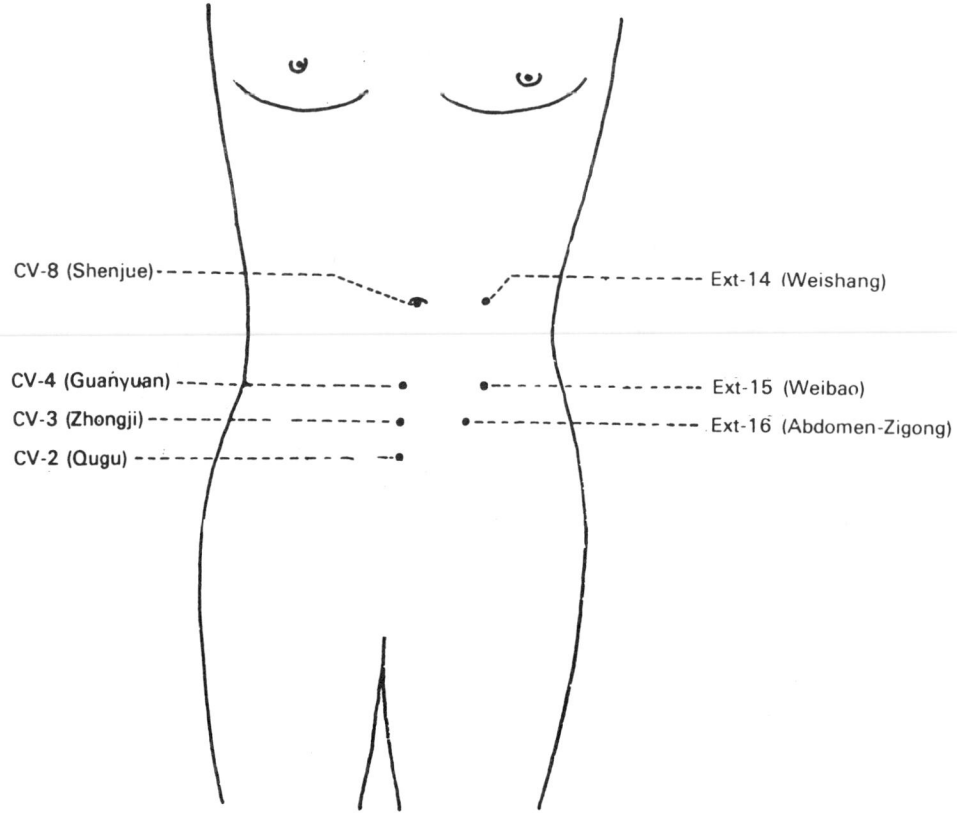

CV-8 (Shenjue) - Ext-14 (Weishang)

CV-4 (Guanyuan) - - - - - - - - - - - - • • - - - - - - - - - - - - Ext-15 (Weibao)
CV-3 (Zhongji) - - - - - - - - - - - - - • • - - - - - - - - - - - Ext-16 (Abdomen-Zigong)
CV-2 (Qugu) - - - - - - - - - - - - - - •

Fig. 15.4

Ex.-15 Weibao
Location	:	3 t-sun lateral to Guanyuan (CV-4).
Indication	:	Prolapse of the uterus.
Needling	:	1.5 to 3 t-sun, slanting towards midline.

Ex.-16 Abdomen-Zigong
Location	:	3 t-sun, lateral to Zhongji (CV-3).
Indications	:	Menstrual disturbances and functional uterine bleeding.
Needling	:	1 to 1.5 t-sun, straight.

Ex.-17 Dingchuan
Location	:	0.5 t-sun lateral to the midline between cervical-7 and thoracic-1 vertebra, 0.5 t-sun lateral to Dazhui (CV-14).
Indications	:	Bronchial asthma.
Needling	:	0.5 to 1 t-sun, towards midline.

Ex.-18 Wuming
Location	:	Below the spinous process of the 2nd thoracic vertebra.

Indication   : Mania.
Needling   : 0.5 to 1 t-sun, slanting upwards.

Ex.-19 Shiqizhui
Location   : Below the spinous process of the 5th lumbar vertebra.
Indications   : Lumbosacral strain, spondylosis, spondylitis and spondylolisthesis.
Needling   : 1 to 2 t-sun, straight.

Ex.-20 Yaoqi
Location   : 2 t-sun above the tip of the coccyx.
Indications   : Epilepsy, muscle relaxation.
Needling   : 1 to 2 t-sun, slanting upwards subcutaneously.

Ex.-21 Huatuojiaji
(Named after the Chinese acupuncturist Huao Tuo)
Location   : This is a series of 28th pairs of points situated on both sides of the
                       spine, about 0.5 t-sun lateral to the midline from the 1st cervical to the
                       4th sacral vertebra (Fig. 15.5).
Peculiarities   : These are the alarm points for the corresponding internal organs.
Indications   : Painful disorders of the back like ankylosing spondylitis, prolapse of
                       disc, spondylolisthesis, myelitis, pott's spine, kyphosis. Diseases of the
                       internal viscera of the corresponding level. Myalgia, fibrositis,
                       backache, stiffness of the back.
Needling   : Lumbosacral region: 1 to 1.5 t-sun, slanting obliquely towards the
                                 spinal column.
                    : Thoraco-cervical region : 1 to 1.5 t-sun, slanting towards the spinal
                                 column.

EXTRA ORDINARY POINTS ON THE UPPER EXTREMITY

Ex.-22 Jianzhong
Location   : Middle of deltoid muscle in the outer aspect of the upper arm.
Indications   : Paralysis of the upper extremity.
Needling   : 1 to 2 t-sun, straight.

Ex.-23 Bizhong
Location   : In the middle of the line joining midpoint of the cubital transverse
                       crease and midpoint of the transverse crease of the wrist on the inner
                       aspect of the forearm.
Indications   : Paralysis of the upper extremity.
Needling   : 1 to 2 t-sun, straight.

Ex.-24 Erbai
Location   : This is a series of four points, on the front of the forearm, 4 t-sun pro-
                       ximal to the midpoint of the transverse crease of the wrist. Two
                       points lie on the right and two on the left side of the tendon of flexor
                       carpi radialis muscle.

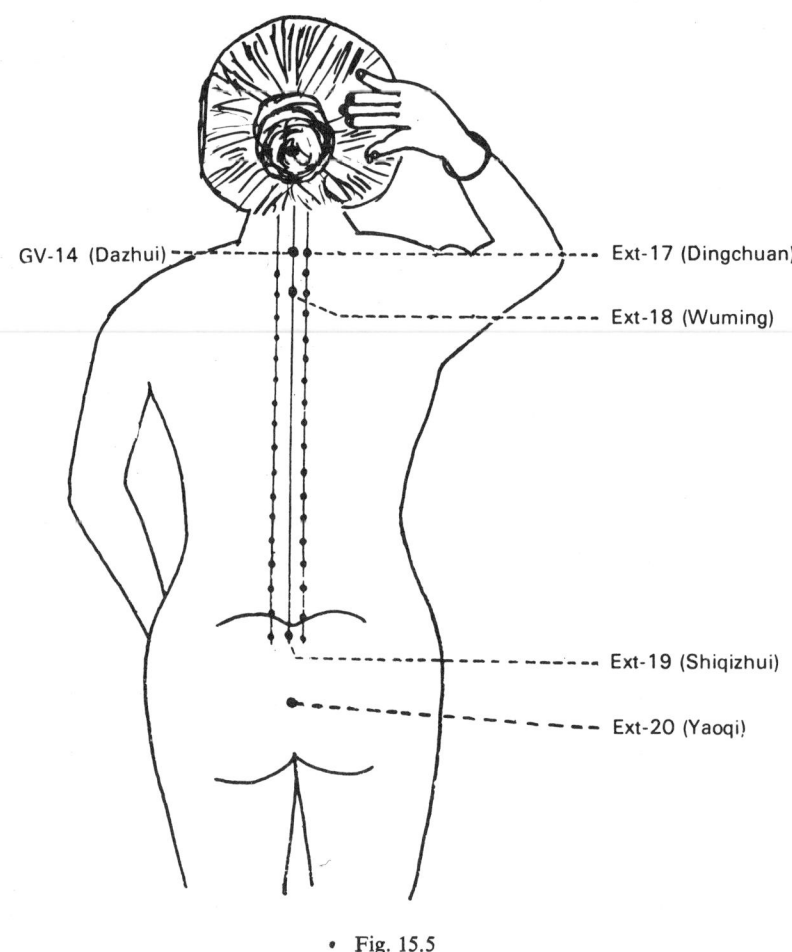

• Fig. 15.5

| Indication | : | Haemorrhoids. |
| Needling | : | 0.5 t-sun, straight. |

Ex.-25 Zhongquan

Location : On the back of the wrist, lateral to the tendon of the extensor digitorum communis muscle.

Indication : Diseases of the wrist joint.

Needling : 0.3 to 0.8 t-sun, straight.

Ex.-26 Luozhen

Location : On the dorsum of the hand, in the 2nd intermetacarpal space, 0.5 t-sun proximal to the metacarpal-phalangeal joints.

Indication : Stiff neck.

Needling : 0.5 t-sun, straight.

Ex.-27 Yatong

Location : On the dorsum of the hand in the 3rd intermetacarpal space, 0.5 t-sun from the metacarpophalangeal joint.
Indication : Toothache.
Needling : 0.5 t-sun, straight.

Ex.-28 Baxie (Pahsieh)

Location : On the dorsum of the hand in the web between the fingers of both hands. They are total 8 points, 4 in each hand.
Indications : Arthritis, pain and paralysis of the fingers, headache, toothache, snake bite.
Needling : 1 t-sun, slanting towards the metacarpal bone.

Ex.-29 Sifeng

Location : This is a series of 4 points in each hand, 8 points in all. They are located on the palmar aspect in the middle of the transverse crease of the proximal interphalangeal joints of the 2nd, 3rd, 4th and little fingers of both hands (Fig. 15.6).
Indications : Whooping cough, indigestion, snake bite in the upper extremity, malnutrition in children.
Needling : Shallow insertion and rotation with 3-edged needle by hand.

Ex.-30 Shixuan

Location : On the tips of the 10 fingers, about 0.1 t-sun away from the free edge of the nail. They are 10 points in all, 5 in each hand.
Indications : Similar to the Jing-well points, these are used in acute emergencies like shock, coma, convulsions, fainting and hyperpyrexia.
Needling : Needling with 3-edged filiform needle, until bleeding.

EXTRA-ORDINARY POINTS ON THE LOWER EXTREMITY

Ex.-31 Heding

Location : On the midpoint of the upper border of the patella.
Indications : Diseases of the knee joint, weakness of the lower limbs.
Needling : 0.5 to 1 t-sun, straight.

Ex.-32 Medial Xiyan

Location : On the medial foramen of the patellar ligament.
Indications : Disorders of the knee joint, weakness of the lower extremity.
Needling : 1 to 1.5 t-sun, straight or slanting towords the opposite foramen.

Ex.-33 Lanwei

Location : 2 t-sun distal to Zusanli (St-36).
Indications : Appendicitis, post-apendicectomy pain. (This is an alarm point for the
: appendix).
Needling : 1 to 2 t-sun, straight.

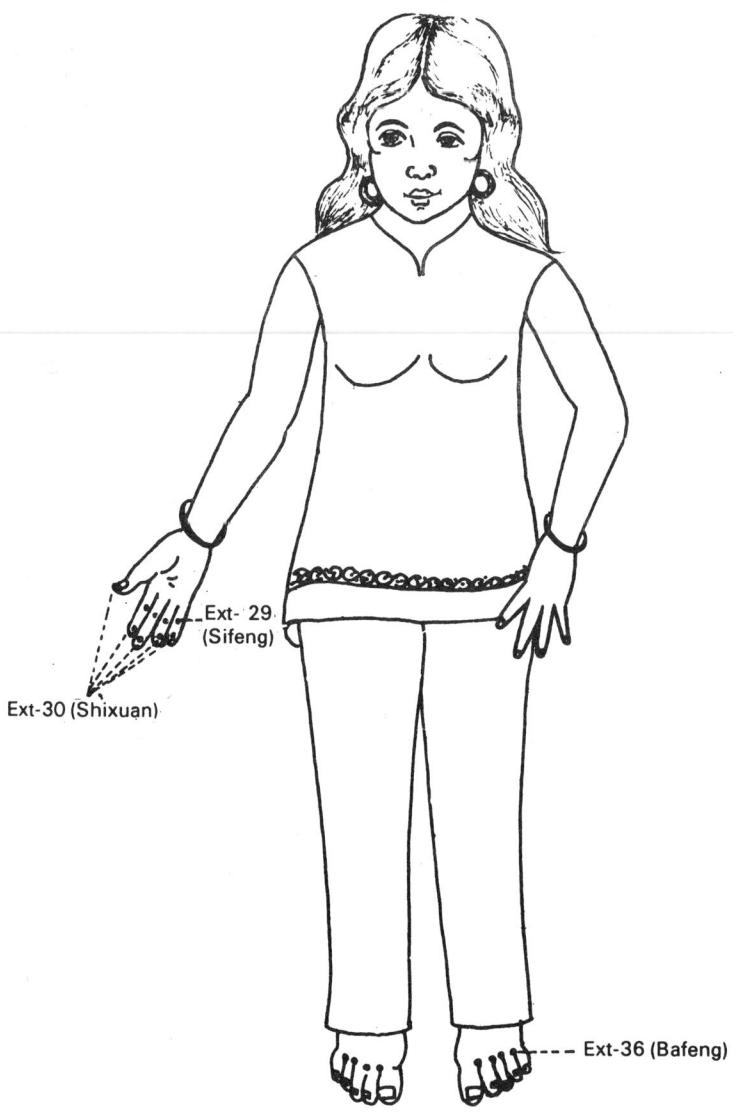

Fig. 15.6

Ex.-34 Linghou

   Location   : Below and behind the head of the fibula opposite Yanglingquan (GB-34).

   Indications   : Sciatica, paralysis of the lower extremity.

   Needling   : 1 to 1.5 t-sun, straight.

Ex.-35 Dannang

   Location   : 1 t-sun below Yanglingquan (GB-34).

Peculiarity	:	Alarm point for gall bladder.
Indications	:	Cholecystitis, diseases of the bile duct, paralysis of the lower extremity.
Needling	:	1 to 1.5 t-sun, straight.

Ex.-36 Bafeng (Chinese ba eight)

Location	:	On the dorsum of the foot, 0.5 t-sun proximal to the free margin of the webs of the toes. There are total 8 points, 4 in each foot, including the points corresponding to Neiting (St-44) and Xingjian (Liv-2).
Indications	:	Rheumatoid arthritis of the small joints of foot and toes. Pain, paralysis, numbness and polyneuropathy of the feet. Cellulitis, lymphangitis, swelling and redness of the foot and toes. Headache and toothache. Snake bite in the feet.
Needling	:	0.5 to 1 t-sun, slanting towards metatarsal bone.

16

RECENT ACUPUNCTURE POINTS

1. Shanken

Location   : On the nose, midway between the inner canthus of the two eyes.

Indications   : Headache, blurring of vision.

Needling   : Slanting, 0.1 to 0.2 t-sun.

2. Shangying Hsiang

Location   : 5 t-sun below the medial angle of the eyes.

Indications   : Rhinitis, nasal polyp.

Needling   : Slanting, 0.3 to 0.5 t-sun deep.

3. Chenming

Location   : Inferior border of the orbit on its inner aspect.

Indications   : Cataract, optic atrophy, night blindness.

Needling   : At the angle of the orbit, 1 to 1.5 t-sun deep.

4. Piliu

Location   : On the outer nostril, in the middle of the line connecting the septum nasi and ala nasi.

Indications   : Acute rhinitis, facial nerve paralysis.

Needling   : Slanting, 0.3 to 0.5 t-sun deep.

5. Piting

Location   : At the upper end of the nasolabial sulcus.

Indications   : Rhinitis, nasal furuncle.

Needling   : Slanting, 0.3 to 0.5 t-sun deep.

6. Houtinghui (Back of listening conference)

Location   : 0.5 t-sun above Yifeng (TW-17) at the level with Tinghui (GB-2).

Indications   : Deafness, tinnitus, vertigo.

Needling   : Slanting, 0.5 to 1 t-sun towards anterior and inferior direction.

7. Tingh Sueh (Listening point)

Location   : In the middle of the line joining Tinggong (SI-19) with Tinghui (GB-2).
Indications   : Deafness, deaf mutism.
Needling   : Straight, 0.5 t-sun.

8. Ting Chung (Listening clever)

Location   : 0.2 t-sun distal Tinghui (GB-2).
Indications   : Deafness, deaf mutism.
Needling   : Straight, 0.5 t-sun.

9. Tingmin

Location   : On the ear, at the lower root of the auricular lobule.
Indication   : Deaf mutism.
Needling   : Straight, 1.5 t-sun deep.

10. Ying Siang

Location   : In the mentolabial sulcus, 0.5 t-sun lateral to ala nasi.
Indications   : Sinusitis, numbness of the face, rhinitis, nasal blocking.
Needling   : 0.2 to 0.3 t-tun, obliquely outwards.

11. Tiho

Location   : On the most prominent part of the middle of the mandible.
Indications   : Lower toothache, facial nerve paralysis.
Needling   : Slanting, 2 to 3 t-sun deep.

12. Pientao

Location   : Lowermost point of the angle of the mandible, in the front of the carotid artery.
Indications   : Tonsillitis.
Needling   : Straight, 1 to 1.5 t-sun deep. Protect the blood vessel.

13. Tienchu

Location   : On the lateral side of the attachment of the trapezius on the back of the head at the level of natural hair line.
Indications   : Occipital headache, nasal congestion.
Needling   : Straight, 0.5 to 1 t-sun.

14. Hsinshih

Location   : On the nape of the neck, 1.5 t-sun lateral to the lower end of the tip of the spinous process of the third cervical vertebra.
Indications   : Stiff neck, back and shoulder pain, cervical spondylosis.
Needling   : Straight, 0.3 to 1 t-sun deep.

15. Chungku

Location   : On the nape of the neck below the spinous process, of the sixth cervical vertebra.
Indications   : Asthma, cervical spondylosis, epilepsy.
Needling   : Slanting, 0.5 to 1 t-sun deep.

16. Shanglienchuan

Location	:	On the middle of the upper border of hyoid bone.
Indications	:	Salivation, pharyngitis, deaf mutism, stiff tongue.
Needling	:	Slanting towards the root of the tongue, 2 t-sun deep.

17. Lung Suen (Deaf point)

Location	:	In between (TW-21) and (SI-19).
Indication	:	Deafness.
Needling	:	Straight 0.2 to 0.3 t-sun.

18. Hungyin (Torrent sound)

Location	:	On the front of the neck, 0.5 t-sun lateral to the laryngeal prominence (extend the neck to locate the point).
Indications	:	Acute and chronic laryngitis, deafness and mutism.
Needling	:	Straight, 0.3 to 0.5 t-sun.

THORAX AND ABDOMEN

19. Shihtsang

Location	:	On the anterior abdominal wall, 3 t-sun lateral to the Chungwan (CV-12).
Indications	:	Nephritis, peptic ulcer, menorrhagia.
Needling	:	Straight, 1.5 to 2 t-sun deep.

20. Chuehyin

Location	:	On the anterior abdominal wall, 0.3 t-sun below Shihmen (CV-5).
Indication	:	Sterility.
Needling	:	No needling. Moxibustion is advised.

21. Weipao

Location	:	On the anterior abdominal wall, 6 t-sun lateral to Guanyuan (CV-4) below and in front of the anterior superior iliac spine.
Indication	:	Prolapse of uterus.
Needling	:	Slanting towards inguinal region, 2 to 3 t-sun deep.

22. Tingtou

Location	:	5 t-sun below Dahe (K-12).
Indication	:	Prolapse of uterus.
Needling	:	Straight, 1.5 to 2 t-sun deep.

23. Chihhsueh

Location	:	On the anterior abdominal wall, 2.5 t-sun below umbilicus.
Indications	:	Enteritis.
Needling	:	Straight, 1.5 to 2 t-sun deep.

24. Tituo

Location	:	On the anterior abdominal wall, 4 t-sun lateral to Guanyuan (CV-4).
Indications	:	Prolapse of uterus, colic, lower abdominal pain.
Needling	:	Straight, 0.5 to 1 t-sun deep.

25. Weipao

Location	:	On the anterior abdominal wall, 6 t-sun lateral to the Guanyuan (CV-4) in the anterio-inferior depression of the anterior superior iliac spine.
Indications	:	Prolapse of uterus, manorrhagia.
Needling	:	Slanting downwards, 2 to 3 t-sun deep, in the direction of inguinal region.

26. Shuhsi (Inguinal point)

Location	:	On the junction of medial two-thirds and lateral one-third of inguinal ligament.
Indications	:	Oedema of foot, impotency, insomnia.
Needling	:	Straight, 1.5 t-sun, slanting downwards.

27. Yiching (Pollution point)

Location	:	On the anterior abdominal wall, 1 t-sun lateral to Guanyuan (CV-4)
Indications	:	Night pollution of urine, impotence.
Needling	:	Straight, 0.5 to 1 t-sun.

28. Chuanhsi (Anti asthma)

Location	:	On the anterior abdominal wall, 1 t-sun lateral to Jujue (CV-14).
Indication	:	Asthma.
Needling	:	Slanting upward, 0.5 to 0.8 t-sun.

29. Chieh Hehsueh (Tuberculosis point)

Location	:	On the anterior abdominal wall, 3.5 t-sun lateral to Jujue (CV-14).
Indications	:	Pulmonary tuberculosis, extra-pulmonary tuberculosis.
Needling	:	Straight, 0.5 t-sun or less.
		Injection of streptomycin and INH 0.2 ml alternate day for 15 days

30. Tsukung

Location	:	On the anterior abdominal wall, 3 t-sun lateral to Zhongji (CV-3).
Indications	:	Prolapse of the uterus, irregular menstruation, endometritis, sterility.
Needling	:	Straight, 1 to 1.5 t-sun.

31. Wuming

Location	:	On the back, below the tip of the spinous process of the second thoracic vertebra.
Indication	:	Insanity.
Needling	:	Slanting, 0.5 to 1 t-sun deep.

32. Chuche

Location	:	On the back, 5 t-sun lateral to the lower end of the tip of the spinous process of the second thoracic vertebra.
Indications	:	Pneumonia, backache, lumbago.
Needling	:	Slanting, 0.5 to 1 t-sun.

33. Chuchuehshu

Location	:	On the back, below the tip of the spinous process of the 4th thoracic vertebra.

Indications	:	Bronchitis, asthma, neurasthenia, intercostal neuralgia.
Needling	:	Slanting, 0.5 to 1 t-sun deep.

34. Chichuan

Location	:	On the back, 2 t-sun lateral to the tip of the spinous process of 7th thoracic vertebra.
Indications	:	Asthma, pleurisy, bronchitis.
Needling	:	Slanting, 0.5 to 1 t-sun deep.

35. Yinkou

Location	:	On the back, at the inferior angle of the scapula.
Indications	:	Haemoptysis, intercostal neuralgia.
Needling	:	Slanting, 0.5 to 1 t-sun deep.

Chuoyu

Location	:	On the back, 2.5 t-sun lateral to the lower end of tip of the spinous process of the 10th thoracic vertebra.
Indications	:	Hysteria, hepatic or gall bladder disorders.
Needling	:	Slanting, 0.5 to 1 t-sun.

37. Piken

Location	:	On the back, 3.5 t-sun lateral to the lower end of the spinous process of the first lumbar vertebra.
Indications	:	Hepatosplenomegaly, nephritis, lumbago.
Needling	:	Straight, 1 to 1.5 t-sun deep.

38. Kuiyang Hsuzh (Ulcer point)

Location	:	On the back, 6 t-sun lateral to the spinous process of L-1 vertebr.
Indications	:	Peptic ulcer, duodenal ulcer.
Needling	:	Slanting, 0.3 to 0.5 t-sun.

39. Houchimen

Location	:	On the middle of the line joining the upper part of the greater trochanter of the femur and tip of the coccyx.
Indications	:	Sciatica, difficult labour.
Needling	:	Straight, 2 to 3 t-sun deep.

40. Yaoyi

Location	:	On the back, 3.8 t-sun lateral to the lower end of the tip of the spinous process of the fourth lumbar vertebra.
Indications	:	Menorrhagia, lumbago.
Needling	:	Straight, 1.5 to 2 t-sun deep.

41. Shihchi Chuihsia

Location	:	On the back, below the tip of the spinous process of the 5th lumbar vertebra.
Indications	:	Lumbago, leg pain, paralysis in the lower extremities, gynaecological disorders.

Needling   : Straight, 1.5 to 2 t-sun deep.

42. Chungkung
Location   : On the back, 3.5 t-sun lateral to the lower end of the tip of the spinous
                         process of the 5th lumbar vertebra.
Indication   : Lumbago.
Needling   : Straight, 1.5 to 2 t-sun deep.

43. Hsiachui
Location   : On the back, below the tip of the spinous process of the 3rd sacral
                         vertebra.
Indications   : Haemorrhoids, urethritis, irregular menstruation.
Needling   : Slanting, 0.5 to 1 t-sun deep.

44. Hsuehy Atien
Location   : On the back, below the tip of the spinous process of the 3rd sacral
                         vertebra.
Indications   : Haemorrhoids, urethritis, irregular menstruation.
Needling   : Slanting, 0.5 to 1 t-sun deep.

45. Wei Jesueh
Location   : On the back of the chest, 5 t-sun lateral to the lower end of the spinous
                         process of the 4th thoracic vertebra.
Indications   : Gingivitis, stomach diseases.
Needling   : Slanting, 0.5 to 1 t-sun.

46. Tiaoyueh
Location   : 2 t-sun below the highest point of the iliac crest.
Indication   : Post-polio residual paralysis.
Needling   : Straight, 1 to 1.5 t-sun deep.

47. Tsuieu
Location   : 1 t-sun below the Houchiemen, on the middle of the line connecting
                         the greater trochanter and the tip of the coccyx.
Indication   : Sciatica.
Needling   : Straight, 2 to 3 t-sun deep.

48. Vishu (Pancreas point)
Location   : On the back, 1.5 t-sun lateral to thoracic 8 and 9 vertebrae.
Indication   : Pancreatitis.
Needling   : 0.5 to 1 t-sun, straight.

49. Shihchi Chui Hsia
Location   : Below the tip of the spinous process of L-5 vertebra.
Indications   : Lumbago, paralysis of the lower limb.
Needling   : Straight, 1.5 to 2 t-sun.

UPPER LIMB

50. Muchi Hchien
Location   : On the back of the thumb, 1 t-sun proximal from the corner of the nail.
Indication : Hydronephrosis.
Needling   : 1 to 2 t-sun deep.

51. Fengkuam
Location   : On the palmar surface of the proximal interphalangeal joint skin crease of the index finger in the middle.
Indication : Infantile convulsions.
Needling   : Shallow insertion till bleeding.

52. Chiutienfeng
Location   : On the palmar surface of the middle finger, in the middle of the skin crease of the distal interphalangeal joint.
Indication : Vitiligo.
Needling   : No needling, moxibustion is advised.

53. Muchihchieh Hengwen
Location   : On the palmar surface of the thumb, in the middle of the interphalangeal joint.
Indication : Corneal opacity.
Needling   : Only moxibustion.

54. Fengyen
Location   : On the lateral side in the crease of metacarpophalangeal joint of the thumb.
Indication : Night blindness.
Needling   : Straight, 1 to 2 t-sun deep.

55. Neiyangchih
Location   : On the front of palm, 1 t-sun below the middle of the distal wrist crease.
Indications : Infantile convulsions, stomatitis.
Needling   : Straight, 3 to 5 t-sun deep.

56. Takukung
Location   : On the back of the thumb, in the middle of the skin crease of the interphalangeal joint.
Indication : Eye diseases.
Needling   : Moxibustion only.

57. Chungkui
Location   : On the back of the hand, middle of the crease of the distal interphalangeal joint of the middle finger.

Indications   : Toothache, gastralgia, vitiligo.
Needling   : Moxibustion only.

58. Hsiaokukung

Location   : On the back of the hand, in the middle of the crease of distal inter-phalangeal joint crease of the little finger.
Indications   : Deafness, eye diseases.
Needling   : Moxibustion only.

59. Luochen

Location   : On the dorsum of the hand, in between the second and third meta-carpal bones, 5 t-sun proximal to the metacarpophalangeal joints.
Indications   : Gastralgia, neck pain, pharyngitis.
Needling   : Straight, 0.5 to 1 t-sun deep.

60. Shouchinmen

Location   : 3.5 t-sun proximal to the middle of the distal wrist crease.
Indications   : Lymphadenitis.
Needling   : Straight, 0.5 to 1.5 t-sun.

61. Chuangwei

Location   : On the front of the elbow in the hollow, slightly lateral to elbow crease when the elbow is flexed.
Indication   : Insanity.
Needling   : Straight, 2 to 3 t-sun deep.

62. Yeling

Location   : 5 t-sun below the anterior axillary fold when the arm is kept by the side of the body.
Indications : Insanity, painful shoulder and arm.
Needling   : Straight, 2 to 3 t-sun deep.

63. Houyeh

Location : At the outer end of the posterior axillary fold.
Indications : Tonsillitis, lymphadenitis.
Needling : Straight, 0.5 to 1 t-sun deep.

64. Nuehmen

Location : On the dorsum of the hand, between the middle and the ring fingers.
Indications : Asthma.
Needling : Slanting, 0.5 to 1 t-sun deep.

65. Yinghsia

Location : On the dorsal surface of the forearm, 3 t-sun distal to the olecranon in between the ulna and radius.
Indications : Deafness, paresis in the upper limb.
Needling : Straight, 1.5 t-sun.

66. Chienming

Location	:	On the outer aspect of the upper arm, 5 t-sun above the insertion of the deltoid muscle, on its posterior part.
Indications	:	Eye diseases, paralysis in the upper limb.
Needling	:	Slanting, 2 to 3 t-sun deep.

67. Yatung (Tooth point)

Location	:	Between the 3rd and 4th metacarpal bones, 1 t-sun proximal to the metacarpal joint in the palm.
Indication	:	Toothache.
Needling	:	Straight, 0.5 t-sun.

68. Chien San Chen (Shoulder three needle)

Location	:	This is a group of three needles, i.e. 1st needle Jianyu (LI-15); 2nd needle—1.5 t-sun above the anterior axillary fold; 3rd needle—1.5 t-sun above the posterior axillary fold.
Indication	:	Frozen shoulder.
Needling	:	1 to 2 t-sun.
NOTE	:	Jianyu (LI-15) should be needled before the two other points.

69. Chupi

Location	:	On the outer aspect of the shoulder, 2 t-sun below the acromion.
Indications	:	Poliomyelitis, paralysis of the upper arm.
Needling	:	Straight, 1 to 2 t-sun.

70. Chen Chen

Location	:	Midpoint of the line joining Jianyu (LI-15) and anterior axillary fold.
Indications	:	Frozen shoulder, pain and paralysis of arm.
Needling	:	Straight, 1 t-sun.

71. Luochen (Stiffness neck)

Location	:	On the dorsum of hand, 0.5 t-sun distal to 1st and 2nd metacarpophalangeal joints.
Indications	:	Neck pain, shoulder pain, laryngeal pain.
Needling	:	Straight or slanting, 0.5 t-sun.

72. Chih Jao (Ulnar radial)

Location	:	6 t-sun above the dorsal wrist crease in between the radius and ulna.
Indications	:	Insanity, numbness of wrist.
Needling	:	Straight, 0.5 to 1 t-sun.

73. Chenshu (Shoulder locus)

Location	:	In front of the arm on the midpoint of the line connecting Jianyu (LI-15) and Yunmen (L-2).
Indication	:	Frozen shoulder.
Needling	:	Straight, 1 to 1.5 t-sun

LOWER LIMB

74. Muchilihengwen
Location   : On the planter aspect of the foot in the middle of the joint crease of the great toe.
Indication   : Orchitis.
Needling   : Straight, 2 to 3 t-sun deep.

75. Shihmien
Location   : On the planter aspect of the foot, in the middle of the heel.
Indications   : Insomnia, planter fascitis.
Needling   : Straight, 2 to 3 t-sun deep.

76. Hsiaochihchien
Location   : At the tip of the distal phalanx of the little toe.
Indication   : Difficult labour.
Needling   : Straight, 1 to 2 t-sun deep.

77. Taiyinchiao
Location   : In the hollow at the tip of the medial malleolus.
Indications   : Prolapse of uterus, menstrual disturbances, sterility, beri-beri.
Needling   : Straight, 3 to 5 t-sun deep.

78. Hsihsia
Location   : On the inferior border of the patella, in the middle of the ligamentum patella.
Indication   : Gastrocnemius spasm.
Needling   : Moxibustion only.

79. Chihchuanchin
Location   : On the inner aspect of the ankle in the middle of the upper border of the medial malleolus.
Indications   : Gastrocnemius spasm, lumbago.
Needling   : Moxibustion only.

80. Shaoyangwei
Location   : On the inner aspect of the ankle, 7.5 t-sun above the centre of the upper border of the medial malleolus.
Indications   : Chronic eczema in the lower leg, lupus, paralysis in the lower limb.
Needling   : Slanting, 0.5 to 1 t-sun deep.

81. Waihuaichien
Location   : On the most prominent point of the lateral malleolus.
Indications   : Toes cramp, tonsilitis, beri-beri, urethritis.
Needling   : Needling till bleeding.

82. Chihping
Location   : On the dorsum of the foot in the middle of each of the metatarsal joint. There are five points in each foot, ten points in all.

Indications   : After effects of infantile paralysis.
Needling   : Slanting, 3 to 5 t-sun deep.

83. Wanli
Location   : 0.5 t-sun below Zusanli (St-36), 3.5 t-sun below the lateral aspect of
                      the patella.
Indication   : Eye diseases.
Needling   : Straight, 2 to 3 t-sun deep.

84. Lanwei
Location   : On the lateral aspect of the knee, 1 t-sun lateral to Zusanli (St-36)
Indication   : Poliomyelitis.
Needling   : Straight, 1 to 2 t-sun deep.

85. Kanyen
Location   : On the inner aspect of the ankle, 2 t-sun above the upper border of
                      the medial malleolus.
Indication   : Hepatitis.
Needling   : Straight, 1 to 2 t-sun deep.

86. Tsuyichung
Location   : On the outer aspect of the leg, directly below the capitulum of fibula.
Indication   : Deafness.
Needling   : Straight, 1.5 to 3 t-sun deep.

87. Linghsia
Location   : 2 t-sun distal to Yanglingquan (GB-34).
Indications   : Deafness, cholecystitis.
Needling   : Straight, 1 to 2 t-sun deep.

88. Yinshang
Location   : 2 t-sun proximal Yinmen (UB-37).
Indication   : Schiatica, cervical spondylosis, headache.
Needling   : Straight, 2 t-sun deep.

89. Chiehshi
Location   : On the front of the thigh, 3 t-sun above the upper border of the
                      patella.
Indications   : Knee joint pain, paralysis of the lower limb, weakness of the lower
                      limb.
Needling   : Straight, 1 to 2 t-sun.

90. Henfing
Location   : On the back of the ankle in midpoint of the line joining medial and
                      lateral malleoli.
Indication   : Post-polio paralysis.
Needling   : Straight, 1 to 2 t-sun.

91. Luoti

Location	:	On the popliteal surface, 9.5 t-sun directly below the central point of the midpopliteal skin crease.
Indication	:	Post-polio paralysis.
Needling	:	Straight, 1 to 2 t-sun.

92. Feiching

Location	:	On the back of the thigh, 1 t-sun above Chengshan (UB-57).
Indication	:	Post-polio paralysis.
Needling	:	Straight, 1 to 1.5 t-sun.

93. Shangyankuan

Location	:	On the outer aspect of the thigh, 1 t-sun above Xiyangguan (GB-33).
Indication	:	Post-polio paralysis.
Needling	:	Straight, 0.5 to 1 t-sun.

94. Szuchiang

Location	:	On the front of the thigh, 4.5 t-sun directly above the midpoint of the upper border of the patella.
Indication	:	Lower limb paralysis and poliomyelitis.
Needling	:	Straight, 1 to 1.5 t-sun.

95. Shenji (Kidney heat)

Location	:	This point corresponds to the Hua-tuo-jiaji point and lies 0.5 t-sun lateral to the thoracic 7 and 8 vertebra.
Indications	:	Kidney disease, bone disease, lumbago, impotence, arthritis.
Needling	:	Straight, 0.5 t-sun.

96. Weiji (Stomach heat)

Location	:	On the bock, 0.5 t-sun lateral to the L-4 and L-5 vertebra.
Indications	:	Peptic ulcer, gastroenteritis, indigestion.
Needling	:	Straight, 0.5 to 1 t-sun.

17

AURICULO THERAPY

Diagnosis and treatment of the diseases by means of the auricle is termed as "auriculo therapy". It is a 2000 years old traditional method based on the concept that all the Zang-Fu organs and twelve meridians are connected with the auricle and the whole body is inversely represented on the auricular surface, just similar to its representation is the brain. This also simulates the position of the universal flexion of an inverted foetus in the womb (Fig. 17.1).

Advantages
1. Almost all the diseases can be treated by this technique.
2. It can be used in combination with all other forms of acupuncture.
3. It brings quick relief.
4. It is economical, convenient, easy to learn and simple.
5. It is used for both prevention and treatment.
6. Specific needles can be safely left *in situ* for many days to obtain desired results.

Indications
1. Diagnosis and differential diagnosis.
2. Prevention of the diseases.
3. Treatment of the diseases.
4. Acupuncture anaesthesia.

Contraindication
None except infections and eczema of both the ears.

Anatomy of the auricle
The auricle is the external part of the special sense organ of hearing. It consists of a fibrocartilaginous elastic plate, covered with skin and presents various elevations and grooves.
The elevations of the one surface form the grooves on other aspect.
There are two surfaces of the auricle—cranial, which faces the skull, and the lateral or outer surface (Fig. 17.2).

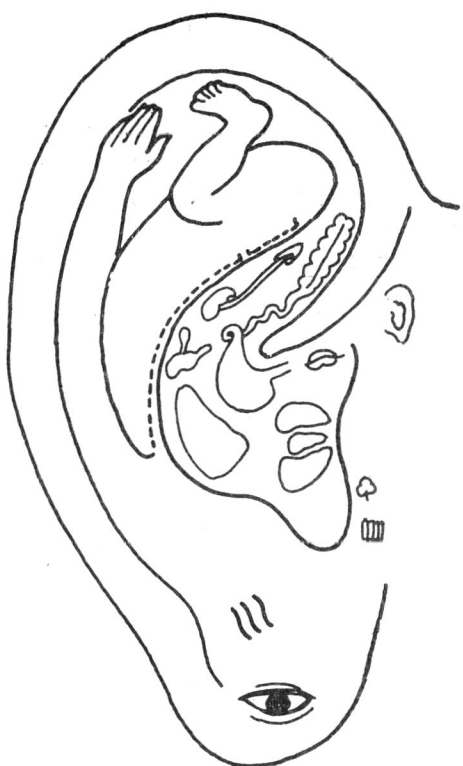

Fig. 17.1   Position of universal flexion of an inverted foetus.

Auricular area

1. Helix   : The exterior-most peripheral curved part of the circumference of the auricle. It is grooved laterally and elevated on the craninal surface. The protusion of its postero-superior part is called auricular tubercle.

2. Crus of helix : It is the part of the helix in the auricular cavity.

3. Antihelix   : This forms the posterior margin of the auricular cavity. It is located as a projection opposite to helix, at its inner side.
                     Its upper end divides into two branches: the superior and inferior crus. The area enclosed by these two branches is called triangular fossa (deltoid fossa).

4. Scapha   : The grooved area between the helix and antihelix is scapha.

5. Tragus   : The lammelar shaped protusion in front of the auricle is called tragus.

6. Antitragus   : It is the protusion opposite the tragus and formed by the lower part of the antihelix.

7. Supratragic   : The depression between the helix and the upper part of the tragus.
    incisure

8. Intertragic   : The depression between the tragus and antitragus.
    incisure

9. Auricular-   : Non-cartilagenous, lobular, hanging, inferior part of the auricle.
    lobule

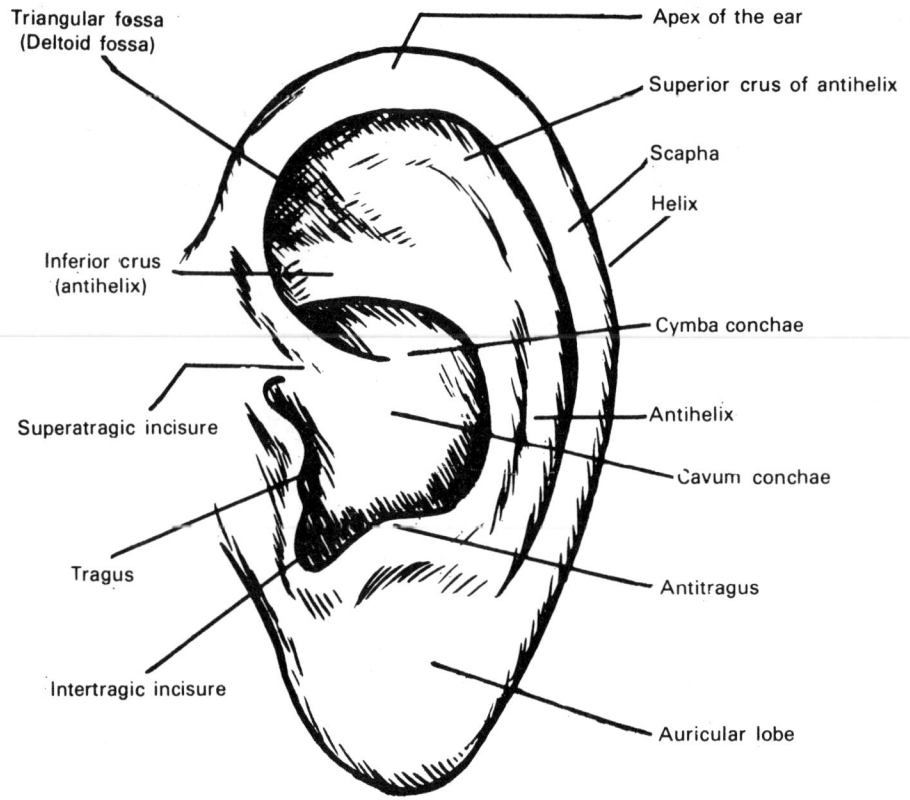

Fig. 17.2   Shows anatomical names of points of the ear.

10. Conchae   :   Auricular cavity is called conchae. The part of this cavity above the crus of the helix is cymba conchae while the part below the crus is cavum conchae.
11. Orifice of the external auditory meatus :
                            It is located inside the cavum conchae.
12. Tail of helix :   This marks the junction of the helix with the auricular lobule.
13. Interhelix   :   It is the groove between the antihelix and tragus.
      incisure

Nerve supply of the auricle

Auricle is peculiar for its abundant nerve supply which is derived from the following sources:

1. Anterior auricular branch of the temporo-auricular nerve.
2. Auricular branch of the vagus nerve.
3. Auricular branch of the facial nerve.
4. Great auricular nerve.
5. Lesser occipital nerve

6.   Branches from the trigeminal nerve.
7.   Branches from the glassopharyngeal nerve.

DISTRIBUTION AND DESCRIPTION OF THE AURICULAR ACUPUNCTURE POINTS

1.   Auricular lobule

It corresponds to the face and is divided into nine areas described below:

One junctional line is drawn horizontally from the brim of the intertragic incisure; two vertical lines from the junctional line so as to divide the lobule into three equal areas; and two horizontal lines are drawn below and parallel to the junctional line so as to divide the vertical lines at equal distances.   This will divide auricular lobule into nine areas as shown in the diagram (Fig. 17.3).

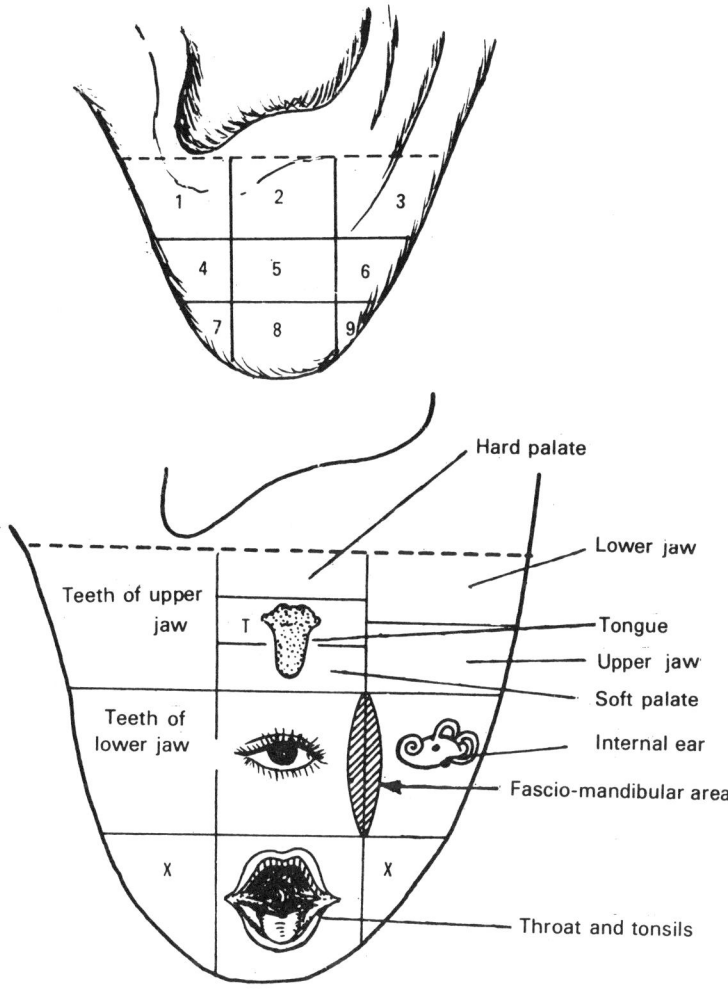

Fig. 17.3   Points on the auricular lobule.

Area-1

Postero-inferior part of this area represents the teeth of the upper jaw. It is the analgesic point for toothache and anaesthetic point for tooth extraction.

Area-2

The upper one-third of this area represents the hard palate. Central one-third represents tongue and lower one-third represents the soft palate.

Area-3

The upper half of this area represents the lower jaw and lower half represents the upper jaw.

Area-4

The central point of this area is the analgesic point for toothache and anaesthestic point for extraction of the teeth of the lower jaw.

Area-5

Central point of this area represents eye.

Area-6

Central point of this area represents internal ear.

Area-7

No acupuncture point.

Area-8

Central point of this area represents tonsils and throat

Area-9

No acupuncture point.

Facio-mandibular area

It is located between area 5 and area 6. It is used in the treatment of trigeminal neuralgia and facial paralysis.

Cheek area

It is located at the junction of 5th and 6th area.

2. Tragus (corresponds to nose and pharynx)

Adrenal gland is located at the lower projection of the tragus pharynx and larynx at the inner surface opposite to the orifice of the external auditory meatus and internal nose at inner surface slightly below the pharynx and larynx area. On the middle of the root of the tragus, point for external nose is located, while the middle of the line connecting the apex of the tragus and external nose represents the thirst point. Hunger point is located in the middle of the line connecting adrenal gland and external nose point. Midpoint of the line connecting adrenal gland and eye-I is hypertension point (Fig. 17.4).

3. Supratragic incisure (heart and external ear)

External ear is located at the depression in front of the supratragic incisure, while the heart is in the depression on the apex of the tragus.

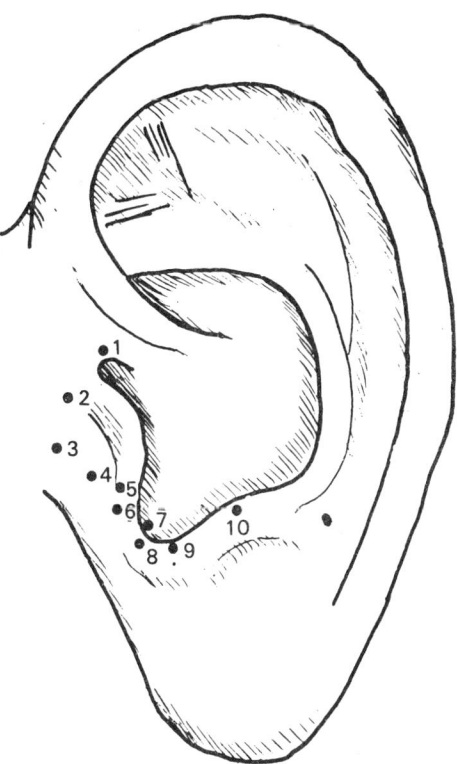

Fig. 17.4   Shows points on tragus, intertragic and supratragic incisure:

1. Heart point   6. Hypertension point
2. Thirst point   7. Internal secretion point
3. External nose   8. Eye I
4. Hunger point   9. Eye II
5. Adrenal gland   10. Ovary

4.   Anti-tragus (head region)

Brain spot is located on the middle of one-third of the superior brim (junction of anti-tragus).   Midpoint of one-third of the middle brim is parotid gland point.   Soothing asthma or Dingchuan point is at the apex of the antitragus.   Forehead is at the antero-inferior part (junction of lobe area-2 with antitragus).   Subcortex is located on the inner surface of the antitragus and in the lower part of the subcortex area testis and ovary are located.

5.   Antihelix (trunk)

The neck is at the notch between the border line of the antihelix and antitragus.   The superior crus corresponds to the lower extremity below the knee.   The inferior crus corresponds to the gluteal region and the thigh.   The anterior margin of the antihelix represents vertebral column (Fig. 17.5).

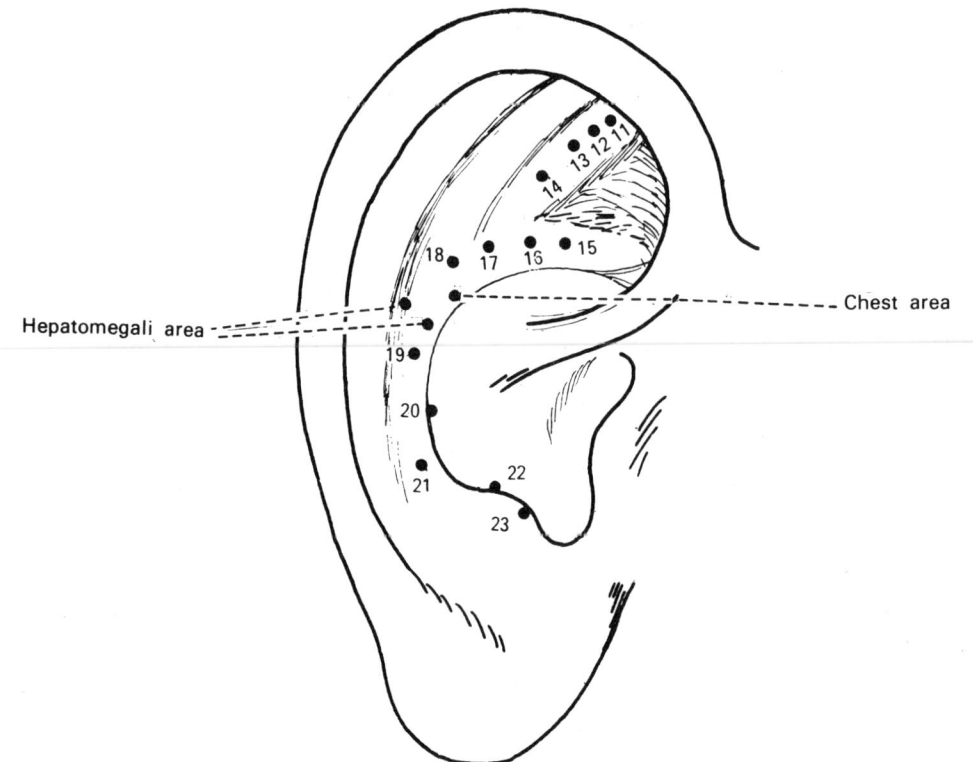

Fig. 17.5 Showing points on anti-tragus and anti-helix.

11.	Toes	18.	Lumbar vertebra
12.	Ankle	19.	Thoracic vertebra
13.	Knee	20.	Neck area
14.	Hip	21.	Cervical vertebra
15.	Lumbago point	22.	Brain spot
16.	Buttock area	23.	Ding chuan (Soothing
17.	Gluteal region		asthma point)

Lying along the curved brim of the cavum conchae on the antihelix and divided into three equal segment.	Cervical vertebra	: Beginning of antihelix on the lower segment.
	Thoracic vertebra	: Above the cervical vertebral area, on the middle segment.
	Lumbar vertebra	: Above the thoracic vertebra on the upper segment.
	Sacrum	: Above the lumbar vertebra, near the bifurcation of the antihelix.

Superior and Inferior Crus of Antihelix

Toes, heel and ankle are located at the postero-superior and antero-superior part of the superior crus of the antihelix.

Knee joint is located on the superior crus with the same level of the superior border of the inferior crus of the antihelix. Hip joint is postero-inferior to the knee joint point.

Midpoint in the superior border of the inferior crus is the ischium and buttock point, the lower projection of the antihelix at the level of coccygeal vertebrae point is lumbago point.

Border line between the brim of the inferior crus of the antihelix and curved brim of the anterior portion of the helix represents sympathetic area.

In between the hip joint and the sympathetic area, on the superior border of the inferior crus, in the middle segment, is the sciatica nerve point.

6. Triangular fossa (deltoid fossa)

Shenmen (point with strong sedative and analgesic effect) is located at the bifurcation of the crura of the antihelix and pelvic cavity at the inner surface of the bifurcation. Uterus is at the midpoint of the triangular fossa just posterior to the anterior portion of the helix.

Point of lowering blood pressure is at the border line between the superior crus of the helix and the antihelix. About 2 mm lateral to the uterus point is the asthma point and hepatitis point. Constipation point is located near the middle section of the antihelix at the antero-superior part of the ischium point. Lines tangential to the inferior border of the superior crus and superior border of the inferior crus meet on a spot on the antihelix known as hot point and is used in treating febrile illness (Fig. 17.6).

7. Crus of helix

The crus of helix represents diaphragm.

8. Helix

External genital organs and urethra are located at the anterior part of the helix with the same level of the inferior crus of antihelix and urinary bladder point respectively. The lower segment of the rectum is at the level with the point of the large intestine on the anterior part of the helix.

Haemorrhoid point is at the apex of the auricle just above lowering blood pressure point. There are four tonsil points:

Tonsils 1 : At the superior margin of the helix.

Tonsils 2 : At the middle of helix, becomes an equilateral triangle with tonsils 1 and 4,

Tonsils 3 : Located between tonsils 2 and 4.

Tonsils 4 : Located on the auricular lobule.

9. Scapha

Clavicle, shoulder, wrists and fingers are located at the scapha with the same level of ear point for the neck, supratragic notch and the auricular tubercle, respectively. Shoulder joint is in between the shoulder and clavicle while the elbow is in between the wrist and the shoulder.

Infero-exterior to the clavicle is the nephritis point.

There are three appendix points on the scapha, located on the superior part of the fingers and shoulder and inferior part of the clavicle. Lying between the fingers and wrist is the urticaria spot (Fig. 17.7).

10. Cymba conchae

The antero-superior part of the cymba-conchae just below the inferior crus of the antihelix is the urinary bladder while kidney is located in the upper part, near the points of the small

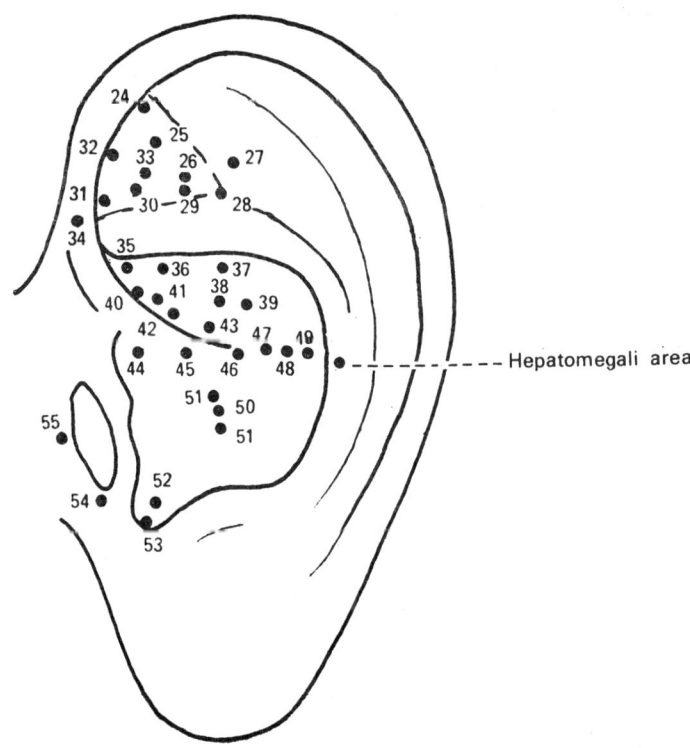

Fig. 17.6 Showing points on triangular fossa, cavum conchae and cymba conchae:

24.	Blood pressure lowering point	40.	Lower segment of rectum
25.	Hepatitis point	41.	Large intestine
26.	Shenmen	42.	Appendix
27.	Hip joint	43.	Duodenum
28.	Hot point	44.	Mouth
29.	Buttock	45.	Oesophagus
30.	Sciatic nerve	46.	Stomach
31.	Sympathy	47.	Gall bladder
32.	Uterus	48.	Liver
33.	Asthma spot	49.	Spleen
34.	External genitalia	50.	Heart
35.	Urethra	51.	Lung
36.	Urinary bladder	52.	Subcortex
37.	Kidney	53.	Internal secretion
38.	Ascites spot	54.	Adrenal
39.	Pancreas	55.	External nose

intestine. Small intestine is at the lower portion of the cymba conchae, above the crus of the helix; ureters are located between the urinary bladder and kidney on the medial side of the urinary bladder and below the sympathetic point is the prostate. Stomach and oesophagus are at the upper portion of the cavum chochae, the former is just below the disappearance of the crus and the later just below the crus of the helix. Behind the oesophagus is the cardiac orifice and opposite the cardiac orifice above the crus in duodenum (Fig. 17.6).

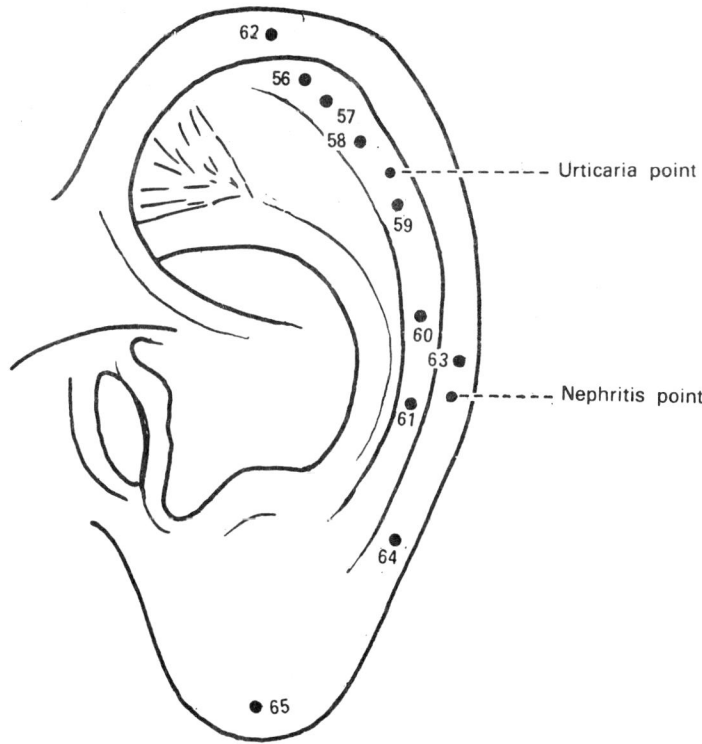

Fig. 17.7 Showing points of scapha and helix:

56.	Fingers	61.	Clavicle
57.	Hand	62.	Tonsils 1
58.	Wrist	63.	Tonsils 2
59.	Elbow	64.	Tonsils 3
60.	Shoulder	65.	Tonsils 4

Large intestine is located at the antero-superior portion of the cymba conchae and just above the crus of the helix. In between the large intestine and small intestine is the appendix point. Liver is located at the postero-superior part of the stomach while the pancreas and gall bladder points are located between the liver and kidney points. Pancreatitis spot is located at the lower two-thirds part between pancreas, gall bladder and duodenum points. In between the kidney, pancreas, gall bladder points and small intestine ascitis point is situated. Analgesic point is located at the upper one-third part between kidney and small intestine.

11. Cavum conchae (Thoracic region)

Heart lies in the deepest part, while lung lies at the circumference of the heart area. Bronchi are located in the lung area. Spleen is at the exterio-inferior part of the stomach area. In the centre of the lung area tuberculosis point is located. Trachea is in between the heart and external auditory meatus. Hepatomegaly spot is located at the lateral side between the stomach and disappearance of the crus of the helix. In the centre of this spot hepatic cirrhosis point is located (Fig. 17.6).

Hepatitis area is slightly below the middle of the stomach and spleen area.

12.   Cranial surface of the auricle

On the cranial surface of the auricle there is a groove which corresponds to the antihelix. This is the lowering blood pressure groove. The remaining of the back of the auricle is divided into three areas—upper middle and lower which correspond to the area of the back and trunk. Back is divided into upper, middle and lower (on the cartilagenous eminence) of the spinal cord is located at the highest point of the root of the auricle (spinal cord I) and in front of the mastoid process (spinal cord II) at the lower margin of the root of the auricle (Fig. 17.8).

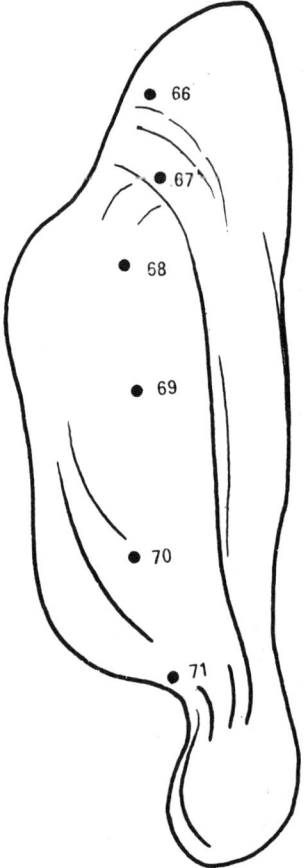

Fig. 17.8   Showing points on the back of the auricle:

66.	Spinal cord	69.	Middle back
67.	Depression groove	70.	Upper back
68.	Lower back	71.	Spinal cord 2

Upper abdomen is at the inferior wall of the orifice of the external auditory meatus while lower abdomen is in its superior wall.

COMMONLY USED AURICULARS POINTS

	Name	Function
1.	Shenmen	Sedation and analgesia.
2.	Sympathetic point	Analgesia and spasmolysis.
3.	Adrenal point	Regulates adrenal gland and cortical hormones.
4.	Subcortex	Regulates excitement and inhibition of the cerebral cortex.
5.	Internal secretion	Regulates endocrinal disturbances.
6.	Heart point	Calms down the heart and mind.
7.	Liver point	Promotes the liver and gall bladder.
8.	Spleen point	Regulates the functions of the spleen.
9.	Lung point	Governs the air and controls respiration.
10.	Kidney point	Strengthening the positive energy, helping the essence, facilitating the "water ways" and increasing the sense of vision and hearing.
11.	Large intestine point	To excrete and carry downwards from small intestine.
12.	Small intestine points	Digestion and separating the nutrient and drugs.
13.	Stomach point	To receive and digest food.
14.	Gall bladder point	To reserve the bile.
15.	Urinary bladder	To contain the fluid.
16.	Brainstem point	Spasmolysis and driving the wind out.
17.	Brain point	Represents pituitary.
18.	Uterus point	Regulates the functions of female internal genital organs.
19.	Dingchuan (Soothing asthma point)	This function's as antiallergic and antipruritic point. It also has antiasthmatic properties.
20.	Ascitic point	Anti-oedema properties.
21.	Eye, Eye-I and Eye-II	Regulate the functioning of the eye.
22.	Internal ear point	Regulates hearing.
23.	Anaesthesia or tooth extraction points	Anaesthetic and analgesic effects on the upper and lower teeth
24.	Points specific for limb joints affect the related area, limbs and the vertebral column.	
25.	Hot spot	Analgesic, antipyretic and vasodilating properties.

RULES FOR THE SELECTION OF THE POINTS

1. Auricular points are of following categories
    i. Those representing particular organs.
    ii. Those possessing special functions. For example.
        a. Blood pressure lowering point for hypertension.
        b. Hot point for fever.
        c. Shenmen for sedation.
        d. Endocrine point for hormonal regulation.
    iii. Specific point for disorders. For example.
        a. Dingchuan for asthma.
        b. Ascitis point for oedema.

In treating diseases, the points can be selected from above categories in various combinations. For example,

Organ affected

Sedation point

Endocrine point.

2. Use of the meridian system—Areas representing the pertaining organ can be used in the treatment of the diseases along the pathway of the meridian.

3. Coupled organ—for example small intestine for heart, spleen and gastric ulcer.

4. Application of the western knowledge of medicine, for example pancreas point for diabetes mellitus.

5. Use of the point detector—low electrical resistance point of the auricle.

6. By examination of the auricle—thorough inspection and palpation.

Procedure

Fine filliform needles and press needles are used. Filliform needles are inserted obliquely, subcutaneously, care being taken not to penetrate the cartilage. Electrical stimulation may be given. Hand stimulation is not advised.

The treatment is carried out for 20 to 30 minutes a day up to 7 to 10 days and then a rest period of one week is given.

Press needles when used are kept in place with the help of the adhensive leucoplast and left *in situ* for 3 to 5 days.

18

SCALP NEEDLING THERAPY

Scalp needling therapy is the gift of Chiao Shun-fa, a Chinese physician, to the world of acupuncture. It is a new method introduced by him and his colleagues in a North China country hospital during 1966-71. In the beginning he made studies on the patients of cerebral stroke and paralysis. He had a thorough knowledge of the ancient Chinese theories of acupuncture as well as modern neurophysiological theories of acupuncture. He applied the knowledge of both the systems in evolving this new technique.

The physiological basis of scalp needle therapy is yet not well understood. It requires an intensive clinical work and laboratory studies for establishing its standing as a modern medical science.

The whole technique of scalp needle therapy is based on the belief that all the parts and centres of the brain are projected on the corresponding part of the scalp in the systematic way and the needle stimulation on the scalp at these specified areas can cause similar stimulation in the corresponding underlying area of the brain. This in turn generates' certain functional changes on the contralateral side of the body.

Division of the areas

A. Main surface lines of the scalp

Two imaginary lines are drawn as follows:

  (i) *Antero-posterior midline* : It is the line connecting the glabella (midpoint between the two eyebrows) and the lower part of external occipital protuberance (Fig. 18.1)
  (ii) *Eyebrow-occipit line* : It is the line connecting the centre of the eyebrow with the tip of the external occipital protuberance. It is drawn on the lateral aspect of the scalp (Fig. 18.2).

The main indications

  1. Post-stroke hemiplegia and after effects of the cerebral concussion.
  2. Intracranial inflammation and their residual effects after the patient has recovered from coma.
  3. Extrapyramidal disord : Chorea, parkinsonism.

271

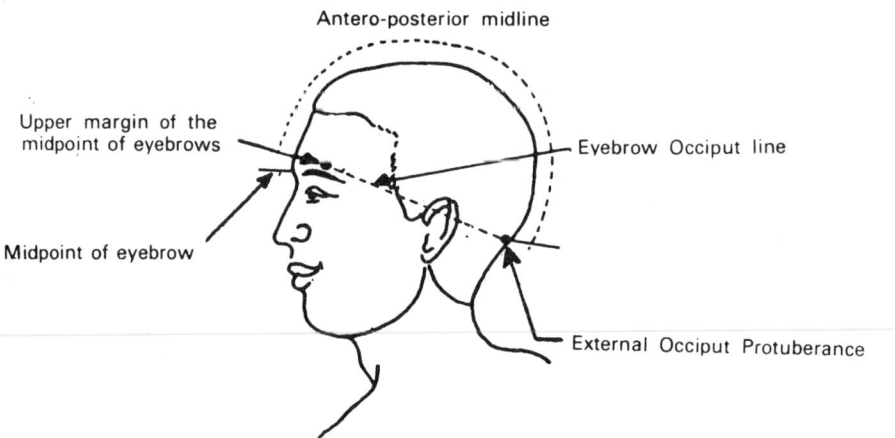

Fig. 18.1 Stimulation area of scalp-needle standard lines.

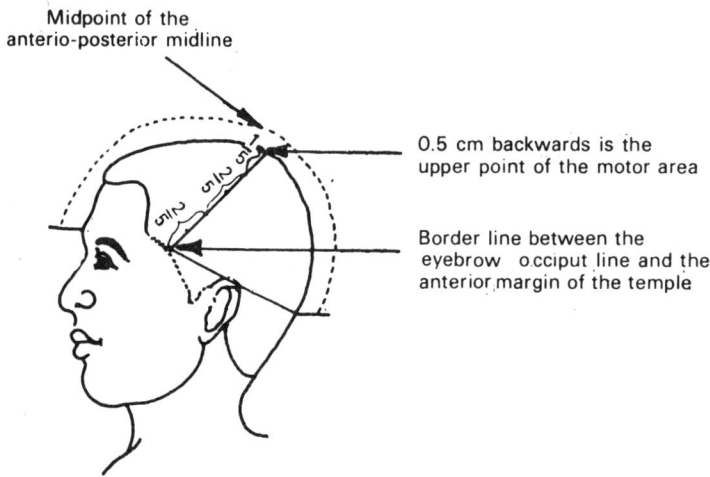

Fig. 18.2 Localisation of motor area.

4. Intracranial parasites : Cystitiserosis.
5. Spinal cord diseases : Multiple sclerosis, urinary incontinence.
6. Peripheral nerve diseases : Trigeminal neuralgia, other neuralgia.
7. Myopathies, muscular atrophy.
8. Visceral diseases, gastric ulcer.
9. Psychological disorders : Nocturnal enuresis in children, impotency, tremors.
10. Cardiovascular disorders : Hypertension, bradycardia and tachycardia.
11. Chest diseases : Cough, asthma, chest pain.
12. Gynaecological disorders : Prolapse of uterus, functional uterine bleeding.
13. Vestibulo-auditory disorders : Deafness, vertigo, earache, tinnitus, labyrinthitis, Meniere's disease.

14. Speech disorders : Aphasia, aphonia.
15. Opthalmic disorders : .Colour blindness and other cortico-visual disturbances.
16. Acupuncture anaesthesia.

B.   Localisation of the brain projection areas

Area 1.   Motor area

Location   :   Motor area corresponds to a line joining a point 0.5 cm behind mid-point of the antero posterior midline with the eyebrow occiput and natural hairline intersecting point—the point where eyebrow occipit and the natural hairline intersect each other on the temple (Fig. 18.3). The representation of the area is as follows:

     I.   Lower two-fifths of the motor area represent contralateral face.

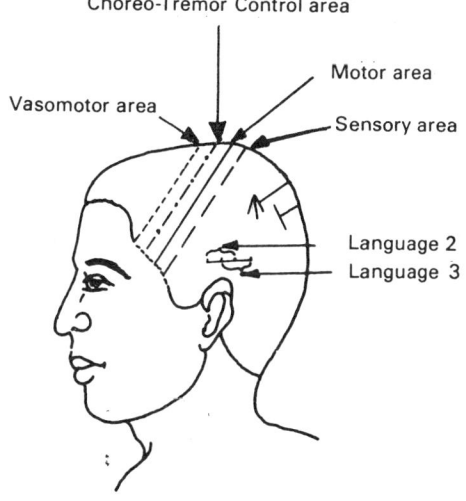

Fig. 18.3 Lateral surface of the stimulation area.

Indications   :   Contralateral central facial palsy, motor aphasia, aphasia, aphonia, excessive salivation.

     II.   Middle two-fifths of the motor area represent contralateral upper limb.

Indications   :   Paralysis of the contralateral arm.

     III. Upper one-fifth of the motor area represents contralateral lower limb and trunk.

Indications   :   Paralysis of contralateral leg.

Area 2 : Sensory area

Location   :   Sensory area corresponds to a line drawn 1.5 cm parallel and behind the motor area.   The representations is as follows:

     I.   Lower two-fifths of the sensory area represent contralateral face.

Indications   :   Contralateral facial numbness, temporal headache, trigeminal neuralgia, trismus, toothache, arthritis of temporomandibular joint.
                         II.   Middle two-fifths of the sensory area represent contralateral upper limb.

Indications   :   Pain, abnormal sensory feeling and numbness of contralateral arm.
                         III. Upper one-fifth of the sensory area represent contralateral leg.

Indications   :   Numbness, parasthesia, abnormal sensory feeling and arthritis of opposite joints, sciatica of lower extremity.

Area 3 : Choreo-tremor controlled area
Location   :   A parallel line, 1.5 cm in front of the motor area.
Indications   :   Infantile chorea, athetosis, spasmodic torticolis, senile tremors, and parkinsonism of the contralateral side. (The regional sub-divisions are similar to the motor and sensory area.)

Area 4 : Vasomotor area
Location   :   A parallel line, 1.5 cm in front of the choreo-tremor controlled area.
Indications   :   Hypertension, hypotension, cerebral oedema.

Area 5 : Foot sensory motor area
Location   :   It is a 3 cm long line running parallel to the anterio-posterior midline. Its midpoint is 1 cm lateral to the midpoint of the anterio-posterior midline (Fig. 18.4).

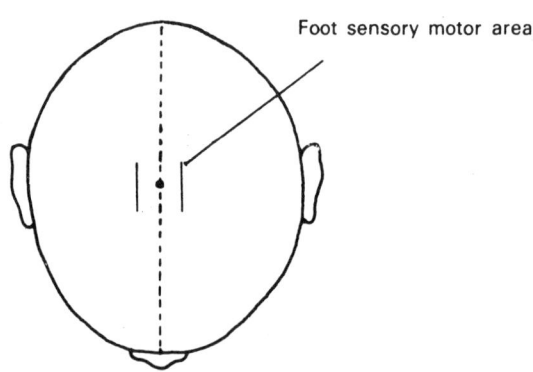
Foot sensory motor area

Fig. 18.4   Parietal surface of the stimulation areas.

Indications   :   Pain, paralysis, parasthesia and numbness of the contralateral lower extremity, uterine bleeding, nocturnal enuresis, acute sprain of lumbar region.

Area 6 : Vertigo-auditory area
Location   :   4 cm horizontal, straight line located 1.5 cm vertically above the auricle.
Indications   :   Deafness, vertigo, oticodinia, tinnitus, Meniere's desease.

Area 7 : Language area 2

Location   : 3 cm straight line situated 2 cm posterio-inferior to the parietal tubercle-parallel to the anterio-posterior midline.

Indication   : Aphasia.

Area 8 : Language area 3

Location   : A 4 cm long line drawn backward from the midpoint of the vertigo auditory area.

Indication   : Sensory aphasia.

Area 9 : Usage area

Location   : Three lines from the parietal tubercle, 3 cm in the forward, backward and downward direction at 40°.
Three separate needles are used in these three different directions, starting from one point at the parietal tubercle.

Indication   : Appraxia.

Area 10 : Visual area

Location   : It is a 4 cm long line drawn upward and parallel to anterio-posterior midline from a point 1 cm lateral to the external occipital protuberance (Fig. 18.5).

Indications   : Colour blindness, cortico visual disturbances.

Area 11 : Equilibrium area

Location   : It is a 4 cm long line drawn downward and parallel to the anterio-posterior midline from a point 3 cm lateral to the external occipital protuberance.

Indication   : Equilibrium disturbances due to cerebellar disorder.

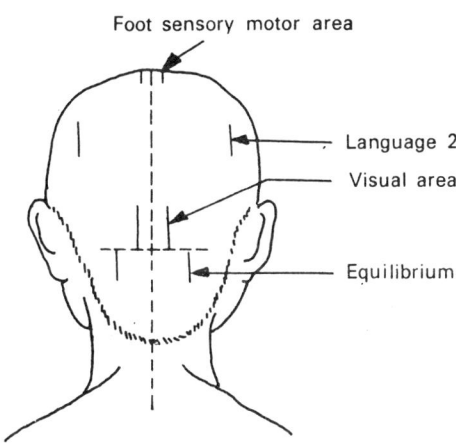

Fig. 18.5 Posterior surface of the stimulation area.

Area 12 : Gastric area

Location   :   2 cm long line, starting directly above the pupil at the natural hairline. It runs backward and parallel to the anterio-posterior midline (Fig. 18.6).

Indication   :   Gastric disorders.

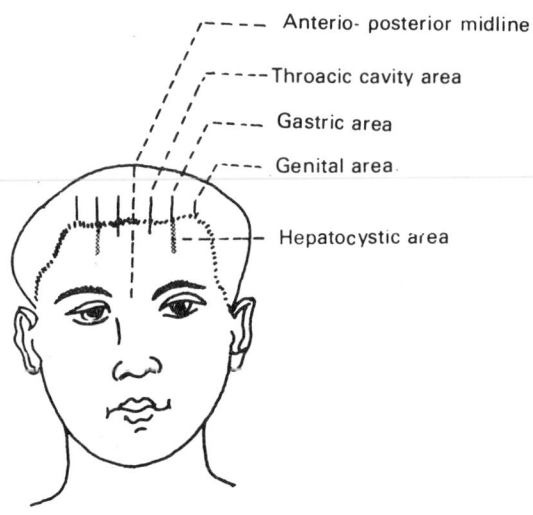

```
,- - - -   Anterio- posterior midline
      ,- - - - -Throacic cavity area
      ,- - - -   Gastric area
      ,- - - -  Genital area
```
Hepatocystic area

Fig. 18.6   Anterior surface of the stimulation areas.

Area 13 : Thoracic cavity area

Location   :   A line drawn from a point on the natural hair line, midway between the gastric area and the anterio-posterior midline. It is 4 cm long forward and backwards from the natural hair line.

Indications   :   Asthma, tachycardia, chest pain, palpitation.

Area 14 : Genital area

Location   :   It is 2 cm long straight line, starting from the natural hair line and running lateral and parallel to the gastric area. The distance between the gastric area and genital area is equivalent to that between the gastric area and thoracic cavity area.

Indications   :   Functional uterine bleeding, prolapse of uterus when used with motor and sensory area for lower limb.

Area 15 : Hepatocystic area

Location   :   2 cm straight line, straight from the gastric area and running forwards.

Indications   :   Epigastric pain, gastric ulcer, chronic hepatitis.

Rules for the selection of the points

1.   For the treatment of the diseases of unilateral limb, the corresponding stimulation area on the opposite side of the scalp is selected. When both the exremities are involved, areas on both the sides are selected.

2. Usually one concerned area is selected but if needed it may be combined with the another area, for example, in gynaecological operations a combination of sensory area and genital area can be used.
3. A combination of body needle points and scalp surface areas can be used for producing acupuncture anaesthesia.

Techniques of manipulation

1. Sterlise the stimulation area nicely with 75% alcohol and 2.5% iodine tincture.
2. No. 26.28, 2.5-3 t-sun fine needle is used.
3. Needle is inserted tangentially into the scalp by twisting and turning subcutaneously, to the required length (approximately $\frac{1}{2}$ to 1 inch).
4. Pushing or lifting of the needle should not be done.
5. Needle is twisted in the frequency of more than 200 times per minute for 3 to 5 minutes. After twisting, the needle is left in place for 5 to 10 minutes. The stimulation is repeated 2 to 3 times and then the needle is withdrawn.
6. Clean the point before insertion with a sterlised cotton wool.
7. Needles may be stimulated electrically instead of the hand manipulation. To achieve good results 200 pulses per minute for 20 to 30 minutes should be given. While stimulating, the needles cross-connection (between right and left sides) should not be made.
8. Needles may be inserted and left in place for half an hour without subjecting them to any type of stimulation (hand or electrical) and good results can be obtained.

19

NOSE HAND AND FOOT ACUPUNCTURE

NOSE ACUPUNCTURE

Acupuncture points on the nose are used to treat all the ailments of the body. There are three imaginary lines on the nose—one in the middle is unpaired and the remaining two are paired and located on the sides of the midline (Fig. 19.1).

First Line—Yin-Solid Organs : It is located in the middle and contains acupuncture points for head and face, throat, heart, lung, liver, spleen, kidney and external genital organs.

Second Line—Yang-Hollow Organs : It is situated lateral to the midline, on both the sides and contains points for gall bladder, stomach, small intestine, large intestine and urinary bladder.

Third Line—It is situated on both lateral sides of the second line and contains points for ear, chest, breast, nape of the neck, loin, upper and lower extremities.

DESCRIPTION OF THE POINTS

The important points are as follows:

First Line

1. *Head and face* : Draw a line from the centre of the forehead at the hair line to a point midway between the eyebrows. Points on the upper third of this line are the head and face points.
2. *Lung point* : Midway between the two eyebrows.
3. *Heart point* : Between the two medial canthus.
4. *Liver point* : At the highest point of the nose bone.
5. *Kidney point* : At the tip of the nose.
6. *Spleen point* : Between the kidney and the liver point.
7. *External genitalia point* : At the tip of the philtrum.
8. *Throat point* : Between the head and face point and lung point.

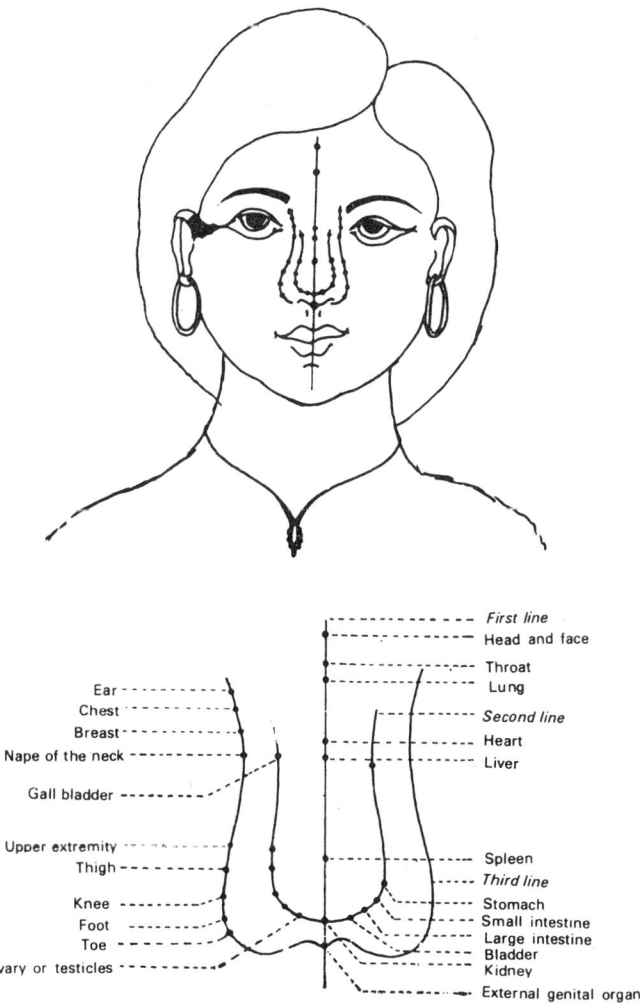

Fig. 19.1 Nose acupuncture.

Second Line
1. *Gall bladder point :* At the level of the liver point.
2. *Stomach point :* At the level of the spleen point.
3. *Small intestine point :* One-third from the centre of ala nasi.
4. *Bladder point :* Lower margin of the ala nasi.

Third Line
1. *Ear point :* Inner end of the eyebrows.
2. *Chest point :* Between the breast point and the ear point.
3. *Breast point :* Just above Jing-ming (UB-1).
4. *Neck point :* Just below Jing-ming (UB-1).

5. *Loin point* : At the level of the gall bladder point.
6. *Upper extremity point* : At the level of the stomach point.
7. *Thigh point* : Outer side of the upper part of the ala nasi.
8. *Knee joint point* : Lateral side of the middle point of the ala nasi.
9. *Foot and toe point* : Outer side of the lower part of the ala nasi.

Extra Points

Testicles or ovary.
Between the external genitalia point and the urinary bladder point.
Indications   : Diseases of the organs which are represented by the points.
Needling   : 0.1 to 0.3 t-sun, slanting on first and second line point. Straight on third line point.

HAND ACUPUNCTURE

Commonly used hand acupuncture points are described below (Figs. 19.2 & 19.3):

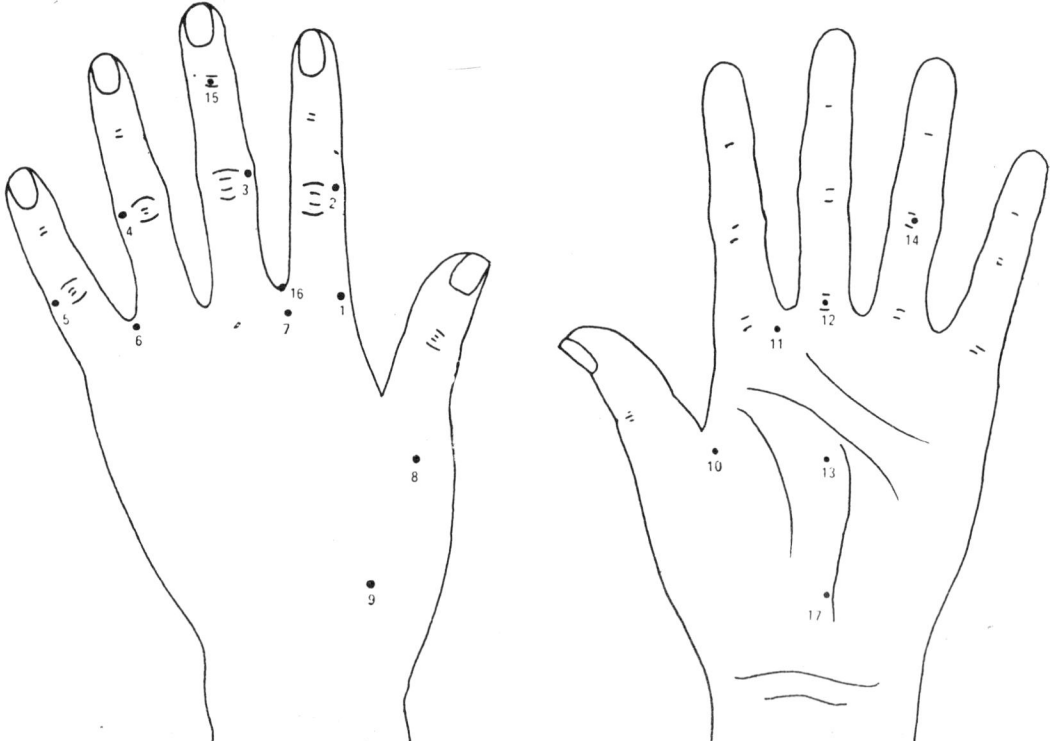

Fig. 19.2 Hand acupuncture (dorsal aspect).   Fig. 19.3 Hand acupuncture (palmar aspect).

1. Shoulder point

Location   : Lateral side of the metacarpophalangeal joint of the index finger.

Indications   : Shoulder pain, frozen shoulder.
Needling   : Slanting insertion, 0.2 to 0.5 t-sun.

2. Forehead point
Location   : Lateral side of the first interphalangeal joint of the index finger.
Indications   : Frontal sinusitis, frontal headache, gastrointestinal spasm.
Needling   : Slanting insertion, 0.2 to 0.5 t-sun.

3. Vertex point
Location   : Lateral side of the first interphalangeal joint of the middle finger.
Indications   : Neurosis and headache.
Needling   : Slanting insertion, 0.2 to 0.5 t-sun.

4. Migraine point
Location   : Medial side of the first interphalangeal joint of the ring finger.
Indications   : Migraine, chest pain, thoracalgia.
Needling   : Slanting insertion, 0.2 to 0.5 t-sun.

5. Occipital point
Location   : Medial side of the first interphalangeal joint of the little finger.
Indications   : Occipital headache, acute tonsillitis, hiccough, pharyngitis.
Needling   : Slanting insertion, 0.2 to 0.5 t-sun.

6. Sciatic nerve point
Location   : Medial side of the metacarpophalangeal joint of the ring finger.
Indication   : Sciatica.
Needling   : Slanting insertion, 0.5 t-sun.

7. Neck and nape point
Location   : Medial side of the metacarpophalangeal joint of the index finger.
Indications   : Stiff neck, cervical spondylosis.
Needling   : Slanting insertion, 0.5 to 1 t-sun.

8. Headache point
Location   : Medial side of the metacarpophalangeal joint of the thumb.
Indications   : Headache, dizziness, abdominal distension.
Needling   : Slanting insertion, 0.2 to 0.5 t-sun.

9. Nose point
Location   : Medial side of the metacarpal bone of the index finger.
Indication   : Nasal pain.
Needling   : Straight insertion, 0.2 to 0.5 t-sun.

10. Hysteria point
Location   : Centre of the crease of the metacarpophalangeal joint of the thumb.
Indications   : Emotional disturbance, hysteria, insanity, psychosis.
Needling   : Straight insertion, 0.2 to 0.5 t-sun.

11. Cough point

Location	:	Medial side of the metacarpophalangeal joint of the index finger.
Indications	:	Chronic bronchitis, asthma.
Needling	:	Straight insertion, 0.2 to 0.5 t-sun.

12. Oral ulcer point

Location	:	Centre of the crease of the metacarpopnalangeal joint of the middle finger.
Indications	:	Thrush, stomatitis, aphthous ulcers.
Needling	:	Slanting insertion, 0.5 t-sun towards the centre of the palm.

13. Polyhidrosis

Location	:	Centre of the palm.
Indication	:	Excessive sweating.
Needling	:	Straight, 1 t-sun deep.

14. Liver point

Location	:	Centre of the first interphalangeal joint of the ring finger.
Indications	:	Jaundice, hepatitis.
Needling	:	Straight insertion or slanting insertion, 0.3–0.5 t-sun.

15. Hiccough point

Location	:	Centre of the second interphalangeal joint of the middle finger.
Indications	:	Hiccough.
Needling	:	Slanting, 0.3 t-sun deep.

16. Antipyretic point

Location	:	Lateral side of the web of the middle finger.
Indication	:	Pyrexia.
Needling	:	Slanting, 0.3 to 0.5 t-sun deep.

17. Anti-convulsion point

Location	:	The junction of the thenar and hypothenar eminences in the palm.
Indication	:	Febrile convulsions.
Needling	:	Straight, 0.5 to 1 t-sun deep.

FOOT ACUPUNCTURE

Commonly used foot acupuncture points are described below (Figs. 19.4, 19.5, 19.6 and 19.7).

Foot point 1

Location	:	Between lateral and medial malleolus at sole.
Indications	:	Neurasthenia, hysteria, insomnia, hypertension.
Needling	:	Straight or slanting, 0.5 to 1 t-sun deep.

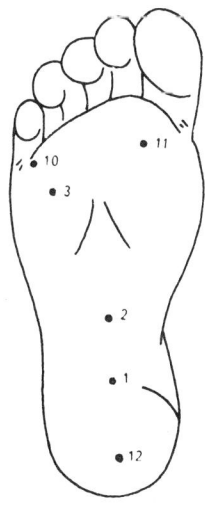

Fig. 19.4 Foot acupuncture.

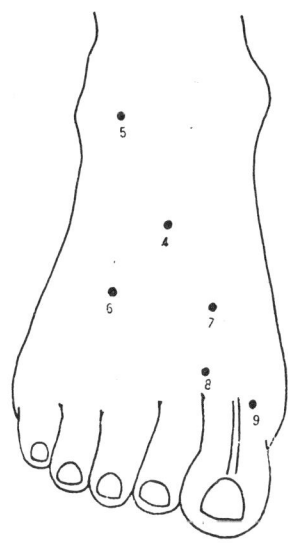

Fig. 19.5 Foot acupuncture.

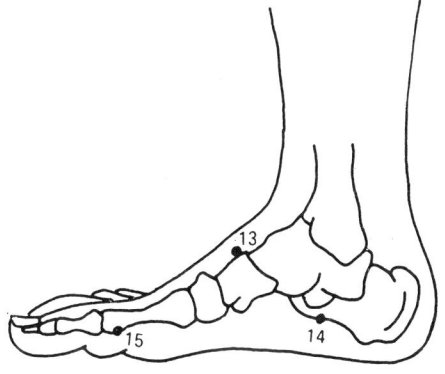

Fig. 19.6 Foot acupuncture.

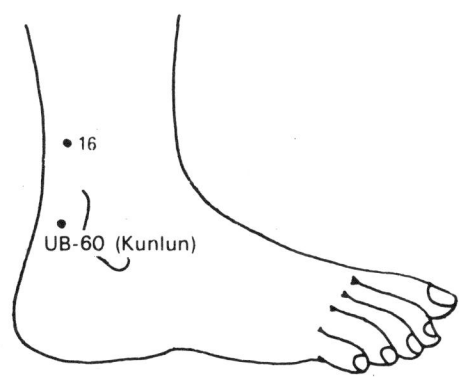

Fig. 19.7 Foot acupuncture.

Foot point 2
Location : 5 t-sun distal from posterior border of heal in the midline.
Indications : Asthenia, hepatitis.
Needling : Straight, 0.5 t-sun deep.

Foot point 3
Location : 1 t-sun proximal to the centre of the 5th toe.
Indication : Toothache.
Needling : Straight, 0.5 t-sun deep.

Foot point 4
Location   : 2.5 t-sun below Jiexi (St-41) on dorsal aspect.
Indication   : Angina pectoris.
Needling   : Spot Prick, 0.1 to 0.6 t sun.

Foot point 5
Location   : 1.5 t-sun proximal to the middle of the fourth and little toe (between Footlinqi (GB-41) and Diwuhui (GB-42).
Indication   : Sciatica.
Needling   : Straight, 0.5 t-sun deep.

Foot point 6
Location   : 2 t-sun proximal to the crease of the 3rd and 4th toe.
Indication   : Wry neck.
Needling   : Straight, 1 t-sun deep.

Foot point 7
Location   : Medial side of the base of metatarsal bone of big toe.
Indication   : Loin sprain.
Needling   : Straight, 1 to 2 t-sun deep.

Foot point 8
Location   : Midway between Xing Jian (Liv-2) and Taichong (Liv-3).
Indication   : Tonsillitis.
Needling   : Slanting, 1 to 2 t-sun.

Foot point 9
Location   : Medial side of the tendon of the big toe.
Indications   : Eczema, urticaria.
Needling   : Straight, 0.1 to 0.2 t-sun deep.

Foot point 10
Location   : Middle of the metatarsophalangeal joint of little toe.
Indications   : Enuresis, frequency of micturition.
Needling   : Slanting, 0.5 t-sun downward.

Foot point 11
Location   : 1 t-sun proximal to the middle of the web of big toe and the second toe at the planter aspect.
Indication   : Toothache.
Needling   : Straight, 0.5 to 1 t-sun.

Foot point 12
Location   : 1 t-sun distal to the posterior border of the heal at the midline.
Indications   : Rhinitis, common cold.
Needling   : Straight, 0.5 t-sun deep.

Foot point 13
Location	:	1 t-sun medial side of Jiexi (St-41), 0.5 t-sun distal to crease of ankle.
Indication	:	Hypertension.
Needling	:	Straight, 0.5 t-sun deep.

Foot point 14
Location	:	2 t-sun below distal end of medial malleolus at the midline of malleolus.
Indication	:	Functional uterine bleeding.
Needling	:	Straight, 1 t-sun deep.

Foot point 15
Location	:	Between Taibai (Sp-3) and Gongsun (Sp-4).
Indications	:	Epilepsy, hysteria, neurasthenia.
Needling	:	Straight, 1 t-sun deep.

Foot point 16
Location	:	1 t-sun above Kunlun (UB-60).
Indications	:	Headache, abdomen pain.
Needling	:	Slanting, 1 to 2 t-sun deep.

ACUPUNCTURE
THERAPY

RULES FOR SELECTION OF POINTS

1. Selection of the points on the basis of their property of influencing their own meridians: A point situated on one particular meridian will treat the diseases of the pertaining organ.

   Points on heart meridian can be selected for the treatment of heart diseases.

   Points on the lung meridian can be selected for the treatment of lung diseases.

2. Use of the knowledge of luo-connection, for example, renal diseases can be treated by selecting the points on the urinary bladder meridian because kidney is lue-connected with urinary bladder.

3. Selection of the points on the pathway of the meridians, for example, points around elbow joints can be taken for the diseases of the elbow joint.

   Points around the shoulder will cure diseases of the shoulder.

4. Selection of the points according to their specific categories.

   Jingwell points: In all acute emergencies, the Jingwell point on the particular meridian will have more potent effect on the disease of the pertaining organ. Jingwell point on heart meridian will have a potent effect in coronary emergencies.

   Xi-cleft point: Used for acute and subacute disorders of the pertaining organ, for example, Kongzui (L-6) can be used for the treatment of bronchial asthma.

   Yuan (source) point: For the chronic diseases of the pertaining organ, for example, Taixi (K-3) can be used for treatment of chronic renal diseases.

   Alarm point: For the treatment of the pertaining organ, for example, Zhongfu (L-I) can be used in the treatment of bronchial asthma.

5. Use of distal points: For example, Hegu (LI-4) is used for the diseases of face and special sense organs. Weizhong (UB-40) is used for low backache.

6. Use of influential points: For example, Dashu (UB-11) is used in the treatment of bone diseases and arthritis.

7. Points used for symptomatic relief: For example, Hegu (LI-4) and Neiting (St-44) for pain, Shenmen (H-7) for sedation.

8. Use of concept of Zang and Fu organ: For example, Liver opens to eye and therefore eye disease can be treated by using a point on liver meridian.

Kidney opens to ear and therefore ear diseases can be treated by using a point on kidney meridian.

9. Use of the knowledge of embryology: For example, Neck Futu (LI-18) can be used in the treatment of thyroid disorders because they belong to the same dematome developmentally.

10. Use of Back-Shu and Mu-front points: Because they represent specific organs, their use can be made in the disease of the organs represented by them.

11. Use of the knowledge of modern medicine for symptomatic relief, for example, hot point on the ear can be used in hyperpyrexia. Pancreatic point on the ear can be used in diabetes.

12. Use of the points, for ear, nose, foot, hand and scalp.

13. Low electric resistance points, because they represent the diseases of the internal organs, can be taken for their treatment.

20
PSYCHIATRIC DISEASES

ANXIETY, NEUROSIS AND NEUROASTHENIA

Anxiety is the most common variety of the psychoneurotic conditions and often results when a person fails to achieve his aspirations. It is characterised by fear, apprehension and restlessness and symptoms and signs resulting from sympathetic excitation. The latter include palpitation, sweating, breathlessness, tightness in the chest and choking. The respiration may be rapid and give rise to tetany due to alkalosis.

Acute attacks last from a few minutes to an hour and are called anxiety neurosis. In between the attacks, patient may experience headache, irritability and tiredness. The chronic variety manifests chiefly in the form of exercise intolerance due to chestpain, palpitation and dyspnoea and is called neuroasthenia.

Anxiety must be differentiated from thyrotoxicosis, pheochromocytoma, angina pectoris and menopausal syndrome by careful history and investigations.

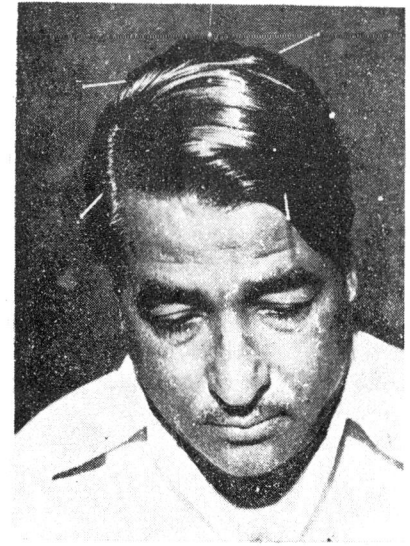

Main points	: Baihui	(GV-20)
	Sishencong	(Ex-6)
	Fengchi	(GB-20)
	Yiming	(Ex-7)
Supplementary points	: Hegu	(LI-4)
	Shenmen	(H-7)
	Neiguan	(P-6)
	Yanglingquan	(GB-34)
	Zusanli	(St-36)
	Shenmai	(UB-62)
	Sanyinjiao	(Sp-6)
Ear points	: Shenmen	
	Subcortex	
	Sympathetic	
	Heart	

Anxiety Neurosis

Stimulation

Mild stimulation 20 to 30 minutes daily for 10 days. Course may be repeated after 5 to 7 days.

TREATMENT OF NEUROASTHENIA

Main points	:	Baihui	(GV-20)
		Sishencong	(Ex-6)
		Anmian I	(Ex-8)
		Anmian II	(Ex-9)
		Shenmen	(H-7)
		Neiguan	(P-6)
		Sanyinjiao	(Sp-6)
		Qihai	(CV-6)
		Zusanli	(St-36)
		Xingjian	(Liv-2)
		Taixi	(K-3)
Ear points	:	Shenmen	
		Subcortex	
		Sympathetic	
		Internal secretion	
		Heart	
		Kidney	
		Spleen	
Scalp needling	:	Motor area	
		Sensory area	
		Foot sensory motor area	
Point Injection	:	Xinshu	(UB-15)
		Pishu	(UB-20)
		Shenshu	(UB-23)
		Zusanli	(St-36)

Points according to symptoms

Headache	:	Baihui	(GV-20)
		Hegu	(LI-4)
Temporal	:	Taiyang	(Ex-2)
headache		Anmian I	(Ex-8)
		Anmian II	(Ex-9)
		Touwei	(St-8)
		Shuaigu	(GB-8)
Occipital	:	Baihui	(GB-20)
headache		Tianzhu	(UB-10)
		Wenliu	(LI-7)
Palpitation	:	Neiguan	(P-6)
		Shenmen	(H-7)

Abdominal   : Neiguan   (P-6)
complaints   Zusanli   (St-36)

Stimulation

Two body points and one ear point should be selected for acupuncture therapy. Mild electrical stimulation should be given daily for 10 days.

Remarks

Acupuncture has been proved quite effective in these conditions.

IMPOTENCE

Impotence implies the presence of sexual desire in a person who cannot obtain peniel erection. This is a common disturbance of sexual function in males, second only to premature ejaculation.

Transient impotence is common and does not indicate an underlying disease. Chronic impotence is of psychogenic origin in 90 per cent cases. The psychological factors responsible may be extreme anxiety, guilt about the sexual act, resentment towards the partner, lack of desire to assume responsiblity of the family and latent homosexuality.

Physical causes are responsible only for 10 per cent cases of impotence. These include chronic debilitating diseases, chronic alcoholism, drug addiction, diabetes, neurological diseases, hypogonadism and local conditions like hydrocoele.

Local points   : Yaoyangguan   (GV-3)
                           Mingmen   (GV-4)
                           Shenshu   (UB-23)
                           Ciliao   (UB-32)
                           Qugu   (CV-2)
                           Guanyuan   (CV-4)
                           Shushi
                           Agrawal's Point*

Supplementary points : Baihui   (GV-20)
                           Shenmen   (H-7)
                           Sanyinjiao   (Sp-6)
                           Ququan   (Liv-8)
                           Zusanli   (St-36)
                           Taixi   (K-3)

Ear points   : Shenmen
                           Heart
                           Kidney
                           Subcortex
                           External genitalia
                           Testes
                           Adrenal gland

---

*Agrawal's point : There is a group of four points situated above and below the penis in conceptional vessel channel and two at 90° right lateral and 90° left letaral to the penis (as shown in photograph). Needling : 0.5 to 1 t-sun straight in the root of penis.

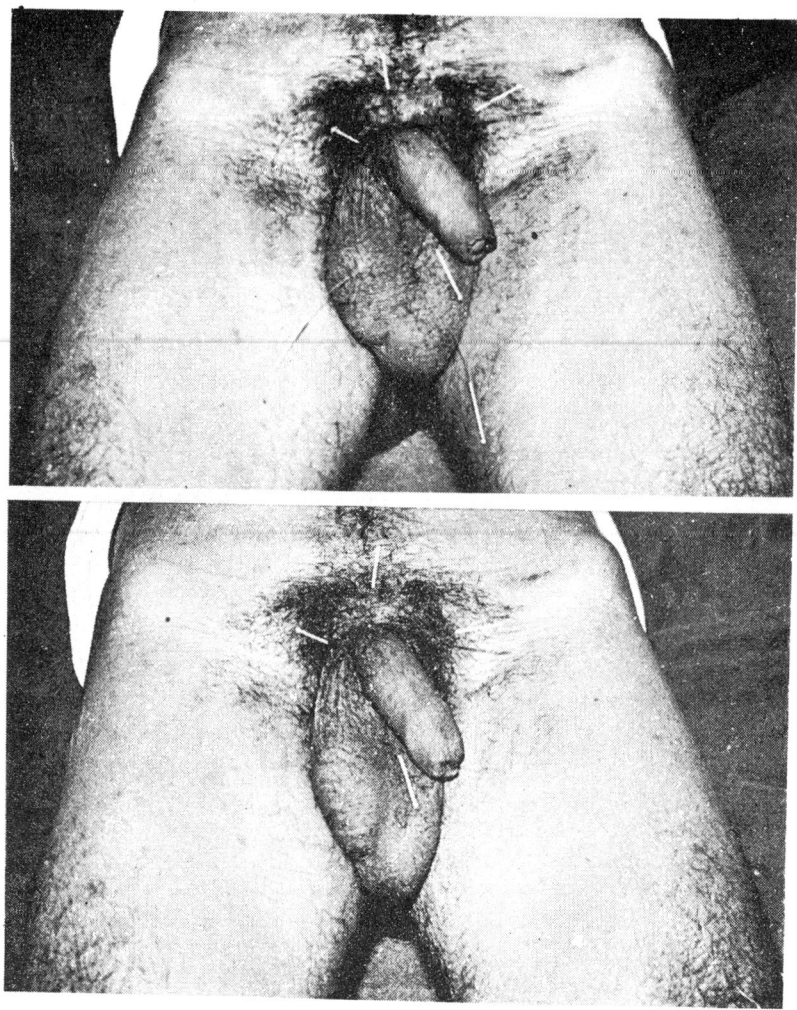

Impotency

Scalp needling   : Genital area—both sides.

Stimulation

Mild electrical stimulation should be given 20 to 30 minutes daily for 10 days. Course may be repeated after 5 to 7 days.

Remarks
1. Complete investigations should be carried out to exclude any underlying causes.
2. If impotence is secondary to a venereal disease, acupuncture should be combined with modern medicine.
3. Prostatic massage is also advised until discharge of prostatic fluid before acupuncture to get good results.

4. By using Agrawal's points, authors have obtained remarkable results.
5. Prognosis is very good.

INSOMNIA

"Peace of mind is an essential preliminary to sleep"—William Mcdougall.

Few common conditions cause more misery and discomfort to the patient than insomnia. The whole mental and physical vigour is impaired, tolerance is reduced, reaction to situations becomes abnormal and the capacity for work is decreased.

In most instances insomnia is due to pain or anxiety. Various painful situations like backache, abdominal pain, restless leg syndrome and acroparasthesia are known to disturb sleep. The psychiatric illnesses which cause insomnia include anxiety neurosis, depression, maniac depressive psychosis and hypochondriasis. Insomnia may occur either in the form of a difficulty in falling asleep and tendency to sleep late or an early morning waking and inability to return to sleep.

Main points	:	Baihui	(GV-20)
		Sishencong	(Ex-6)
		Anmian I	(Ex-8)
		Anmian II	(Ex-9)

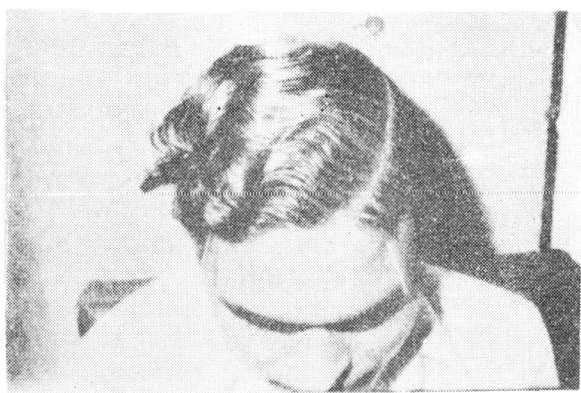

Insomnia

Supplementary			
points	:	Shenmen	(H-7)
		Neiguan	(P-6)
		Shenmai	(UB-62)
		Yanglingquan	(GB-34)
Ear points	:	Shenmen	
		Subcortex	
		Sympathic	
		Heart	

Stimulation

Mild stimulation should be given for 20 to 30 minutes daily for 7 to 10 days.

Remarks

Authors have found excellent results in all the cases of insomnia treated so far.

ANOREXIA NERVOSA

Anorexia nervosa is characterised by a voluntary and marked reduction in the intake of food, leading to weight loss and malnutrition. The condition may so severe as to lead to death from starvation. The disease generally affects women in their early adulthood. There are no signs of organic illness and the patient is usually physically active inspite of the poor nutritional status. Amenorrhoea is commonly present.

Anorexia nervosa is a manifestation of mental abnormality and occurs in those who are excessively concerned about obesity and physical appearance, who have a hysterical personality, who are depressed, and who are overcared for. Before the diagnosis of anorexia nervosa is made, carcinoma, diabetes, malabsorption syndrome and panhypopituitarism should be excluded.

Main points	:	Baihui	(GV-20)
		Sishencong	(Ex-6)
		Qihai	(CV-6)
		Zhongwan	(CV-12)
		Shenmen	(H-7)
		Neiguan	(P-6)
		Zusanli	(St-36)
		Sanyinjiao	(Sp-6)
Ear points	:	Shenmen	
		Subcortex	
		Heart	
		Stomach	
		Spleen	

Stimulation

Mild stimulation should be given daily for 20 to 30 minutes for two weeks.

Remarks

Acupuncture shows good result.

ADDICTION

Addiction to a wide variety of drugs may occur including opium and its derivatives, synthetic narcotic analgesics, barbiturates, other hypnotic drugs, tranquilisers, amphetamine and psychodeleptic agents like L.S.D. and marijuana. Addiction is likely to develop in emotionally unstable persons following the treatment of anxiety with drugs, in those who have free access to the drugs (doctors, nurses), and antisocial persons who utilise these drugs for "pleasure trips".

The basic problems with the use of addictive drugs are physiologic and psychic dependence, tolerance (increase in dose to produce same effect), and addiction (compelling need to continue taking it).   All of these are most marked with opium and its derivatives.

When the drug is suddenly stopped, withdrawal symptoms appear which are usually in the form of motor and psychic overactivity.

The problem of dependence, tolerance and withdrawal are also seen with alcohol addiction. Smoking is associated only with psychological dependence.

DRUG ADDICTION

Main points	:	Baihui	(GV-20)
		Sishencong	(Ex-6)
		Hegu	(LI-4)
		Shenmen	(H-7)
		Waiguan	(TW-5)
		Neiguan	(P-6)
		Houxi	(SI-3)
		Lieque	(L-7)
		Shenmai	(UB-62)
		Yanglingquan	(GB-34)
		Zusanli	(St-36)
Ear points	:	Lung area	
		Stomach	
		Shenmen	
		Subcortex	
		Heart	

Press needle therapy

Round body press needle should be inserted in any of the above ear points alternatively and patient should be trained to massage the needle when he gets withdrawal symptoms.

Stimulation

Mild electrical stimulations should be given for 30 to 45 minutes daily for 5 to 10 days. Course may be repeated after a rest of 5 to 7 days.

ALCOHOL ADDICTION

Main points	:	Baihui	(GV-20)
		Sishencong	(Ex-6)
		Shenmen	(H-7)
		Neiguan	(P-6)
		Lieque	(L-7)
		Tianshu	(St-25)
		Zusanli	(St-36)
		Shenmai	(UB-62)

Ear points   :   Shenmen
                               Subcortex
                               Mouth area
                               Stomach
                               Liver
                               Lung
                               Heart

SMOKING

Baihui	(GV-20)
Sishencong	(Ex-6)
Nose Heliao	(LI-19)
Yingxiang	(LI-20)
Suliao	(GV-25)
Shenmen	(H-7)
Lieque	(L-7)
Neiguan	(P-6)
Shenmai	(UB-62)
Zusanli	(St-36)

Ear points   :   Lung
                               Large intestine
                               Shenmen
                               Subcortex
                               Heart

Stimulation

Mild stimulation should be given for 20 to 30 minutes 2 to 3 times a day for two weeks.

Remarks
1. Treatment can be given 3 to 4 times daily in the beginning.
2. During the rest, press needle should be continuously used.
3. Motivation of the patient to accept acupuncture therapy is very essential.
4. A heavy dose of vitamins and high protein diet should also be advised to the patient.
5. Prognosis depends on cooperation and willingness of the patient.

TICS (Habit Spasms)

Many individuals throughout their life are prone to habitual movements such as sniffing, clearing the throat, protruding the chin, or blinking whenever they become tense. The movements are voluntary and the patient feels compelled to make them in order to relieve tension. They can be inhibited for a time by an effort but reappear when attention is diverted. Children between 5 and 10 years of age are more prone to develop tics. The movements are coordinated acts produced subconsciously. Convulsive tic is the severest variety in which the whole body is thrown into a generalised vigorous muscular activity.

Main points	:	Baihui	(GV-20)
		Shishencong	(Ex-6)
		Yiming	(Ex-7)
Supplementary	:	Hegu	(LI-4)
points		Shenmen	(H-7)
		Neiguan	(P-6)
		Yanglingquan	(GB-34)
		Zusanli	(St-36)
Ear points	:	Shenmen	
		Subcortex	
		Heart	
		Brain area	
		According to part effected	

POINTS ACCORDING TO SYMPTOMS

Tics of the eye

		Baihui	(GV-20)
		Yangbai	(GB-14)
		Fengchi	(GB-20)
		Yintang	(Ex-1)
		Taiyang	(Ex-2)
		Yuyao	(Ex-3)
		Touwei	(St-8)
Supplementary	:	Hegu	(LI-4)
points		Shenmen	(H-7)
		Yanglingquan	(GB-34)
		Fciyang	(UB-58)
		Xingjian	(LIV-2)
Ear points	:	Eye area	
		Shenmen	
		Subcortex	
		Heart	

Tics of the face

		Baihui	(GV-20)
		Dicang	(St-4)
		Jiachengjiang	(Ex-5)
		Yifeng	(TW-17)
		Quanliao	(SI-18)
		Tinggong	(SI-19)
Supplementary	:	Hegu	(LI-4)
points		Shenmen	(H-7)
		Neiguan	(P-6)
		Yanglingquan	(GB-34)
		Zusanli	(St-36)

Ear points	:	Faciomandibular area	
		Heart	
		Shenmen	

Tics of the neck

Main points	:	Baihui	(GV-20)
		Fengchi	(GB-20)
		Jianjing	(GB-21)
		Dashu	(UB-11)
		Huoto's points	
Supplementary	:	Lieque	(L-7)
points		Shenmen	(H-7)
		Neiguan	(P-6)
		Yanglingquan	(GB-34)
		Shenmai	(UB-62)
		Zusanli	(St-36)
Ear points	:	Neck area	
		Sympathetic	
		Shenmen	
		Heart	

Stimulation

Mild electrical stimulation should be given for 20 to 30 minutes daily for 10 days. Course may be repeated after a rest of 5 to 7 days.

Remarks

Results are good but the effectiveness of therapy depends upon the duration of illness.

NOCTURNAL ENURESIS

Also commonly known as bed wetting, this condition is characterised by unintentional urination during sleep. The condition is common in children. Before the diagnosis is made, any gross urologic abnormality should be ruled out. The intermittent passage of urine in infancy is governed by a spinal reflex. The control of micturition by higher cerebral centres is achieved in the second year of life. Bed wetting after the age of 3 years is considered abnormal. The incidence of this condition is 12.5 per cent at the age of 5 years, 5 per cent at the age of 9 years, and less that 1 per cent at puberty. The condition usually occurs in those children who receive toilet training at the later age. The organic conditions which should be excluded are diabetes mellitus, diabetes insipidus, chronic renal failure, urinary tract infection and mental retardation.

Main points	:		
	Group A	Qugu	(CV-2)
		Zhongji	(CV-3)
		Guanyuan	(CV-4)
		Guilai	(St-29)

Group B	Yaoyangguan	(GV-3)
	Shenshu	(UB-23)
	Dachangshu	(UB-25)
	Ciliao	(UB-32)
Supplementary	: Baihui	(GV-20)
points	Shenmen	(H-7)
	Neiguan	(P-6)
	Weizhong	(UB-40)
	Zusanli	(St-36)
	Sanyinjiao	(Sp-6)
	Taixi	(K-3)
Ear points	: Kidney	
	Urinary bladder	
	Shenmen	
	Subcortex	
	Sympathetic	
	Urethera	
Scalp needling	: Foot sensoro-motor area	
	Genital area	

Stimulation
1. Mild electrical stimulation should be given for 20 to 30 minutes daily for 10 to 15 days. Course may be repeated after a rest of 5 to 7 days.
2. Moxibustion can be done on the Guanyuan (CV-4), Zhongwan (CV-12) and Mingmen (GV-4) for 5 to 10 minutes daily.
3. Tapping with seven star needle on Huato's point on lumbosacral region on alternate day.
4. Injection of vitamin B_1, B_{12}, 0.5 to 1 ml can be given on any of the following points: Shenshu (UB-23), Dachangshu (UB-25), Guanyuan (CV-4), and Sanyinjiao (Sp-6) on alternate days.

Remarks
1. Prognosis is good.
2. Proper investigations should be carried out to exclude any organic cause.

MENTAL RETARDATION

Mental retardation may accompany cerebral palsy or may occur alone. The problem is one of the most difficult of all for the physician and one of the most dreadful of all for the parents. The milestones of development are delayed, the intelligence quotient is below 70, the development of speech and motor functions is slow, physical growth is usually retarded and the sphincter control may be absent. Associated craniovertebral or neurologic abnormalities may be seen.

Mental retardation may be a manifestation of chromosomal abnormalities like mangolism, Turner's syndrome or Kleinfelter's syndrome. On the other hand it may form part of the clinical picture of certain hereditary disorders like aminoacidurias. Cranial defects like microcephaly may characterise such hereditary conditions. Cretinism, due to the deficiency of thyroxin, should always be ruled out in cases of mental retardation. Cretins have a stunted growth, thick rough skin, big tongue, and croaky voice. More common than all these conditions is a variety called simple mental retardation in which there is no structural defect in the skeletal or nervous system. The condition is thought to be familial. These patients show an increased tendency for convulsions.

Main points	:	Baihui	(GV-20)
		Sishencong	(Ex-6)
		Yiming	(Ex-7)
		Touwai	(St-8)
Supplementary	:	Shendao	(GV-11)
points		Xianshu	(UB-15)
		Shenmen	(H-7)
		Neiguan	(P-6)
		Yanglingquan	(GB-34)
		Zusanli	(St 36)
		Sanyinjiao	(Sp-6)
		Qihai	(CV-6)
Ear points		Subcortex	
		Symathetic	
		Brain stem	
		Heart	
		Gall bladder	

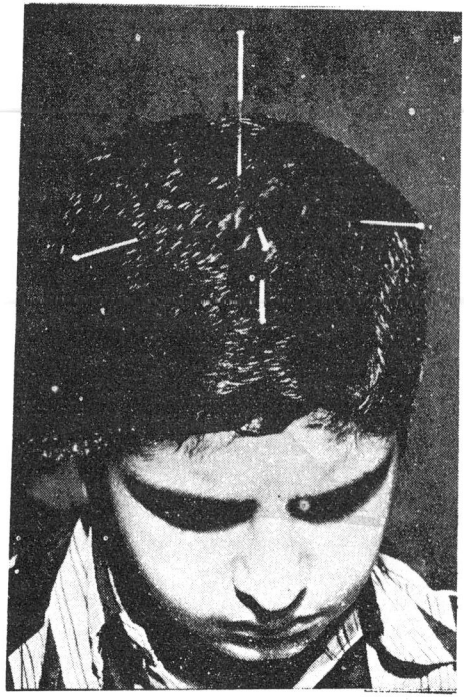

Mental retardness

Stimulation

Mild stimulation should be given for 20 to 30 minutes daily for one month. Course may be repeated after a rest of two weeks.

Remarks

1. A long term acupuncture therapy is advised.
2. Improvement is slow.

HYSTERIA

In hysteria symptoms of illness are represented by the patient for some advantage without being fully conscious of this motive. Poor sexual adjustment, mental stress, disagreeable circumstances and suppression of ideas may precipitate hysteria. A probable hereditary background is also considered to be present.

The sensory and motor symptoms of hysteria mimic organic neurologic diseases and include blindness, deafness, hypoaesthesia, paralysis spasm, tremors, difficulty in swallowing (globus hystericus) and aphonia. A careful neurologic examination can easily prove them to be of hysterical origin. The quasipsychotic symptoms include delirium, confusion, stupor and loss of memory.

Hysteria, where the patient is indifferent to and unaware of his symptoms, has to be differentiated from malingering in which the patient is aware of his symptoms and the motive.

Main points	:	Baihui	(GV-20)
		Sishencong	(Ex-6)
		Anmian I	(Ex-8)
		Anmian II	(Ex-9)
		Tianzhu	(UB-10)
Supplementary points	:	Tongli	(H-5)
		Shenmen	(H-7)
		Neiguan	(P-6)
		Hegu	(LI-4)
		Waiguan	(TW-5)
		Taixi	(K-3)
		Sanyinjiao	(Sp-6)
		Shenmai	(UB-62)
		Femur zhongdu	(GB-32)
Points during attack	:	Yongquan	(K-1)
		Renzhong	(GV-26)
		Jing-well points	

POINTS ACCORDING TO SYMPTOMS

Globus hystericus	:	Tiantu	(CV-22)
		Leique	(L-7)
Aphonia	:	Lianquan	(CV-23)
		Yinxi	(H-6)
Loss of vision	:	Yintang	(Ex-1)
		Taiyang	(Ex-2)
		Yuyao	(Ex-3)
		Qiuhou	(Ex-4)
		Chengqi	(St-1)
		Yangbai	(GB-14)
Ear points	:	Heart	
		Kidney	
		Shenmen	
		Subcortex	
		Sympathetic	

Stimulation

1. During the acute attack all Jing-well points should be given strong hand stimulation.
2. During the routine therapy body points can be given mild electrical stimulation.

Remarks

1. Apart from acupuncture, efforts must be made to abolish the precipitating factors.
2. Prognosis is good.

SCHIZOPHRENIA

The condition is characterised by a slow, steady deterioration of the personality, particularly involving thinking, conduct, and depth of insight. The precise aetiology is not known. Hereditary factors are thought to be responsible for some of the cases. There is a slowly progressive withdrawal from reality. Alteration of mood may manifest in the form of euphoria or depression. Speech and behaviour become irrelevant, irrational or delusional. Delusions of grandeur or persecution are often present. Logical reasoning becomes impossible. Disturbances of consciousness, memory and orientation are present.

Main points	:	Baihui	(GV-20)
		Renzhong	(GV-26)
		Sishencong	(Ex-6)
		Anmian I	(Ex-8)
		Anmian II	(Ex-9)
Supplementary points	:	Dazhui	(GV-14)
		Shenmen	(H-7)
		Daling	(P-7)
		Shenmai	(UB-62)
		Fenglong	(St-40)
		Yanglingquan	(GB-34)

POINTS ACCORDING TO SYMPTOMS

For auditory hallucinations	:	Tinchui	(GB-2)
		Quanliao	(SI-18)
		Waiguan	(TW-5)
		Yifeng	(TW-17)
		Ermen	(TW-21)
		Hegu	(LI-14)
For visual hallucinations	:	Xingjian	(Liv-2)
		Jingming	(UB-1)
		Yuyao	(Ex-3)
		Hegu	(LI-4)
Ear points	:	Shenmen	
		Subcortex	
		Brainstem	
		Sympathetic	
		Heart	
		Liver	
Point injection		Xinshu	(UB-15)
		Geshu	(UB-17)
		Jianshi	(P-5)
		Shenmen	(H-7)
		Zusanli	(St-36)

Doses : 1 to 2 mg of diazepam can be injected in any of the above points.

Stimulation

1. For the meniac type of patient continuous stimulation should be given until the patient becomes quiet.
2. For the depressive type of patient regular treatment can be given for 10 to 15 days and course can be repeated after a rest of 7 to 10 days.
3. Mild electrical stimulation can be given to the body points.

Remarks

1. Psychotherapy should be combined with acupuncture.
2. The improvement is slow but satisfactory results are often achieved.

21
NEUROLOGICAL DISEASES

HEADACHE

Headache, along with fatigue, hunger and thirst, represent man's most frequent discomforts. The significance of headache is dual. It may be benign and represent symptomatic expression of the affairs of the day or it may be symptom of a potentially malignant diseases like intracranial tumour.

MECHANISMS OF HEADACHE

Headache occurs due to stretching, irritation, or inflammation of various pain sensitive structures in the cranium. The mechanisms include :
1. Dilation of cranial arteries, e.g. migrane.
2. Muscular spasm, e.g. tension headache.
3. Stretching or inflammation of delicate structures of eye, ear, nasal cavity and paranasal sinuses, e.g. sinusitis.
4. Stretching or irritation of sensory cranial and cervical nerves, e.g. osteoarthritis of cervical spine.
5. Irritation of meninges, e.g. meningitis, subarachnoid haemorrhage.
6. Increased intracranial pressure, e.g. brain tumour.

DIFFERENTIAL DIAGNOSIS

Tension headache is the most common variety of headache. It occurs in the presence of psychological stress, is located over the top of the head or in the occipital region, and lasts for a period of days to weeks. Premenstrual and menopausal headache is of this variety. Eye strain headache, due to errors of refraction, is precipitated by acts like reading, driving, or watching a movie and is situated over forehead or temples and sometimes in the occipital region. Headache due to sinusitis is more severe in the morning and increases on stooping.

Unilateral headache of migraine has been discussed later. Severe headache of sudden onset is characteristic of subarachnoid haemorrhage. The CSF is haemorrhagic. Similar headache of less sudden onset occurs in meningitis.   It is associated with vomiting, fever, neck rigidity and characteristic CSF picture (raised pressure, proteins and cells).

Pain in the occipital region and neck rigidity, not uncommonly occur due to irritation of cervical nerves in diseases of the cervical spine like osteoarthritis and tuberculosis.   X-ray of the cervical spine is confirmatory.

Intracranial tumours are characterised by headache, projectile vomiting, papilloedema, and localising neurological signs.   Headache following head injury may occur due to subdural haematoma or as a part of posttraumatic nervous irritability.

Main points	:	Baihui	(GV-20)
		Yiming	(Ex-7)
Supplementary points	:	Hegu	(LI-4)
		Yanglingquan	(GB-34)
		Zusanli	(St-36)

FRONTAL HEADACHE

Main points	:	Baihui	(GV-20)
		Touwei	(St-8)
		Yintang	(Ex-1)
		Sishencong	(Ex-6)
Supplementary points	:	Hegu	(LI-4)
		Neiting	(St-44)
		Yanglingquan	(GB-34)
Ear points	:	Shenmen	
		Subcortex	
		Sympathetic	
		Heart	

Scalp needling
1.   Faciomandibular area
2.   Sensory area, lower two-fifths (both sides)

TEMPORAL HEADACHE

Main points	:	Baihui	(GV-20)
		Touwei	(St-8)
		Shuaigu	(GB-8)
		Fengchi	(GB-20)
Supplementary points	:	Taiyang	(Ex-2)
		Hegu	(LI-4)
		Yemen	(TW-2)
		Waiguan	(TW-5)
		Yanglingquan	(GB-34)
Ear points	:	Same as above	

OCCIPITAL HEADACHE

Main points	:	Baihui	(GV-20)	
		Fengchi	(GB-20)	
		Tianzhu	(UB-10)	
		Dazhui	(GV-14)	
		Anmian I	(Ex-8)	
		Anmian II	(Ex-9)	
Supplementary points	:	Hegu	(LI-4)	
		Lieque	(L-7)	
		Yanglao	(SI-6)	Strong manual Stimuli
		Yanglingquan	(GB-34)	

HEADACHE AT VERTEX

Main points	:	Baihui	(GV-20)
		Sishencong	(Ex-6)
		Touwei	(St-8)
		Fengchi	(GB-20)
Supplementary points	:	Hegu	(LI-4)
		Zhiyin	(UB-67)
		Taichong	(Liv-3)
		Neiting	(St-44)
Ear points	:	Same as above.	

Stimulation

Mild electrical stimulation should be given to all the body points. Strong manual stimulation to Hegu (LI-4) should be given, in case of severe headache.

Remarks
1. Proper investigations should be carried out to exclude any pathological cause for headache.
2. Prognosis with acupuncture is excellent in cases of tension headache.
3. Even when headache is due to an organic condition relief can be obtained with acupuncture but the underlying pathology should be simultaneously treated.

MIGRAINE

Migraine is a condition characterised by attacks of hemicranial pain associated with nausea, vomiting, visual disturbances, and less often, other neurological abnormalities. During the episode there is initial vasoconstriction followed by dilatation of extracranial, and sometimes intracranial, arteries. These changes are induced by the release of serotonine, adrenaline and noradrenaline, to which the arteries of migranous individuals are particularly sensitive. A hereditary background exists.

The episodes begin in second decade of life and diminish in frequency as the age advances. Each episode usually begins in the morning with throbbing unilateral headache which lasts upto a day or two and is relieved by sleep. Visual disturbances are common at the onset and include bright spots, scotomas, homonymous hemianopia, diplopia, ptosis and extracular palsies. Other neurological abnormalities like paresis, aphasia, staggering, confusion, etc. are less common. Nausea and vomiting are present throughout the attack. As contrasted to this, "classic" variety, "common" migraine may present with headache alone.

Migraine should be differentiated from cluster headache which has an onset at night and lasts for an hour or two. The attacks reoccur each night for a few weeks or months followed by relief for many years.

Main points	: Baihui	(GV-20)
	Touwei	(St-8)
	Shuaigu	(GB-8)
	Fengchi	(GB-20)
Supplementary points	: Hegu	(LI-4)
	Quchi	(LI-11)
	Taichong	(Liv-3)
	Ququan	(Liv-8)
	Yanglingquan	(GB-34)
	Guangming	(GB-37)
	Jingqu	(L-8)
	Waiguan	(TW-5)
Ear points	: Shenmen	
	Subcortex	
	Kidney	
	Gall bladder	
	Liver	
Scalp needling	: Sensory area, lower two-fifths (both sides)	

Migraine

TREATMENT ACCORDING TO SYMPTOMS

Insomnia

Main points	: Baihui	(GV-20)
	Sishencong	(Ex-6)
	Pishu	(UB-20)
	Anmian I	(Ex-8)
	Anmian II	(Ex-9)
	Yamen	(GV-15)
Supplementary points	: Shenmen	(H-7)
	Hegu	(LI-4)
	Zusanli	(St-36)

Headache with loss of appetite and nausea

Main points	: Baihui	(GV-20)
	Sishencong	(Ex-6)
	Touwei	(St-8)
	Shuaigu	(GB-8)
	Fengchi	(GB-20)

Supplementary points	:	Zhongwan	(CV-12)
		Zusanli	(St-36)
		Hegu	(LI-4)

Headache with Vomiting

Main points	:	Baihui	(GV-20)
		Sishencong	(Ex-6)
		Fengchi	(GB-20)
		Touwei	(St-8)
Supplementary points	:	Neiguan	(P-6)
		Zusanli	(St-36)
		Zhongwan	(CV-12)
		Hegu	(LI-4)
		Shenmen	(H-7)

Stimulation

Mild electrical stimulation should be given to body points only for 20 to 30 minutes daily for 10 days. Course may be repeated after a rest of 5 to 7 days.

Remarks

Acupuncture has been proved quite effective in cases of migraine.

TRIGEMINAL NEURALGIA

A functional disorder of the sensory ganglion of the trigeminal nerve, trigeminal neuralgia is characterised by attacks of severe pain over face. The condition mostly occurs in the middle aged persons. The frequency may vary from many attacks in a day to a few every year. Each attack begins abruptly, lasts for a few seconds to two minutes, and is characterized by severe piercing, burning, or constricting pain in the cheeks, gums and lips. Chin is less often affected and the forehead rarely. An attack may be precipitated by the stimulation of "trigger zones" in the area affected by pain. Such stimuli may be chewing, movements of facial muscles during speech, or a cold wind. There is no sensory loss.

This clinical picture is so typical that there is no difficulty in distinguishing other types of facial pain as are caused by the diseases of the teeth and paranasal sinuses. Pain similar to that of trigeminal neuralgia may occur due to tumours pressing on the nerve but it is associated with a sensory loss. Trigeminal neuralgia may occur as a part of the clinical picture of multiple sclerosis.

PAIN IN THE REGION OF OPHTHALMIC BRANCH

Main points	:	Tongziliao	(GB-1)
		Tinghui	(GB-2)
		Yangbai	(GB-14)
		Taiyang	(Ex-2)
		Touwei	(St-8)
		Sizhukong	(TW-23)
		Ah-shi points	

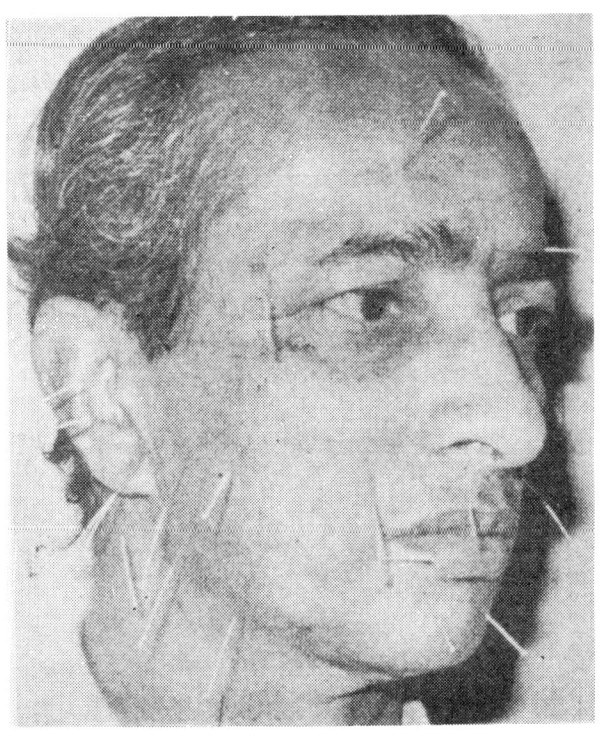

Trigeminal neuralgia

Supplementary	:	Baihui	(GV-20)
points		Hegu	(LI-4)
		Quchi	(LI-11)
		Neiting	(St-44)
		Yifeng	(TW-17)
		Yanglingquan	(GB-34)

PAIN IN THE REGION OF MAXILLARY BRANCH

Main points	:	Sibai	(St-2)
		Juliao	(ST-3)
		Jiache	(St-6)
		Renzhong	(GV-26)
		Quanliao	(SI-18)
		Yingxiang	(LI-20)
		Ah-shi points	
Supplementary	:	Baihui	(GV-20)
points		Hegu	(LI-4)
		Quchi	(LI-11)
		Neiting	(St-44)
		Yifeng	(TW-17)
		Yanglingquan	(GB-34)

PAIN IN THE REGION OF MANDIBULAR BRANCH

Main points	:	Dicang	(St-4)
		Daying	(St-5)
		Jiache	(St-6)
		Chengjiang	(CV-24)
		Jiachengjiang	(Ex-5)
		Tinghui	(GB-2)
		Yifeng	(TW-17)
		Ah-shi points	
Supplementary	:	Hegu	(LI-4)
points		Quchi	(LI-11)
		Neiting	(St-44)
		Yanglingquan	(GB-34)
Ear points			
for head area	:	Maxilla	
		Mandible	
		Sympathetic	
		Shenmen	
		Faciomandibular area	
Scalp acupuncture	:	Lower to one-fifth of the motor and sensory area	
Point injection	:	For ophthalmic branch : Zanzhu	(UB-2)
		For maxillary branch : Sibai	(St-2)
		For mandibular branch : Jiache	(St-6)

1.0 ml of procain 2% with 5 ml of analgin with 0.5 ml of vitamin B_{12} can be injected into the respective point on the effected site.

Stimulation

Mild to moderate electrical stimulation for 20 to 30 minutes once or twice a day for 10 to 20 days. Course may be repeated after a rest of 7 to 10 days.

Remarks

Excellent results have been recorded in all the cases treated by the authors.

BELL'S PALSY

The seventh cranial (facial) nerve is basically a motor nerve that supplies all the muscles of facial expression. It also carries the taste sensation from anterior two-thirds of the tongue after the chorda tympani joins it in the middle ear. Though it may be affected by various pathological processes anywhere in its course, the term Bell's Palsy is reserved for its affection at the stylomastoid foramen (through which it emerges out of the cranium) by a nonspecific inflammatory process.

The onset is acute. Pain behind the ear for a day or two may precede the paralysis. The affected side of the face shows absence of wrinkling on the forehead, widening of the palpabral fissure, smoothening of the nasolabial furrow and drooping of the angle of mouth. On attempted closure of the eyes the eyeball rolls upwards (Bell's phenomenon). Food collects under the involved cheek and saliva dribbles out of the mouth. The taste sensation is not impaired. 80 per cent cases recover fully within a few weeks.

Main points

Group I :	Sibai	(St-2)
	Dicang	(St-4)
	Zanzhu	(UB-2)
	Yangbai	(GB-14)
Group II	Jingming	(UB-1)
	Quchi	(LI-11)
	Yingxiang	(LI-20)
	Sizhukong	(TW-23)
Group III	Yifeng	(TW-17)
	Daimai	(GB-26)
	Taiyang	(Ex-2)
	Jiachengjiang	(Ex-5)
	Jujue	(CV-14)
Supple- :	Baihui	(GV-20)
mentary	Hegu	(LI-4)
points	Quchi	(LI-11)
	Yanglao	(SI-6)
	Yanglingquan	(GB-34)
	Zusanli	(St-36)

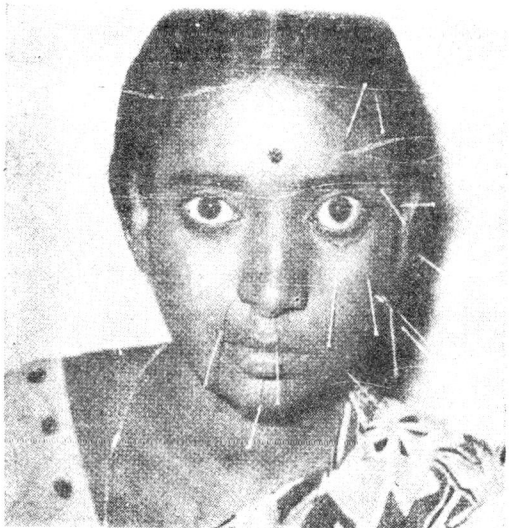

Bell's Palsy

POINTS ACCORDING TO SYMPTOMS

A. If the nasolabial : us is slanting obviously the saliva can drop from the angle of mouth. In this c dition following points may be used :

Renzhong	(GV-26)
Jiache	(St-6)
Dicang	(St-4)
Jiachengjiang	(Ex-5)
Chengjiang	(CV-24)

B. Pain in the mastoid region :

Yifeng	(TW-17)

Ear Acupuncture Therapy

Shenmen

Fascio mandibular area

Scalp Acupuncture Therapy

Lower one-fifth of the motor area.

Technique

Select the point from the group described above acupuncture points to the part affected Supplementary points should also be taken in all the cases.

Stimulation

In all the cases of facial paralysis electrostimulator is advisable. Mild to moderate electrical stimulation of adjustable type of current should be given for 10 days.

The therapy can be repeated after a rest of 5 to 7 days.

Point injection therapy

Daying	(St-5)
Xiaguan	(St-7)
Taiyang	(Ex-2)
Yifeng	(TW-17)
Hegu	(LI-4)

Injection of 50 to 100 mg of vitamin B_1 can be given in any of the above points on alternate days.

Prognosis

Complete cure can be expected with 2 to 3 course of the therapy.

Remarks

1. Moxibustion can also be applied on the same side.
2. Other causes of facial palsy should be excluded.
3. Prognosis is good.

SQUINT

Binocular vision is dependent upon a parallel axis of both the eyes. Squint refers to an ocular imbalance that results in an improper alignment of the two eyes. This may be due to the paralysis of the muscles which move the eyes (paralytic squint). The extraocular muscles which move the eye are supplied by 3rd, 4th and 6th cranial nerves. These nerves and their nuclei in the brainstem may be affected by conditions like tumours, meningitis, cerebrovascular disease, and degenerative diseases. If the eye movements are tested, that performed by the affected muscle will be found to be impaired. Squint not due to the paralysis of the extraocular muscles is called concomitant squint. The eye movements, if tested separately for each eye, will be found to be normal. Concomitant squint usually accompanies dimness of vision in one eye. Squint is associated with diplopia (seeing two images of one object) as the images of an object fall on noncorresponding parts of the two retinas.

Main points	:	Touwei	(St-8)
		Dazhui	(GV-14)
		Yintang	(Ex-1)
		Taiyang	(Ex-2)
		Yuyao	(Ex-3)
		Sizhukong	(TW-23)
Supplementary points	:	Baihui	(GV-20)
		Feiyang	(UB-58)
		Hegu	(LI-4)
		Taichong	(Liv-3)
		Yanglingquan	(GB-34)

Ear points	:	Eye area
		Eye I
		Eye II
		Shenmen
		Subcortex
Scalp needling	:	Motor area lower two-thirds (both side)

Stimulation

Mild electrical stimulation may be given 20 to 30 minutes daily for 10 days. Course may be repeated after a rest of 5 to 7 days.

Remarks

1. Concomitant squint should be treated on the lines of treatment for the underlying cause of dimness of vision.
2. Paralytic squint responds very well to acupuncture therapy.

PTOSIS

Drooping of the upper eyelid, ptosis, results from paralysis of the levator palpabrae superioris which lifts the eyelid. This muscle is innervated by the oculomotor nerve which may be affected by various conditions—traumatic, inflammatory, neoplastic, etc.—at the base of the skull. Ptosis is also a feature of Horner's syndrome which occurs due to sympathetic paralysis.

Main points	:	Touwei	(St-8)
		Yangbai	(GB-14)
		Sizhukong	(CV-23)
		Zanzhu	(UB-2)
		Yintang	(Ex-1)
		Yuyao	(Ex-3)
Supplementary points	:	Baihui	(GV-20)
		Sishencong	(Ex-6)
		Waiguan	(TW-5)
		Shenmen	(H-7)
		Zusanli	(St-36)
		Feiyang	(UB-58)
		Yanglingquan	(GB-34)
Ear points	:	Eye area	
		Faciomandibular area	
		Subcortex	
		Shenmen	

Stimulation

Mild electrical stimulation should be given 20 to 30 minutes daily for 10 days. Course may be repeated after a rest of 5 to 7 days.

Remarks

Results are very good.

HEMIPLEGIA

Weakness of one half of the body (hemiplegia) is almost always occurs due to the lesions of the corticospinal tract. This tract which begins from the motor cortex and supplies all the muscles on the opposite side may be involved at different sites. The site or level of the lesion can be assessed from the accompanying neurological signs.

Cortical and subcortical lesions produce incomplete hemiplegia and disorders of speech. In addition, cortical lesions also produce convulsions. Lesions in the internal capsule produce complete hemiplegia with involvement of the face on opposite side. Lesions in the midbrain are associated with hemiplegia on the opposite side and oculomotor paralysis on the same side. Pontine lesions give rise to crossed hemiplegia in which the limbs are paralysed on the opposite side and facial and abducent nerves on the same side. In medullary lesions contralateral hemiplegia is associated with ipsilateral vagus or hypoglossal paralysis. In lesions of the cervical spinal cord hemiplegia is on the same side and cranial nerves are spared.

The commonest cause of hemiplegia is cerebrovascular disease (haemorrhage, embolism, thrombosis) in which the onset is acute. Trauma (cerebral contusion, subdural haematoma) is another common cause of hemiplegia. Other conditions which may cause hemiplegia of a comparatively slow onset are cerebral abscess, encephalitis, tuberculous meningitis, brain tumours and demyelinating diseases.

PARALYSIS OF UPPER EXTREMITY

Main points

Group	I	: Hegu	(LI-4)
		Quchi	(LI-11)
		Binao	(LI-14)
		Jianyu	(LI-15)
		Jianjing	(GB-21)
Group	II	: Yemen	(TW-2)
		Waiguan	(TW-5)
		Zhigou	(TW-6)
		Tianjing	(TW-10)
		Jianliao	(TW-14)
Group	III	: Yanggu	(SI-5)
		Yanglao	(SI-6)
		Jianzhen	(SI-9)
		Naoshu	(SI-10)
		Baxie	(Ex-28)
Group	IV	: Shenmen	(H-7)
		Shaohai	(H-3)
		Yunmen	(L-2)
		Taiyuan	(L-9)
		Chize	(L-5)
		Daling	(P-7)
		Neiguan	(P-6)

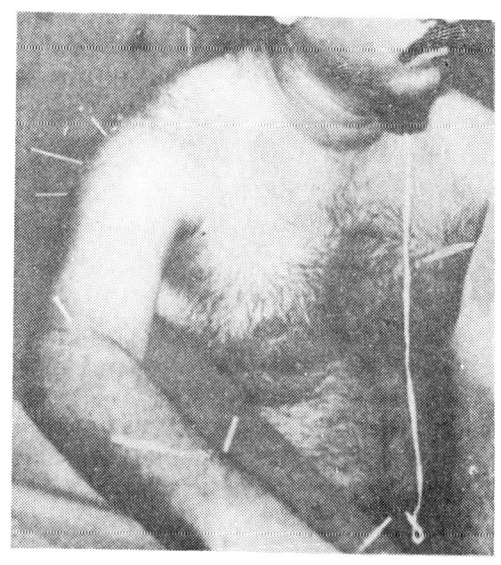

Hemiplegia

Supplementary points	:	Baihui	(GV-20)
		Zusanli	(St-36)
		Yanglingquan	(GB-34)

PARALYSIS OF LOWER EXTREMITY

Main points			
Group I	:	Chengfu	(UB-36)
		Yinmen	(UB-37)
		Weizhong	(UB-40)
		Chengshan	(UB-57)
		Shenmai	(UB-62)
Group II	:	Fengshi	(GB-31)
		Yanglingquan	(GB-34)
		Xuanzhong	(GB-39)
Group III	:	Baiguan	(St-31)
		Femerfutu	(St-32)
		Zusanli	(St-36)
		Fenglong	(St-40)
		Jiexi	(St-41)
		Neiting	(St-44)
Group IV	:	Sanyinjiao	(Sp-6)
		Yinlingquan	(Sp-9)
		Taixi	(K-3)
		Shuiquan	(K-5)
		Zhongdu	(Liv-6)

Supplementary points	:	Baihui	(GV-20)
		Hegu	(LI-4)
		Quze	(P-3)
		Taiyuan	(L-9)
Ear points		Upper extremity	
		Lower extremity	
		Shenmen	
		Subcortex	
		Brain area	
Scalp Needling	:	Motor area and sensory area, opposite site.	

Stimulation

Electro-acupuncture therapy once daily for 20 to 30 minutes for 10 days.

Mild to moderate electricity with adjustable or dense and disperse variety of the current should be used.

Remarks

1. Indirect moxibustion can be used.
2. Active physiotherapy should be advised.
3. Underlying diseases like hypertension and diabetes should be treated simultaneously.
4. If spasticity is more electrical stimulation should be given only at the following points:
       Yaoqi   (Ex-20)
       Jizhong   (GV-6)
5. Prognosis depends upon the underlying cause.

PARAPLEGIA

Weakness of both the lower limbs (paraplegia) occurs in diseases of the spinal cord, nerve roots and the peripheral nerves. Lesions of the spinal cord produce spastic paraplegia in which the muscle tone is increased (spasticity), muscle wasting is absent or late, reduction of muscle power in affected muscles is uniform, jerks are exaggerated, plantars are extensor, and the bladder is involved causing retention of urine. As opposed to this, lesions of the peripheral nerves and roots produced flaccid paraplegia in which muscle tone is reduced (flaccidity), muscle wasting is early, decrease in muscle power is more in the distal muscles, jerks are reduced, plantars are flexor, bladder is not involved, and root pains may be present.

Spastic paraplegia is more common than flaccid paraplegia. Pott's paraplegia is one of the common varieties of spastic paraplegia. Examination of the spine reveals gibbus and localised tenderness, and X-ray of the spine shows reduction of the intervertebral spaces and destruction of the vertebral bodies. Other common causes of spastic paraplegia are lathyrism and transverse myelitis. Fracture dislocation of the spine, tumours of the spinal cord, disseminated sclerosis, subacute combined degeneration of the cord, syphilis, motor neurone disease and syringomyelia are some of the uncommon conditions causing spastic paraplegia. Flaccid paraplegia may occur due to prolapsed intervertebral disc, epidural tumours, spinal epidural abscess and peripheral neuropathy.

Main points	:		
Group I		Huantiao	(GB-30)
		Fengshi	(GB-31)
		Yanglingquan	(GB-34)
		Guangming	(GB-37)
Group II		Biguan	(St-31)
		Femerfutu	(St-32)
		Zusanli	(St-36)
		Xiajuxu	(St-39)
		Jiexi	(St-41)
		Bafeng	(Ex-36)
Group III	:	Chengfu	(UB-36)
		Yinmen	(UB-37)
		Weizhong	(UB-40)
		Chengshan	(UB-57)
		Kunlun	(UB-60)
Supplementary points	:	Yaoshu	(GV-2)
		Yaoyangguan	(GV-3)
		Xuanshu	(GV-5)
		Shenshu	(UB-23)
		Dachangshu	(UB-25)
		Huatuojiaji points	(Ex-21)
		Baihui	(GV-20)
Ear points	:	Lumbo sacral area	
		Buttock area	
		Lower extremity area	
		Shenmen	
		Subcortex	
		Brainstem	
Scalp needling	:	1. Motor area upper one-fifth (both sides)	
		2. Sensory area upper one-fifth (both sides)	
		3. Foot sensoro-motor area	

POINTS ACCORDING TO SYMPTOMS

For retention of urine :

Local points	:	Shenshu	(UB-23)
		Dachangshu	(UB-25)
		Yaoyangguan	(GV-3)
		Qugu	(CV-2)
		Guanyuan	(CV-4)
		Guilai	(St-29)
Supplementary points	:	Taixi	(K-3)
		Sanyinjiao	(Sp-6)
		Weizhong	(UB-40)
		Yanglingquan	(GB-34)

Ear points	:	Sympathetic
		Shenmen
		Kidney
		Urinary bladder
Scalp needling	:	Foot sensoro-motor area, genital area.

For retention of stools

Local points	:	Tianshu	(St-25)
		Guilai	(St-29)
		Ciliao	(UB-32)
		Yaoyangguan	(GV-3)
Supplementary points	:	Zusanli	(St-36)
		Yanglingquan	(GB-34)
		Hegu	(LI-4)
		Baihui	(GV-20)
Ear points	:	Large intestine area	
		Shenmen	
		Subcortex	
		Heart	
Scalp needling	:	Foot sensoro-motor area	
		Gastric area	

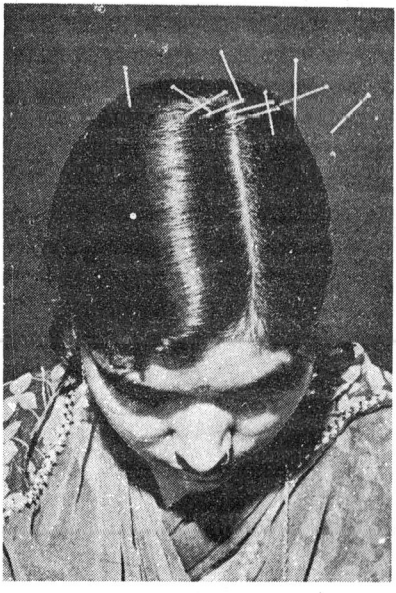

Paraplegia (scalp needling)

Stimulation

Moderate electrical stimulation can be given dally for 20 to 30 minutes for 2 weeks and course should be repeated after 5 to 7 days.

Remarks
1. Acupuncture should be combined with physiotherapy.
2. Electrical stimulation should not be used in spastic paraplegia.
3. Response is slow in spastic paraplegia

POLIOMYELITIS

Poliomyelitis is a viral infection which may produce involvement of the central nervous system. The neurological features of the disease are due to the involvement of anterior horn cells in the spinal cord and cells of the motor nuclei of the cranial nerves in the brainstem. Incidence of poliomyelitis is found all over the world. The disease is more common during the rainy season. The virus is present in the pharynx and intestines of the patient, transmission from where occurs by faecal-oral route.

In 95 per cent cases the infection is subclinical. Prodromal symptoms consist of fever, sorethroat, coryza, nausea and abdominal discomfort. In nonparalytic polio, only these features, along with neck rigidity and abnormal CSF picture, are present. In cases of paralytic polio paralysis ensues over these prodromal symptoms. Depending upon the site of motor weakness, paralytic polio may be classified into bulbar polio (cranial nerve involvement), spinal polio (spinal nerve involvement) and a combination of these two. The paralysed muscles are flaccid and undergo wasting and the concerned jerks are diminished. Sensory changes and signs of pyramidal involvement are never present.

In the acute stage death may occur due to respiratory paralysis, myocarditis, or pulmonary oedema. The overall mortality is 5 per cent. In those who survive, recovery is likely upto 2 years but 80 per cent improvement occurs in first six months. Lack of recovery from polio-paralysis is not an uncommon cause of permanent disability and deformities like wrist-drop-and foot drop.

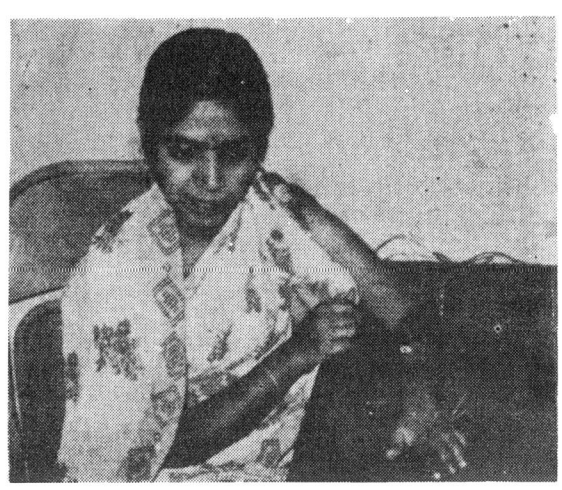

Poliomyelitis (U.E.)

PARALYSIS OF UPPER EXTREMITY

Main points

Group I	:	Hegu	(LI-4)
		Quchi	(LI-11)
		Binao	(LI-14)
		Jianyu	(LI.15)
		Jianjing	(GB-21)
Group II	:	Yemen	(TW-2)
		Waiguan	(TW-5)
		Tianjing	(TW-10)
		Jianliao	(TW-14)
Group III	:	Yanglao	(SI-6)
		Jianzhen	(SI-9)
		Naoshu	(SI-10)
		Baxie	(Ex-28)
Group IV	:	Shenmen	(H-7)
		Chize	(L-5)
		Taiyuan	(L-9)
		Quze	(P-3)
		Daling	(P-7)

Supplementary points   :   Yanglingquan   (GB-34)

PARALYSIS OF LOWER EXTREMITY

Group I   :   Chengfu   (UB-36)
                         Yinmen   (UB-37)
                         Weizhong   (UB-40)
                         Chengjin   (UB-56)
                         Kunlun   (UB-60)

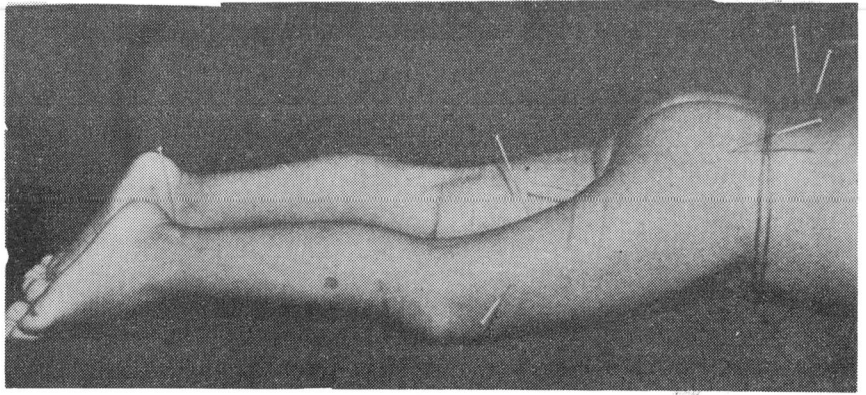

Poliomyelitis (lower extremity)

Group II   :   Huantiao   (GB-34)
                         Fengshi   (GB-31)
                         Yanglingquan   (GB-34)

Group III   :   Femurfutu   (ST-32)
                         Zusanli   (St-36)
                         Fenglong   (St-40)
                         Jiexi   (St-41)
                         Neiting   (St-44)

Group IV   :   Sanyinjiao   (Sp-6)
                         Yinlingquan   (Sp-9)
                         Xuehai   (Sp-10)
                         Taixi   (K-3)
                         Shuiquan   (K-5)
                         Ligou   (Liv-5)

Paralysis of diaphragm

                         Geshu   (UB-17)
                         Binao   (LI-14)
                         Yanglingquan   (GB-34)

Paralysis of abdominal muscles

Pishu	(UB-20)
Weishu	(UB-21)
Liangmen	(St-21)
Tianshu	(St-25)
Zusanli	(St-36)
Huangshu	(K-16)
Daheng	(Sp-15)
Yanglingquan	(GB-34)

POINTS ACCORDING TO SYMPTOMS

1.	Diarrhoea	Tianshu	(St-25)
		Zusanli	(St-36)
2.	Sorethroat	Tianrong	(SI-17)
		Quchi	(LI-11)
3.	Headache and vomiting	Yintang	(Ex-1)
		Neiguan	(P-6)

SEQUELAE OF POLIOMYELITIS

Hyperextension of Knee Joint

Main points

Group I	:	Fuxi	(UB-38)
		Weiyang	(UB-39)
		Weizhong	(UB-40)
		Chengjin	(UB-56)
Group II	:	Dubi	(St-35)
		Zusanli	(St-36)
		Yanglingquan	(GB-34)
		Heding	(Ex-31)
Group III	:	Heding	(Ex-31)
		Medial-Xiyan	(Ex-32)
		Ququan	(Liv-8)
		Yinlingquan	(Sp-9)
		Xuehai	(Sp-10)

Foot drop

Shangjuxu	(St-37)
Jiexi	(St-41)
Neiting	(St-44)
Yanglingquan	(GB-34)
Kunlun	(UB-60)

Extroversion of foot

Taixi	(K-3)
Sanyinjiao	(Sp-6)
Jiexi	(St-41)
Yanglingquan	(GB-34)

Introversion of foot

Kunlun	(UB-60)
Shenmai	(UB-62)
Jiexi	(St-41)
Yanglingquan	(GB-34)
Xuanzghong	(GB-39)

Facial paralysis

Jiache	(St-6)
Xiaguan	(St-7)
Yifeng	(TW-17)
Hegu	(LI-4)

Paralysis of neck muscles

Tianzhu	(UB-10)
Dashu	(UB-11)
Fengchi	(GB-20)
Tianrong	(SI-17)
Huato's point	(Ex-21)

Stimulation

During the actue stage points should be selected according to symptom and electrical stimulation should be avoided. After the active stage of disease has subsided the electro-stimulation should be given.

Electrical stimulation

Mild electrical stimulation for 20 minutes daily for 10 to 20 days and then the seeond course may be repeated after 7 to 10 days. The electricity may be started in adjustable wave and then it would be the ripple or saw tooth type.

After acupuncture massage to the affected area is also indicated.

Cat-gut therapy

Yanglingquan	(GB-34)
Zusanli	(St-36)
Sanyinjiao	(Sp-6)

Cat-gut should be used for any of the above points in the affected site. It can be repeated after 10 days.

Point injection

Chengshan	(UB-57)
Femurfutu	(St-32)
Zusanli	(St-36)

0.5 to 1.0 ml vitamin B complex can be injected in any of the above points on alternate days.

Remarks

1. Active acupuncture treatment with electrical stimulator should be used 3 weeks after the initial attack.

2.   Active exercise and physiotherapy should also be advised after acupuncture.
3.   In old cases corrective surgery can be advised after getting the muscle power with acupuncture therapy.

WRIST DROP

Wrist drop occurs due to paralysis of the extensors of the wrist which are innervated by the radial nerve. Radial nerve palsy is one of the commonest peripheral nerve afflictions due to its long course, its position in relation to the humerus and its vulnerability to compression when it winds around the humerus.

Radial nerve supplies the triceps muscle, supinators of the forearm, the extensors of the wrist and fingers, and the extensor and abductor muscles of the thumb. Its paralysis results into wrist drop, flexion of the fingers at metacarpophalangeal joints and inability to extend and abduct the thumb. Sensory changes are rarely found and may be in the form of hypoasthesia over the posterior aspect of forearm and a small area on the radial side of the dorsum of the hand. The most common site where the nerve is involved is behind the humerus where it might be affected by fracture of the middle third of humerus, pressure during sleep, an injection abscess and rarely, leprosy.

If radial nerve is involved in the axilla (e.g. "crutch palsy"), the triceps muscle is also paralysed resulting into inability to extend the elbow and loss of triceps jerk in addition to the wrist drop. Apart from radial nerve lesions wrist drop may occur due to involvement of anterior horn cells in poliomyelitis.

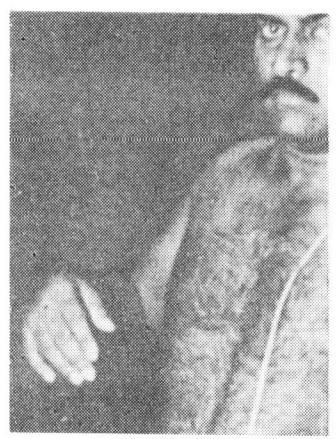

Wrist drop

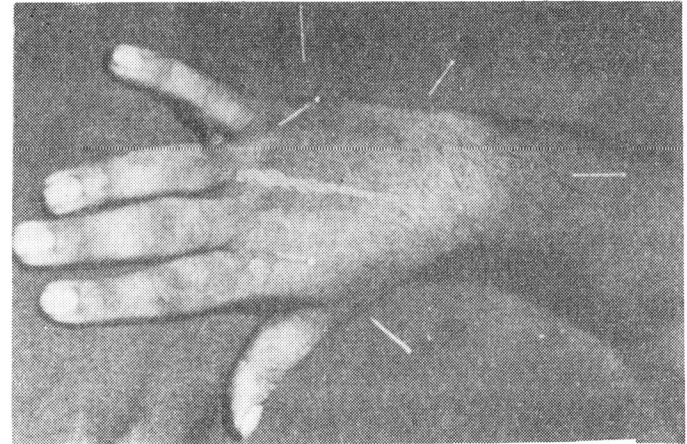

Wrist drop

Main points

Group I	:	Yemen	(TW-2)
		Zhongzhu	(TW-3)
		Waiguan	(TW-5)
Group II	:	Hegu	(LI-4)
		Yangxi	(LI-5)
		Quchi	(LI-11)

Group III	:	Shenmen	(H-7)
		Daling	(P-7)
		Taiyuan	(L-9)
Supplementary points	:	Yanglingquan	(GB-34)
Ear points	:	Wrist area	
Scalp acupuncture	:	Motor area	
		Sensory area	
		Middle to one-fifth opposite site	

Stimulation

Mild electrical stimulation 20 to 30 minutes daily for 10 to 15 days, second course may be repeated after a rest of 7 days.

Remarks

Physiotherapy should be advised.

Wrist drop splint may be used.

FOOT DROP

Foot drop results from paralysis of the dorsiflexors of ankle which are innervated by the common peroneal nerve. It is a branch of the sciatic nerve and supplies everters of the foot and dorsiflexors of the ankle and the toes. Its paralysis results into foot drop, eversion of the foot and flexion of the toes. Because of foot drop, the gait is of high stepping type. There is a sensory loss in the region of the lateral aspect of lower half of the leg and middle of dorsum of the foot.

Where it winds around the fibula, the nerve is involved by wounds, fracture of the upper end of the fibula, tight bandage and pressure in bedridden patients. The nerve is also affected in diabetes mellitus and leprosy. The roots which constitute the nerve (L-4, 5, S-1) may be affected by conditions causing sciatica. Poliomyelitis may be responsible for some cases of foot drop. Foot drop is also a feature in cases of hemiplegia and paraplegia due to upper motor neurone lesions because of the physiological increase in the tone of plantar flexors.

Main points			
Group I	:	Zusanli	(St-36)
		Fenglong	(St-40)
		Jiexi	(St-41)
		Neiting	(St-44)
Group II	:	Kunlun	(UB-60)
		Shenmai	(UB-62)
		Yanglingquan	(GB-34)
		Bafeng	(Ex-36)
Group III	:	Taixi	(K-3)
		Dazhong	(K-4)
		Sanyinjiao	(Sp-6)

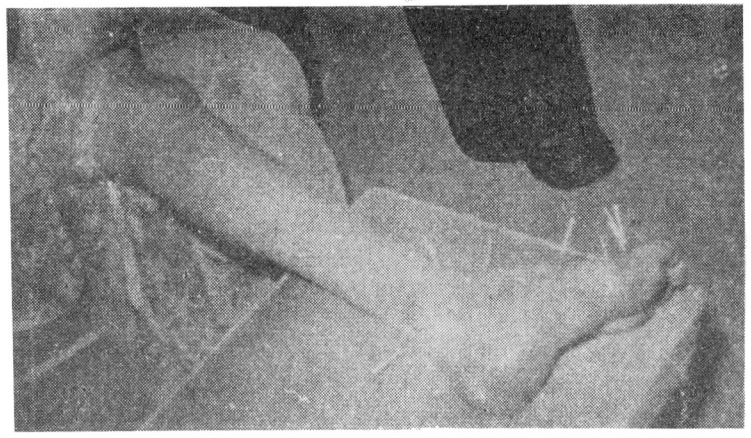

Foot drop

Ear acupuncture : Ankle area
Foot area
Scalp acupuncture : Motor area
Sensory area
Upper one-fifth of the above area is opposite site foot sensory area.

Stimulation
Electrical stimulation for 20 to 30 minutes daily for 10 days. Second course may be repeated after a rest of 7 to 10 days.

Remarks
Splints and physiotherapy should be advised simultaneously.

CEREBRAL PALSY

This name is employed to describe those conditions which are characterised by a major, usually nonprogressive disturbance of motor function since infancy or childhood. The aetiology and the distribution of motor weakness are varied. The disorder is broadly classified into spastic paralytic conditions, flaccid paralytic conditions and extrapyramidal disorders.

Conditions characterised by spastic weakness of the muscles
1. Infantile hemiplegia : Paralysis of one half of the body; usually follow birth trauma or encephalitis. There is a tendency for convulsions.
2. Double hemiplegia : Weakness involves all the limbs and the face. Arms are more affected than the legs.
3. Cerebral spastic diplegia : In this condition also all the limbs are affected but the weakness is more in the legs than in the arms. This usually results from foetal asphyxia.

4. Quadriplegic state : All the limbs are affected but the face is spared. A common cause is fracture or dislocation of the cervical spine during a difficult breech delivery.

Conditions characterised by flaccid weakness of the muscles

This group includes conditions like infantile spinal muscular atrophy, amyotonia congenita, and different types of plexus and nerve palsies.

EXTRAPYRAMIDAL DISORDERS

Though not always classified under the category of cerebral palsy, these disorders include double athetosis and congenital ataxia.

Cerebral palsy is usually accompanied by some degree of mental retardation.

Main points	:	Baihui	(GV-20)
		Sishencong	(Ex-6)
		Neiguan	(P-6)
		Shenmen	(H-7)
		Xinshu	(UB-15)
		Shendao	(GV-11)
		Shenmai	(UB-62)
Ear points	:	Shenmen	
		Subcortex	
		Brainstem	
		Heart	
		Gall bladder	
Scalp needling	:	Motor area	
		According to symptoms	

Stimulation

Mild stimulation should be given daily 20 to 30 minutes for 2 weeks. Course may be repeated after 10 days.

Remarks

1. The points described above are basically for mental retardation. The accompanying paralysis and other symptoms should be treated with appropriate points discussed in the respective chapters.
2. Because of the multitude, the symptoms have to be treated one by one according to the severity consequently, the recovery is slow.
3. Long-term acupuncture therapy is needed.

PERIPHERAL NEUROPATHY

This is a group of disorders characterised by inflammatory or degenerative changes in single or multiple motor or sensory nerves which manifest as muscular weakness, tingling, numbness, burning, or loss of sensation in the region of the affected nerve. The most common variety involves pepripheral nerves symmetrically causing sensory and motor symptoms in the distal parts of the limbs. This distribution is conventionally called glove and stocking. Generalised peripheral neuropathy is a result of systemic disorders like deficiency of certain vitamins (B_1 B_{12}, etc.) diabetes mellitus, and carcinoma. The condition is generally chronic, but one variety called Guillan Barre syndrome presents in acute manner. Involvement of the single peripheral nerve may be the result of injury, prolonged pressure, ischaemia, or leprosy.

FOR UPPER EXTREMITY

Main points

Group I   :   Hegu   (LI-4)
                              Quchi   (LI-11)
                              Jianyu   (LI-15)
                              Jianjing   (GB-21)
                              Waiguan   (TW-5)
                              Tianjing   (TW-10)

Group II   :   Shenmen   (H-7)
                              Quze   (P-3)
                              Daling   (P-7)
                              Lieque   (L-7)
                              Yunmen   (L-2)

Scalp needling   :   Sensory area middle two-fifths opposite side

Supplementary points   :   Yanglingquan   (GB-34)
                              Zusanli   (St-36)
                              Sanyinjiao   (Sp-6)
                              Taixi   (K-3)

Ear points   :   Heart
                              Upper extremity area
                              Internal secretion
                              Adrenaline

FOR LOWER EXTREMITY

Main points

Group I   :   Huantiao   (GB-30)
                              Fengshi   (GB-31)
                              Yanglingquan   (GB-34)
                              Guangming   (GB-37)
                              Chengfu   (UB-36)
                              Yinmen   (UB-37)
                              Weizhong   (UB-40)

Group II   :   Biguan   (St-31)
                              Femurfutu   (St-32)
                              Zusanli   (St-36)
                              Jiexi   (St-41)

Group III	:	Taixi	(K-3)
		Taichong	(Liv-3)
		Ququan	(Liv-8)
		Sanyinjiao	(Sp-6)
		Xuehai	(Sp-10)
Supplementary points	:	Baihui	(GV-20)
		Quchi	(LI-11)
Ear points	:	Lower extremity area	
		Shenmen	
		Subcortex	
		Heart	
		Internal secretion	
Scalp needling	:	Sensory area upper one-fifth opposite side.	

Stimulation

Mild electrical stimulation can be given 20 to 30 minutes daily for 10 days and the course may be repeated after a rest of 5 to 7 days.

Remarks

The underlying cause of the disease should be treated through modern medicine.
Prognosis is good.

POSTHERPETIC NEURALGIA

Herpes zoaster is a viral disease characterised by unilateral segmental inflammation of the posterior root ganglia or the sensory ganglia of the cranial nerves.

There is a vesicular eruption of the skin in the distribution of the involved nerve. When the ophthalmic nerve is involved, the condition is called herpes zoaster ophthalmicus and when the intercostal nerves are affected it is called herpes zoaster intercostalis. Apart from the vesicles, the involved area shows erythema and is intensely painful.

Postherpetic neuralgia is a serious complication of herpes zoaster which is usually limited to older patients suffering from arteriosclerosis. Severe incapacitating pain persists for weeks or months after the acute episode.

Following herpes zoaster ophthalmicus

Main points	:	Baihui	(GV-20)
		Touwei	(St-8)
		Shuaigu	(GB-8)
		Yangbai	(GB-14)
		Fengchi	(GB-20)
		Sizhukong	(TW-23)
		Quanliao	(SI-18)
		Tinggong	(SI-19)

Supplementary points	:	Hegu	(LI-4)
		Quchi	(LI-11)
		Dazhui	(GV-14)
		Waiguan	(TW-5)
		Yanglingquan	(GB-34)
		Zusanli	(St-36)
Ear points	:	Faciomandibular area	
		Shenmen	
		Subcortex	
		Internal secretion	
Scalp needling	:	Sensory area	
		Lower two-fifths (opposite side)	

Following herpes zoaster intercostalis

Main points	:	Zhongfu	(L-1)
		Shanzhong	(CV-17)
		Rugen	(St-18)
		Qimen	(Liv-14)
		Daimai	(GB-26)
		Huatuojiaji	(taping with seven star needles)
Supplementary points	:	Dazhui	(GV-14)
		Baihui	(GV-20)
		Hegu	(LI-4)
		Quchi	(LI-11)
		Yanglingquan	(GB-34)
		Zusanli	(St-36)
Ear points	:	Shenmen	
		Subcortex	
		Thoracic spine	
Scalp needling	:	Sensory area	
		Middle two-fifths (opposite side)	

Stimulation

Mild electrical stimulation should be given for 20 to 30 minutes daily for 10 days. Course may be repeated after a rest of 5 to 7 days.

Remarks

Acupuncture shows excellent results.

DISORDERS OF SPEECH

Speech is a highly developed and recently evolved function of man. For expression of ideas and emotions man remains dependent upon speech especially when he is affected by disease, the loss is probably much more than that due to blindness, deafness or lameness. Disorders of speech are often associated with mental disturbances.

When a person is not able to produce voice, it is called aphonia.   This is always hysterical. Disorders causing inability to understand or execute speech are called aphasia.   Aphasia is of various types:

1. Motor aphasia—inability to speak,
2. agraphia—inability to write,
3. word deafness—inability to understand spoken words,
4. word blindness—inability to understand written words,
5. nominal aphasia—gross inability to recall familiar words or names.

All these disorders are a result of affection of the speech centres situated in the dominant cerebral hemisphere.

Speech disorders in which the defect is in the articulation are called dysarthrias. Dysarthria may occur due to lesions of the pyramidal tracts or of cerebellum.   By far the commonest of this type of disorders is stammering.   Stammering is a spasmodic defect of articulation leading to a sudden check in the utterance of words or to a rapid repetition of the consonental sounds.   Spasmodic movements of face and head are also often present. There is no structural change in the organs of articulation.   It is more common in left handers, particularly if an attempt is made to change the handedness.

The individuals are of nervous temperament and the fault increases in presence of nervousness.   The defect becomes less with increase in age.   Hereditary background may be present in some of cases.

Aphasia

Main points	: Lianquan	(CV-23)
	Chengjiang	(CV-24)
	Jiachengjiang	(Ex-5)
	Tianrong	(SI-17)
	Neck Futu	(LI-18)

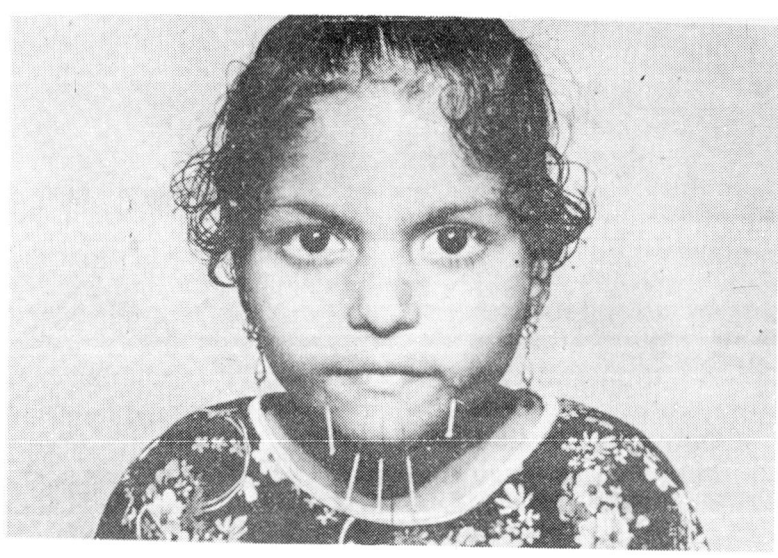

Aphasia

Supplementary points	:	Yamen	(GV-15)
		Baihui	(GV-20)
		Tongli	(H-5)
		Yinxi	(H-6)
		Hegu	(LI-4)
Ear points	:	Shenmen	
		Subcortex	
		Pharynx area	
		Laryinx	
		Heart	
Scalp needling	:	Language area 2	
		Language area 3	

Stammering Speech

Main points	:	Lianquan	(CV-23)
		Chengjiang	(CV-24)
		Jiachengjiang	(Ex-5)
		Neck Futu	(LI-18)
Supplementary points	:	Hegu	(LI-4)
		Tongli	(H-5)
		Waiguan	(TW-5)
		Neiguan	(P-6)
Ear points	:	Shenmen	
		Mouth area	
		Heart area	
		Sympathetic	

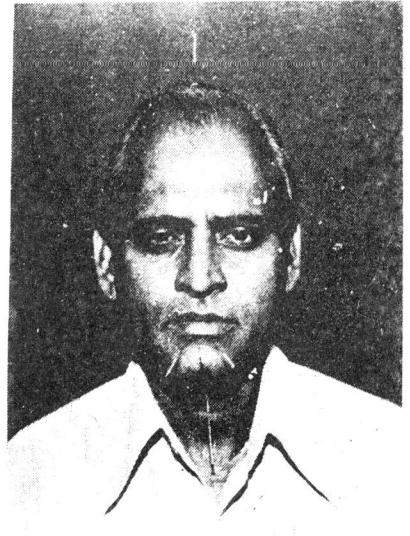

Stammering

Stimulation

Mild stimulations for 20 to 30 minutes daily for 10 days. Course may be repeated after a rest of 5 to 7 days.

Remarks

Acupuncture has been proved quite effective.

EPILEPSY

Epilepsy is the expression of a sudden. excessive, disorderly discharge of cerebral neurones resulting into instantaneous disturbances of sensation, loss of consciousness and convulsive movements. Epilepsy is of various types. Grand mal epilepsy is characterised by occurrence of aura (premonitory symptoms), generalised tonic and clonic convulsions, and unconsciousness. When such seizures occur so frequently that the patient remains unconscious till the next seizure the condition is called status epilepticus. Petit mal epilepsy is characterised by a brief loss of consciousness with the absence of all motor activity (akinetic seizure) or a single jerky movement of a limb (myoclonic seizure). Psychomotor epilepsy is characterised by complex abnormality of behaviour and movement. In jacksonian (focal) epilepsy convulsive movements involve only a part of the body and there is no loss of consciousness.

Most of the cases of epilepsy show no demonstrable structural defect in the cerebral cortex (idiopathic epilepsy). Secondary epilepsy, where a cause can be detected, may occur in the presence of organic lesions causing cerebral cortical irritation, such as encephalitis, cerebral abscess, cerebral tumours, head injury and cerebrovascular disease. Presence of papilloedema, neurological deficit, abnormal CSF picture or focal fits favours the diagnosis of secondary epilepsy which should be further investigated to find out the type of lesion.

Certain systemic diseases are associated with convulsions. These are hypoglycaemia, hypertensive encephalopathy, uraemia, hypoxia, hyponatraemia and sudden high fever.

Hysterical convulsions can be differentiated from epilepsy by the absence of history of tongue bite, injury or incontinence of urine.

Main points

Group 1	:	Baihui	(GV-20)
		Sishencong	(Ex-6)
		Zusanli	(St-36)
		Fenglong	(St-40)
		Xinshu	(UB-15)
Group 2	:	Bathui	(GV-20)
		Fengchi	(GB-20)
		Pushen	(UB-61)
		Zusanli	(St-36)
		Neiguan	(P-6)
		Yintang	(Ex-1)
Group 3	:	Dazhui	(GV-14)
		Baihui	(GV-20)
		Yanglingquan	(GB-34)
		Fenglong	(St-40)
		Taichong	(Liv-3)
Group 4	:	Yongquan	(K-1)
		Neiguan	(P-6)
		Touwei	(St-8)
		Shenmen	(H-7)
		Shenmai	(UB-62)
		Anmian I	(Ex-8)
		Anmian II	(Ex-9)
Ear points	:	Shenmen	
		Subcortex	
		Sympathetic	
		Heart	
		Kidney	
Scalp needling	:	Motor area	
		Sensory area	
		Foot sensory motor area	

Stimulation

Mild stimulation should be given for 20 to 30 minutes daily for 10 days. Course may be repeated after rest of 5 to 7 days.

Remarks
1. A slow withdrawal of the antiepileptic drugs is recommended.
2. Response is slow.

PARKINSONISM

Parkinsonism is one of the degenerative disorders of the basal ganglia. Pathological changes are seen in substantia nigra (situated in the midbrain) which shows a lack of dopamine, serotonine and acetylcholine, which act as neurotransmitters,. Most of the cases are of unknown aetiology and are spoken of as paralysis agitans. A few cases have been observed to occur following encephalitis (postencephalitic parkinsonism).

The characteristic symptoms are pill rolling tremor, rigidity and akinesia. The rigidity is constant, of lead pipe or cogwheel type, as opposed to claspknife rigidity of pyramidal disease which occurs only at the beginning of the passive action. Akinesia means a lack of activity without a loss of muscle power and is responsible for the mask-like facies. While standing or walking the patient adopts a stooping position. Motor system, sensory system and the reflexes are normal.

Recently a syndrome indistinguishable from parkinsonism has been observed following the long-term ingestion of reserpine and phenothiazines. The symptoms disappear after the drug is withdrawn.

Main points	: Baihui	(GV-20)
	Sishencong	(Ex-6)
	Anmian I	(Ex-8)
	Anmian II	(Ex-9)
	Touwei	(St-8)
	Fengchi	(GB-20)
Supplementary points	: Shenmen	(H-7)
	Neiguan	(P-6)
	Hegu	(LI-4)
	Quchi	(LI-11)
	Yanglao	(SI-6)
	Waiguan	(TW-5)
	Chengshan	(UB-57)
	Shenmai	(UB-62)
	Yanglingquan	(GB-34)
	Neiting	(St-44)
Ear points	: Shenmen	
	Subcortex	
	Sympathetic	
	Heart	
	Kidney	

Scalp needling	:	1. Chorea-tremor control area
		2. Equilibrium area
Point injection	:	Quchi	(LI-11)
		Yanglingquan	(GB-34)
		Zusanli	(St-36)

Vitamin B_1, in doses of 50-100 mg can be injected in any of the above points on alternate day.

Stimulation

Mild electrical stimulation can be given to body points once a day for 15 days and course can be repeated after a rest of 7 to 10 days.

Remarks

1. Response to acupuncture is slow.
2. A longer course of treatment is advised.

22
MUSCULO-SKELETAL DISEASES

RULES FOR THE SELECTION OF THE POINTS FOR MUSCULO-SKELETAL DISEASES

1. Use of Ah-shi points
   Needling
   Cupping
   Moxibustion

2. Use of influential points

Dashu	(UB-11)
Yanglingquan	(GB-34)

3. Use of analgesic point

Hegu	(LI-4)
Neiting	(St-44)

4. Use of sedative point

Baihui	(GV-20)
Ear Shenmen	

5. Use of immunity improving point

Quchi	(LI-11)
Dazhui	(GV-14)

6. Use of oedema points to relieve swelling around the joint

Taixi	(K-3)
Yinlingquan	(Sp-9)

7. Ear Acupuncture
   According to part affected
   Shenmen
   Kidney (kidney controls the bone)
   Internal secretion
   Sympathetic

8. Physiotherapy and active exercises

RHEUMATOID ARTHRITIS

Rheumatoid arthritis is an autoimmune disease characterised by symmetrical peripheral polyarthritis and extra-articular manifestations. The disease usually occurs in the age group of 35 to 50 years and affects females thrice as often as males.

Arthritis is symmetrical and involves the small joints of hands and feet and the wrist joints first. The joints are stiff, painful, tender and swollen. Destruction of the joints and muscular wasting consequent to immobility lead to deformities. Constitutional symptoms like fever and malaise are present.

Extra-articular manifestations include anaemia, rheumatoid nodules, entrapment neuropathy, pleural effusion, splenomegaly and myopathy. Amyloidosis occurs in 25 per cent cases.

Erythrocyte sedimentation rate (ESR) is raised and X-ray shows joint destruction and bony changes. Serological tests (latex test, L.E. cell) are positive in 80 per cent cases.

If untreated, the disease is progressive and leads to irreversible destruction of the joints and deformities.

FINGER

Main points	:	Baihui	(GV-20)
		Houxi	(SI-3)
		Yanggu	(SI-5)
		Shaofu	(H-8)
		Daling	(P-7)
		Yuji	(L-10)
		Zhongzhu	(TW-3)
		Hegu	(LI-4)
		Baxie	(Ex-28)
		As-shi points	
Ear Points	:	Finger area	
		Shenmen	
		Internal secretion	

WRIST JOINT

Main points			
Group I	:	Hegu	(LI-4)
		Yangxi	(LI-5)
		Waiguan	(TW-5)
		Yanglao	(SI-6)
Group II	:	Taiyuan	(L-9)
		Shenmen	(H-7)
		Daling	(P-7)
		As-shi point	
Supplementary points	:	Neiting	(St-44)
		Yanglingquan	(GB-34)
		Baihui	(GV-20)

Ear points   : Wrist joint
                              Shenmen
                              Internal secretion

ELBOW JOINT

Main Points
Group I   : Quchi   (LI-11)
                              Zhouliao   (LI-12)
                              Tianjing   (TW-10)
                              Ah-shi point
Group II   : Shaohai   (H-3)
                              Quze   (P-3)
                              Chize   (L-5)
                              Ah-shi points
Supplementary points   : Baihui   (GV-20)
                              Hegu   (LI-4)
                              Yanglingquan   (GB-34)
Ear points   : Elbow joint
                              Shenmen

SHOULDER JOINT

Main points   : Jianyu   (LI-15)
                              Jianliao   (TW-14)
                              Jianzhen   (SI-9)
                              Jianjing   (GB-21)
                              Ah-shi points
Supplementary points   : Baihui   (GV-20)
                              Hegu   (LI-4)
                              Quchi   (LI-11)
                              Yanglingquan   (GB-34)
                              Tiaokou   (St-38) (Same side)
Ear points   : Shoulder joint area
                              Shenmen

TOES

Main points   : Jiexi   (St-41)
                              Xiangu   (St-43)
                              Neiting   (St-44)
                              Bafeng   (Ex-36)
                              Ah-shi points
Supplementary points   : Baihui   (GV-20)
                              Hegu   (LI-4)
                              Yanglingquan   (GB-34)
Ear points   : Toes area
                              Shenmen

ANKLE JOINT

Main points

Group I   :   Yanglingquan (GB-34)
                Xuanzhong (GB-39)
                Foot linqi   (GB-41)
                Jiexi   (St-41)
                Kunlum   (UB-60)
                Shenmai   (UB-62)
                Ah-shi points

Group II   :   Taixi   (K-3)
                Gongsun   (Sp-4)
                Shanqiu   (Sp-5)
                Sanyinjiao (Sp-6)
                Zhongfeng (Liv-4)
                Ah-shi points

Supplementary :   Baihui   (GV-20)
points   Hegu   (LI-4)

Ear points :   Ankle area
                Shenmen

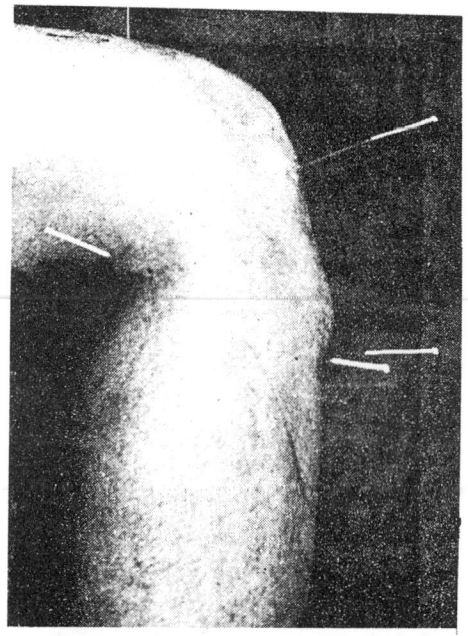

KNEE JOINT

Main points

Group I   Liangqaiu   (St-34)
                Dubi   (St-35)
                Zusanli   (St-36)
                Yanglingquan (GB-34)
                Ah-shi points

Group II   :   Fengshi   (GB-31)
                Weiyang   (UB-39)
                Chengjin (UB-56)
                Ah-shi points

Group III :   Yinlingquan (Sp-9)
                Xuehai   (Sp-10)
                Heding   (Ex-31)
                Xiyan   (Ex-32)
                Ququan   (Liv-8)
                Ah-shi points

Supplementary points :   Baihui   (GV-20)
                          Sanyinjiao (Sp-6)
                          Liangqiu (St-34)
                          Hegu   (LI-4)

Ear points   :   Knee joint
                        Shenmen

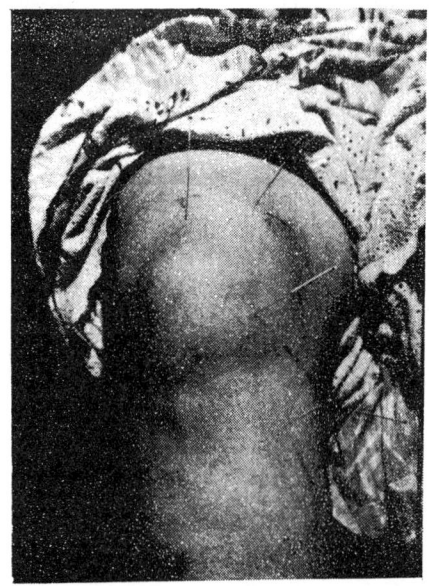

Arthritis of the Knee Joint

HIP JOINT

Main points	:	Femur Juliao	(GB-29)
		Huantiao	(GB-30)
		Chengfu	(UB-36)
		Zhibian	(UB-54)
		Biguan	(St-31)
		Ah-shi points	
Supplementary points	:	Baihui	(GV-20)
		Weizhong	(UB-40)
		Neiting	(St-44)
		Hegu	(LI-4)
Ear points	:	Hip joint	
		Shenmen	

TEMPROMANDIBULAR ARTHRITIS

		Quanliao	(SI-18)
		Tinggong	(SI-19)
		Tinghui	(GB-2)
		Xiaguan	(St-7)
		Ah-shi points	
Supplementary points	:	Baihui	(GV-20)
		Hegu	(LI-4)
		Neiting	(St-44)
		Yanglingquan	(GB-34)
Ear points	:	Fasciomandibular area	
		Shenmen	

Stimulation

Mild to moderate electrical stimulation should be given for 20 to 30 minutes for 10 days. Course may be repeated after a rest of 5 to 7 days.

Remarks
1. Moxibustion should be given on Ah-shi points.
2. Massage and physiotherapy should also be advised.
3. Response is good if deformities have not occurred.

DE QUERVAIN'S DISEASE

This is a condition in which the tendons of abductor pollicis longus and extensor pollicis brevis are entrapped by thickening of their common sheath. Patient complains of pain at the posterior aspect of the root of the thumb, and limitation of its extension and abduction movements.

Main points	:	Hegu	(LI-4)
		Yangxi	(LI-5)
		Taiyuan	(L-9)
		Shaoshang	(L-11)

Supplementary points	:	Baihui	(GV-20)
		Yanglingquan	(GB-34)
		Neiting	(St-44)
Ear points	:	Wrist joint	
		Shenmen	

Stimulation

Mild electrical stimulation should be given for 20 to 30 minutes daily for 10 days.   Course may be repeated after a rest of 5 to 7 days.

Remarks

Prognosis is good.

CARPAL TUNNEL   SYNDROME

This is a variety of entrapment neuropathy in which the median nerve is compressed as it passes through the carpal tunnel formed by the carpal bones and the flexor retinaculum, The compression is caused by thickening of the   sheathe of flexor tendons which also pass through the carpal tunnel. Some cases may be associated with rheumatoid disease, myxoedema and pregnancy but in most of the cases no obvious cause is evident. Patient feels pain and parasthesia in the thumb and lateral three fingers and examination may reveal hyposthesia in the distribution and wasting and weakness of the abductor pollicis brevis, muscel.

Local points	:	Neiguan	(P-6)
		Daling	(P-7)
		Laogong	(P-8)
		Shenmen	(H-7)
		Taiyuan	(L-9)
Supplementary points	:	Baihui	(GV-20)
		Hegu	(LI-4)
		Neiting	(ST-44)
		Yinlingquan	(Sp-9)
Ear points	:	Wrist joint	
		Shenmen	

Stimulation

Mild electrical stimulation 20 to 30 minutes daily for 7 to 10 days.

Remarks

Prognosis is good.

TENNIS ELBOW

This condition is characterised by pain in the elbow at rest and on extension of wrist and fingers.   The attachment of the extensors of the forearm to the lateral epicondyle is tender.

Main points	: Shousanli	(LI-10)
	Quchi	(LI-11)
	Sidu	(TW-9)
	Tianjing	(TW-10)
	Xiaohai	(SI-8)
	Ah-shi points	
Supplementary points	: Baihui	(GV-20)
	Hegu	(LI-4)
	Neiting	(St-44)
	Yanglingquan	(GB-34)
	Yangjiao	(GB-35)
Ear points	: Elbow joint	
	Shenmen	
Scalp needling	: Sensory area, middle two-fifths, opposite side.	

Stimulation
1. Moderate electrical stimulation should be given 20 to 30 minutes daily for 10 days. Course may be repeated after a rest of 5 to 7 days.
2. Indirect moxibustion 5 to 10 minutes daily on Ah-shi point and Quchi (LI-11) daily.
3. Point injection of 0.5 to 1 ml analgin on Quchi (LI-11) can be given.

Remarks
Prognosis is good.

GOLFER'S ELBOW   (Pulled elbow)

This condition is similar to tennis elbow except that it effects the attachment of the flexor muscles of the forearm to the medial epicondyle.

Main points	: Shousanli	(LI-10)
	Quchi	(LI-11)
	Sidu	(TW-9)
	Ah-shi point	
Supplementary points	: Hegu	(LI-4)

Stimulation
Mild electrical stimulation 20 to 30 minutes daily for 3 to 5 days.

Remarks
Results are excellent.

FROZEN SHOULDER AND SHOULDER HAND SYNDROME

Inflammation of the periarticular structures around the shoulder joint is termed as frozen shoulder. The rotator cuff is most affected. Pain in the shoulder is associated with restriction, particularly of rotation and abduction.

When frozen shoulder is accompanied by pain and swelling in the hand due to sudek's atrophy, the condition is termed shoulder hand syndrome. Both the entities are often of neurovascular aetiology and may occur as a complication of myocardial infarction and hemiplegia.

Main points	:	Jianyu	(LI-15)
		Jianjing	(GB-21)
		Jianliao	(TW-14)
		Jianzhen	(SI-9)
		Naoshu	(SI-10)
		Tianzong	(SI-11)

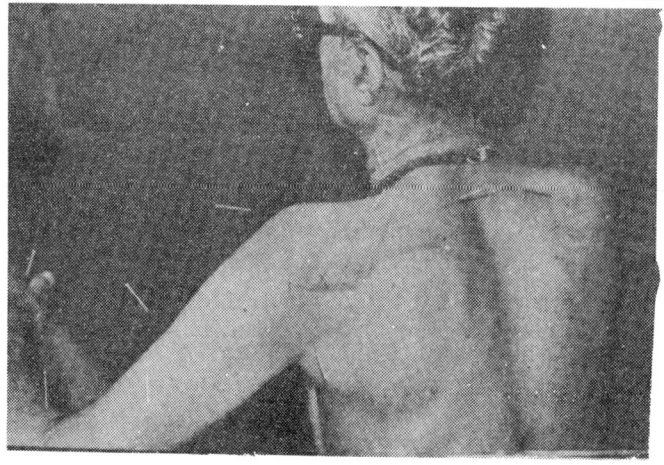

Frozen shoulder

Supplementary points	:	Hegu	(LI-4)
		Quchi	(LI-11)
		Tiaokou	(St-38) same side
		Yanglingquan	(GB-34)
		Foot Linqi	(GB-41) opposite side
		Dashu	(UB-11)
		Chengshan	(UB-57)
		Baihui	(GV-20)
Ear points	:	Shoulder	
		Shenmen	
		Subcortex	
		Internal secretion	
Scalp needling	:	Sensory area, middle to fifth (opposite side).	

Stimulation

1. Moderate electrical stimulation can be given for 20 to 30 minutes daily for 10 days. Course may be repeated after a rest of 5 to 7 days.
2. Indirect moxibustion should be done over the Ah-shi points and Hegu (LI-4).

3. Cupping in the Ah-shi points is also advised.

Remarks

1. Acupuncture is quite effective.
2. Active exercises and physiotherapy should also be combined.

PLANTER FASCITIS

This is an inflammatory process that affects the fascia and soft connective tissue at the site of attachment of the planter fascia to the inferior aspect of the tuberosity of the calcanium. The precise cause of the inflammation is not known.

The main clinical features are pain beneath the heel on standing or walking. On examination there is marked tenderness over the site of attachment of the planter fascia to the calcanious.

Main points	:	Yongquan	(K-1)
		Taixi	(K-3)
		Gongsun	(Sp-4)
		Sanyinjiao	(Sp-6)

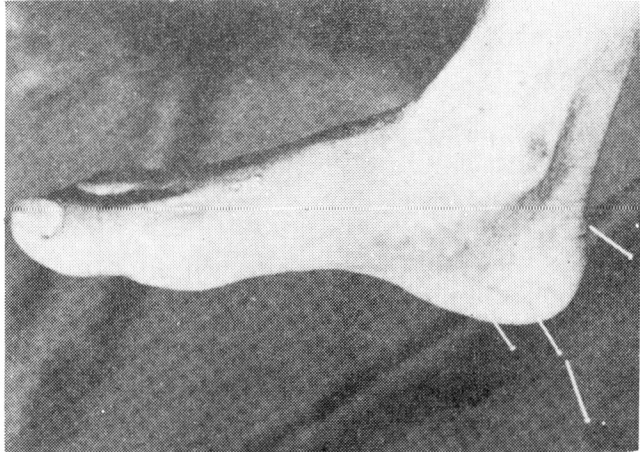

Planter Fascitis

Supplementary points	:	Baihui	(GV-20)
		Yanglingquan	(GB-34)
		Hegu	(LI-4)
		Quchi	(LI-11)
Ear points	:	Foot area	
		Shenmen	
Scalp needling	:	Foot sensoro-motor area	

Stimulation

Mild electrical stimulation should be given for 20 to 30 minutes daily for 10 days. Course may be repeated after a rest of 5 to 7 days.

Remarks

Prognosis is good.

ANKYLOSING SPONDYLITIS

This is an inflammatory arthropathy, primarily involving the sacroiliac joints and the spine with a marked tendancy to ankylosis (fusion). The precise aetiology is not known. A large number (96 per cent) of patients show the presence of HLA-B27 antigen. Patients are commonly young men in the third decade. The initial symptom is a low backache with morning stiffness due to involvement of sacroiliac joints. Later on the spine is involved from below upwards (sparing the cervical spine). At a still later stage the proximal joints of the limbs, particularly the hip joints are affected. The disease is progressive and leads to crippling deformities. Iritis and prostatourethritis are commonly associated. The diagnosis can be confirmed by radiography which shows obliteration of the sacroiliac joints in the early stage and the characteristic bamboo spine at a later stage.

Main points
1. Should be selected on the governing vessels and urinary bladder meridian.
2. Huato's points (Ex-21).
3. Ah-shi points.

Supplementary points	:	Shendao	(GV-11)
		Baihui	(GV-20)
		Sanyangluo	(TW-8)
		Hegu	(LI-4)
		Weizhong	(UB-40)
		Kunlun	(UB-60)
		Neiting	(St-44)
Ear points	:	Shenmen	
		Subcortex	
		Internal secretion	
		According to the part affected	

Stimulation
1. Moderate to strong stimulation should be given 20 to 30 minutes daily for 10 days. Course may be repeated after a rest of 5 to 7 days.
2. Tapping with 7 star needle on the Huotuo's point should be done daily.
3. Indirect moxibustion should be done on Ah-shi point and Huoto's point.
4. Cupping on the Ah-shi points should also be done.

Remarks
1. A long course of treatment is often required.
2. Active exercises and physiotherapy should also be advised.

BACKACHE

Low backache is a common ailment affecting the middle aged and elderly persons, and a diagnostic problem because the parts affected are not accessible to inspection and palpation. An X-ray of the lumbosacral spine is often necessary for the diagnosis.

"Low back strain" is the commonest cause of backache. A history of trivial injury to the spine, like weightlifting or jumping, is often obtained. Local pain and tenderness are present. The pain increases on movement and is relieved by rest. More severe injury may give rise to fracture of the body of a vertebra in which case the cause of backache is obvious. Pathological fracture may occur in the absence of injury.

Prolapsed intervertebral disc is another important cause of low backache and sciatica and has been discussed in the next chapter.

Osteoarthritis of the spine gives rise to pain and stiffness and the X-ray shows osteophytic overgrowth with spur formation. Ankylosing spondylitis affects young men and has already been discussed.

Osteoporosis may give rise to sudden, severe pain in the back. Osteomalacia, on the other hand, produces a dull ache. Pott's spine is not an uncommon cause of backache.

Backache may occur in the form of referred pain from diseases of the abdominal and pelvic viscera.

In any case of backache the pain may be self-perpetuated due to the protective muscular spasm that occurs.

Main points	: Yaoshu	(GV-2)
	Yaoyangguan	(GV-3)
	Mingmen	(GV-4)
	Shenshu	(UB-23)
	Dachangshu	(UB-25)
	Ciliao	(UB-32)
	Zhibian	(UB-54)
	Huato's points	(Ex-21)
Supplementary points	: Baihui	(GV-20)
	Hegu	(LI-4)
	Weizhong	(UB-40)
	Kunlun	(UB-60)
	Neiting	(St-44)
Ear points	: Lumber vertebra	
	Kidney	
	Shenmen	
	Subcortex	
Scalp needling	: Foot sensory motor area	
	Sensory area, upper one-fifth (both sides)	

Stimulation

1. Moderate to strong electrical stimulation should be given for 20 to 30 minutes daily for 10 days. Course may be repeated after rest of 5 to 7 days.
2. Tapping with seven star needle on the Hualuo's point on lumbosacral region is also advised.

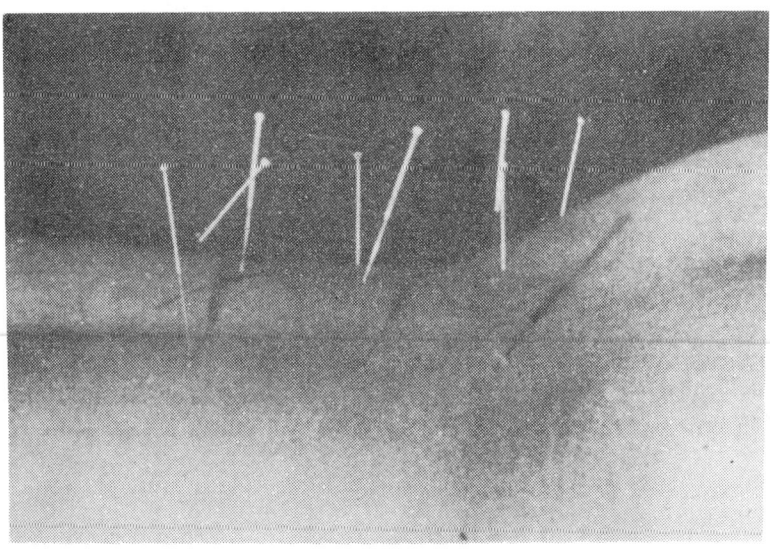

Backache

3. Indirect moxibustion should also be done.
4. Use of vacuum cup on the Ah-shi point gives good result.
5. Injection of 0.5 to 1 ml analgin and 0.5 to 1 ml 1 per cent procain can also be given on As-shi points.

Remarks
1. Patients should be advised to use a hard bed.
2. Stooping and weightlifting should be forebidden.
3. Spinal exercises should be combined with acupuncture.
4. Results are good.

SCIATICA

The term sciatica is employed when pain is experienced in the distribution of the sciatic nerve, that is, in the buttock, back of the thigh, outer side and back of the leg and the outer border of the foot. The condition is usually unilateral. Mechanical irritation that produces rootpain in the sciatic nerve distribution may also give rise to hypoaesthesia in the same distribution, paralysis of the muscles supplied by sciatic nerve (flexors of the knee and all the muscles below the knee) and absence of ankle jerk.

Most of the cases are due to irritation of the roots of the sciatic nerve (lumbar 4, 5, sacral 1, 2, 3,). The commonest cause of such irritation is prolapsed intervertebral disc (PID). The patients are generally under 40 years of age, a history of minor injury or sprain of the back is present, the straight leg raising (SLR) test is positive, and the spine is painful and stiff, apart from the neurological signs which may be present to a greater or lesser extent. Myelography is useful to confirm the diagnosis.

Other conditions which may cause sciatica include osteoarthritis of the spine, vertebral tumour, and the pelvic tumours.

It must be remembered that pain may be referred in the distribution of the sciatic nerve in conditions like arthritis of the hip joint and sacroiliac joint, trauma of the gluteal muscles, and lesions of the vertebral ligaments.

Main points

Group I	Yaoyangguan	(GV-3)	Chengfu	(UB-36)
	Mingmen	(GV-4)	Huantiao	(GB-30)
	Ciliao	(UB-32)	Huato's points	(Ex-21)

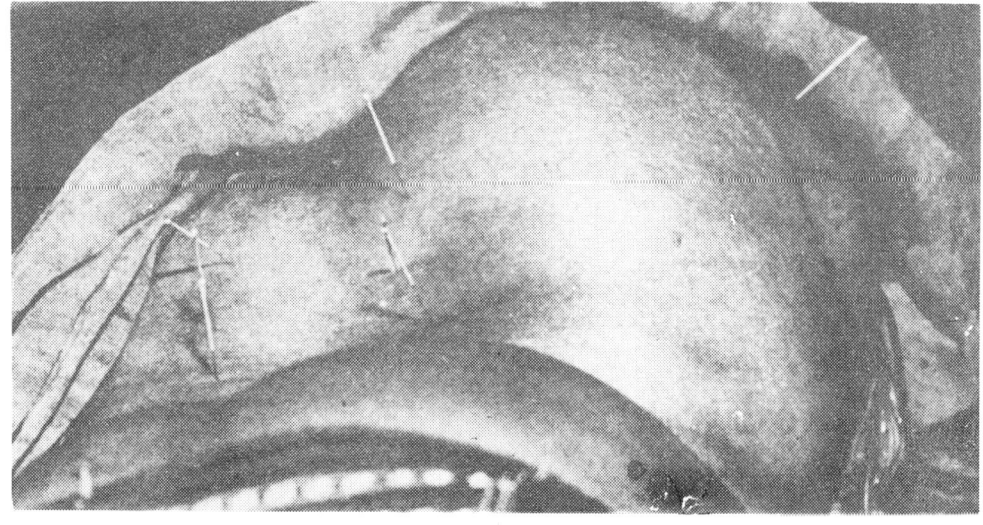

Sciatica

Group II	:	Shenshu	(UB-23)
		Dachangshu	(UB-25)
		Weizhong	(UB-40)
		Fengshi	(GB-31)
Group III	:	Huiyang	(UB-35)
		Chengshan	(UB-57)
		Fenglong	(St-40)
		Huato's points	(Ex-21)
Group IV	:	Yinmen	(UB-37)
		Chengshan	(UB-57)
		Yanglingquan	(GB-34)
		Huato's points	(Ex-21)
Supplimentary points	:	Baihui	(GV-20)
		Hegu	(LI-4)
		Neiting	(St-44)
		Dashu	(UB-11)

		Weizhong	(UB-40)
		Kunlun	(UB-60)
Ear points	:	Lumbar vertebra	
		Sacral vertebra	
		Shenmen	
		Adrenal gland	
Scalp needling	:	Foot sensory motor area	
		Sensory area upper one-fifth (opposite side)	

Stimulation

1. Moderate electrical stimulation should be given for 20 to 30 minutes daily for 10 days. Course may be repeated after a rest of 5 to 7 days.
2. Point injection.
    0.5 to 1 ml of 1% procaine can be injected on the following points Huantiao (GB-30), Shenshu (UB-23).
3. Tapping around the Huato's point on the lumbosacral region should also be done.
4. Cupping on the ah-shi points can also be done.

Remarks

1. General precautions like use of hard bed, spinal extension exercises and hot fomentation should be advised.
2. Response is excellent.

WRY NECK (TORTICOLLIS)

Spasmodic torticollis (wry neck) is a condition characterised by tonic and clonic spasm of sternomastoid, scalenus and trapezius muscles resulting into turning of the hand to one side tilting of the face upwards. Continuous spasm of these muscles give rise to pain in the neck. The onset is insidious and there are remissions and exacerbations. Those affected belong to the middle age group. Strees and upright posture aggravate the involuntary movements.

Previously considered to be of psychogenic origin, the condition is a degenerative disorder of the basal ganglia.

Main points	:	Dazhui	(GV-14)
		Yamen	(GV-15)
		Tianzhu	(UB-10)
		Dashu	(UB-11)
		Fengchi	(GB-20)
		Huato's points	(Ex-21)
		Ah-shi points	
Supplementary points	:	Baihui	(GV-20)
		Hegu	(LI-4)
		Houxi	(SI-3)
		Yanglao	(SI-6)
		Lieque	(L-7)
		Yanglingquan	(GB-34)

	Xuanzhong	(GB-39)
	Shenmai	(UB-62)
	Neiting	(St-44)
Ear points	: Cervical vertebra	
	Shenmen	
	Neck area	
	Subcortex	

Stimulation
1. Mild electric stimulation should be given for 20 to 30 minutes daily for 10 days. Course may be repeated after the rest of 5 to 7 days.
2. Tapping with 7 star needle along the Huato's points is also advised.
3. Use of vaccum cup in Ah-shi point shows a good result.

Remarks
1. Response is very good.

OSTEOARTHRITIS OF THE CERVICAL SPINE
(Cervical spondylosis, cervical spondylarthrosis)

The degenerative changes are common in cervical spine. In the beginning intervertebral disc shows the primary degenerative changes and leads to pain and stiffness of the neck. Sometime the pain is referred to the upper extremity also.

In the later stage osteophytes commonly encroach upon the intervertebral foramina, reducing the space for transmission of the cervical nerves and leading to manifestations of nerve pressure, sometime the spinal cord may suffer damage due to encroachment of osteophytes within the spinal canal.

The main symptoms are pain in the neck (in the trapezius area) and stiffness of the neck. There may be referred pain of the dull nature on the shoulder joint and radiating pain on the upper extremity.

Main points	: Fengchi	(GB-20)
	Tianzhu	(UB-10)
	Dashu	(UB-11)
	Dazhui	(GV-14)
	Yamen	(GV-15)
	Yiming	(Ex-7)
	Huoto's point	
	Ah-shi points	
Supplementary points	: Baihui	(GV-20)
	Lieque	(L-7)
	Houxi	(SI-3)
	Waiguan	(TW-5)
	Hegu	(LI-4)
	Yanglingquan	(GB-34)
	Xuanzhong	(GB-39)
	Neiting	(St-44)

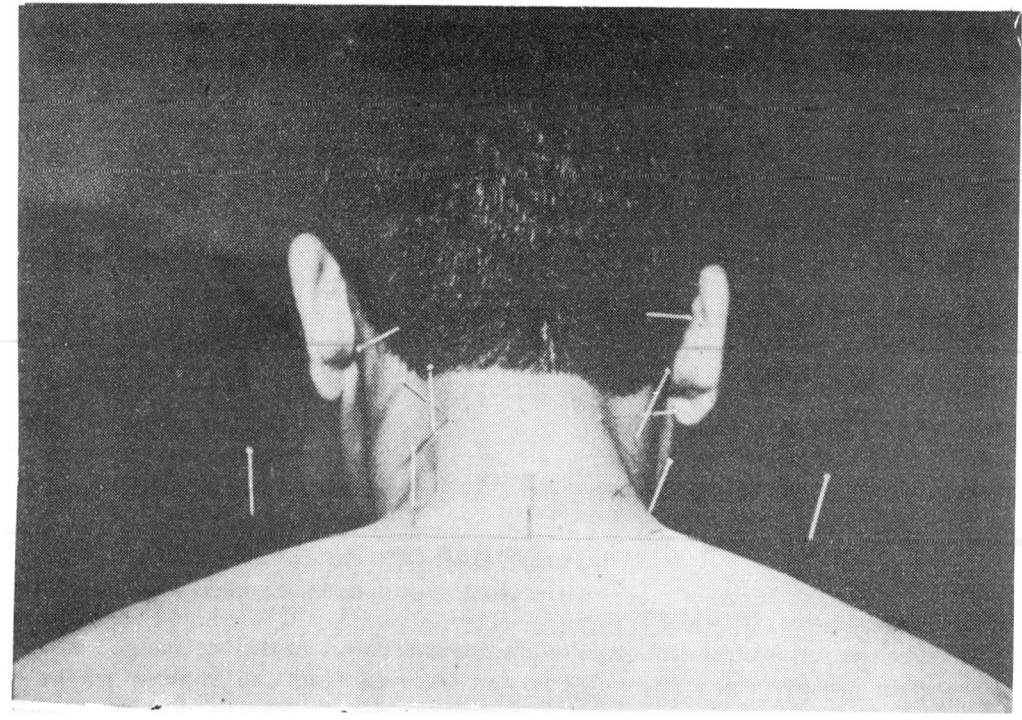

Osteoarthritis of cervical spine

Ear points   :   Neck area
                              Shenmen

Stimulation

Moderate electrical stimulation 20 to 30 minutes daily for 10 days. Course may be repeated after a rest of 5 to 7 days.

Remarks

Prognosis is good.

MYALGIA CHEST

Neuromuscular pain is the commonest veriety of chest pain. It is often confused with ischaemic heart disease. Myalgia chest occurs due to the rupture of muscle fibres by an unaccostomed exercise. The pain is superficial and is associated with local tenderness and sometimes swelling. Movements involving the affected muscle increases the pain.

Main points   :   Jiuwei   (CV-15)
                             Shanzhong   (CV-17)
                             Huagai   (CV-20)
                             Qimen   (Liv-14)
                             Rugen   (St-18)

Supplementary points	:	Baihui	(GV-20)
		Hegu	(LI-4)
		Neiguan	(P-6)
		Sanyangluo	(TW-8)
		Yanglingquan	(GB-34)
		Neiting	(St-44)
Ear points	:	Thoracic cavity
		Shenmen
		Internal secretion
Scalp needling	:	Sensory area, middle to fifth both side.

Stimulation

Mild electrical stimulation can be given to the body point 20 to 30 minutes daily for 10 days. Course may be repeated after a rest of 5 to 7 days.

Remarks

1. During severe pain strong hand stimulation should be given to Hegu (LI-4).
2. Tapping with 7 star needle on Huato's point can also be done.
3. Response is very good.

23

SPECIAL SENSE ORGANS

DISEASES OF THE EYE

MYOPIA

Vision is possible when the images of what we see fall on the retinas. In myopia the images from distant objects fall in front of the retina due to increased convergence of the rays by the lens or the cornea. Myopia is also produced by a long eyeball. The distant objects are blurred. This may result in eyestrain.

Main points
Group I	:	Baihui	(GV-20)
		Jingming	(UB-1)
		Chengqi	(St-1)
		Tongziliao	(GB-1)
		Hegu	(LI-4)
		Qiuhou	(Ex-4)
Group II	:	Yiming	(Ex-7)
		Fengchi	(GB-20)
		Guangming	(GB-37)
Supplementary points	:	Hegu	(LI-4)
		Guangming	(GB-37)
		Taichong	(Liv-3)
		Feiyang	(UB-58)
Ear points	:	Liver	
		Kidney	
		Shenmen	
		Eye	
		Eye I	
		Eye II	
Scalp needling	:	Visual area	

Stimulation

Point should be selected from the local group and from supplementary points. Mild electrical stimulation can be given for the supplementary points.

Remarks

Low degree of myopia shows better results.

CATARACT

Cataract is the result of the opacification of lens. Such opacification is a normal ageing process but the age of onset is variable. Premature cataract formation is a feature of certain systemic diseases such as diabetes mellitus and hypercalcaemia. Cataract leads to progressive dimness of vision and can be seen as the normally transparent lens becomes white and opaque. When the opacification is incomplete, the cataract is said to be immature, and when the opacification is completed it is said to be a mature cataract.

Main points	:	Chengqi	(ST-1)
		Yangbai	(GB-14)
		Zanzhu	(UB-2)
		Yintang	(Ex-1)
		Qiuhou	(Ex-4)
Supplementary points	:	Hegu	(LI-4)
		Baihui	(GV-20)
		Taichong	(Liv-3)
Ear points	:	Eye	
		Eye I	
		Eye II	
		Liver	
		Shenmen	
Scalp needling	:	Visual area	

Stimulation

Mild stimulation should be given to the body point for 20 to 30 minutes daily. Course may be repeated after a rest of 5 to 7 days.

Remarks

Further opacification of the lens can be prevented with acupuncture.

GLAUCOMA

This is a condition in which the intraocular pressure is raised. It is one of the common causes of headache in older individuals. Glaucoma is of two varieties—narrow angle and wide angle—depending upon the angle of the anterior chamber. Wide angle glaucoma is usually symptomatic. The diagnosis of glaucoma can be confirmed by tonometry.

Main points			
Group I	:	Baihui	(CV-20)
		Tongziliao	(GB-1)

		Fengchi	(GB-20)
		Zanzhu	(UB-2)
		Chengqi	(St-1)
Group II	:	Sibai	(St-2)
		Yintang	(Ex-1)
		Yuyao	(Ex-3)
		Qiuhou	(Ex-4)
		Yangbai	(GB-14)
Supplementary points	:	Hegu	(LI-4)
		Taixi	(K-3)
		Xingjian	(Liv-2)
		Taichong	(Liv-3)
		Guangming	(GB-37)
		Ganshu	(UB-18)
		Feiyang	(UB-58)
		Zusanli	(St-36)

Points according to symptoms

1. Headache	:	Baihui	(GV-20)
		Hegu	(LI-4)
		Neiting	(St-44)
2. Nausea and vomiting	:	Neiguan	(P-6)
		Zhongwan	(CV-12)
		Zusanli	(St-36)
Ear points	:	Eye	
		Eye I	
		Eye II	
		Liver	
		Shenmen	
		Endocrine	
		Oedema points	

Scalp needling
1. Vaso motor area (both sides)
2. Visual area

Stimulation

Mild stimulation should be given for 20 to 30 minuts daily for 10 days. Course may be repeated after rest of 5 to 7 days.

Remarks

In early cases acupuncture gives good results. In chronic cases it should be combined with modern medicine.

ACUTE CONJUNCTIVITIS

This is the commonest eye disease. Most of the cases are due to exogenous agents like foreign bodies, exposure to wind or intense light, fumes, bacteria or viruses. The affected eye is red. The eyelids are swollen. Conjunctival oedema (chemosis) may be present. The patient may have photophobia. Ophthalmia neonatorum is a particularly severe variety of conjunctivitis affecting the newborn infants. It is caused by gonococcal or staphylococcal infection. Conjunctivitis should be differentiated fron glaucoma, keratitis and corneal ulcer. In these conditions, the conjuctiva shows ciliary congestion which is maximum around the cornea.

Main points			
Group A	:	Baihui	(GV-20)
		Fengchi	(GB-20)
		Chengqi	(St-1)
		Taiyang	(Ex-2)
Group B	:	Jingming	(UB-1)
		Zanzhu	(UB-2)
		Tongziliao	(GB-1)
		Yangbai	(GB-14)
		Sizhukong	(TW-23)
Supplementary points	:	Hegu	(LI-4)
		Quchi	(LI-11)
		Dazhui	(GV-14)
		Baihui	(GV-20)
		Taichong	(Liv-3)
		Sanyinjiao	(Sp-6)
Ear points	:	Liver	
		Eye	
		Spleen	
		Shenmen	

Stimulation

Mild stimulation can be given for 3 to 5 days.

Remarks

Acupuncture is beneficial in preventing further attacks in recurrent acute conjunctivitis.

NIGHT BLINDNESS

Also known as nyctalopia, this is a manifestation of vitamin A deficiency. Vision in subdued light is dependent upon the activity of the rods. The rods contain a pigment called rhodopsin which breaks into retinine and opsin when light falls on the rods. Vitamin A is necessary for the normal metabolism of this pigment. Deficiency of vitamin A leads to dryness of the conjunctiva and the cornea, corneal ulcers, keratomalacia, and changes in the skin, apart from night blindness.

Main points	:	Tongziliao	(GB-1)
		Yangbai	(GB-14)
		Fengchi	(GB-20)
		Chengqi	(St-1)
		Sizhukong	(TW-23)
		Jingming	(UB-1)

Supplementary points	:	Hegu	(LI-4)
		Taichong	(Liv-3)
		Guangming	(GB-37)
Ear points	:	Eye	
		Eye I	
		Eye II	
		Liver	
		Shenmen	
Scalp needling	:	Visual area	

Stimulation

Mild stimulation can be given for 15 to 20 minutes daily for 10 days.   Acupuncture can be repeated after a rest of 5 to 7 days.

Remarks

High doses of vitamin A should be given simultaneously.

OPTIC NEURITIS

Optic neuritis includes papillitis in which the optic nerve head is affected, and retrobulbar neuritis in which the proximal portion of the optic nerve is involved. The effect of both these conditions on the vision is similar. There is a gradual diminution of vision until it is completely lost. This may be unilateral or bilateral. In case of papillitis, examination of the optic fundus shows swollen optic disc which is also slightly hyperaemic. This has to be differentiated from paplloedema in which the loss of vision is less. Retrobulbar neuritis presents in the form of primary optic atrophy on fundoscopic examination. The optic disc is pale. Optic neuritis may occur as a part of the picture of demyelinating diseases like disseminated sclerosis, due to the nutritional deficiency, or due to the toxic effects of chemicals like methyl alcohol.

Main points			
Group I	:	Jingming	(UB-1)
		Zanzhu	(UB-2)
		Chengqi	(St-1)
		Sibai	(St-2)
		Yintang	(Ex-1)
		Yuyao	(Ex-3)
Group II	:	Tongziliao	(GB-1)
		Yangbai	(GB-14)
		Fengchi	(GB-20)
		Taiynag	(Ex-2)
		Qiuhou	(Ex-4)
Supplementary :		Hegu	(LI-4)
points		Quchi	(LI-11)
		Yangbai	(GB-14)
		Baihui	(GV-20)
		Taichong	(Liv-3)

Ear points	:	Eye
		Eye I
		Eye II
		Liver
		Subcortex
Scalp needling	:	Visual area

Stimulation

Electric stimulation should not be given at the points around the eye.   Above two groups should be taken on alternate days.   Moderate stimulation to the body points can be given for 10 to 20 minutes daily for 10 days.   Course may be repeated after a rest of 5 to 7 days.

Remarks

1. A long-term acupuncture therapy is required.
2. Vitamin supplements should be given simultaneously.

DETACHMENT OF RETINA

This may be spontaneous or traumatic.   Spontaneous detachment usually occurs after the age of 50.   The conditions which predispose the detachment of retina after progressive myopia and diabetic retinopathy.   There is blurring of vision in one eye which is gradually progressive.   The,e is no pain or redness.   Detachment can be confirmed by ophthalmoscopic examination.

Main points	:	Chengqi	(St-1)
		Taiyang	(Ex-2)
		Yuyao	(Ex-3)
		Qiuhou	(Ex-4)
		Yiming	(Ex-7)
		Zanzhu	(UB-2)
Supplementary points	:	Baihui	(GV-20)
		Hegu	(LI-4)
		Ganshu	(UB-18)
		Shenshu	(UB-23)
		Guangming	(GB-37)
		Taichong	(Liv-3)
		Sanyinjiao	(Sp-6)
Ear points	:	Eye
		Eye I
		Eye II
		Shenmen
		Liver
		Kidney
		Adrenal
Scalp needling	:	Visual on both sides

Stimulation

Mild stimulation should be given daily for 20 to 30 minutes for 10 days. Course may be repeated after a rest of 5 to 7 days.

Remarks

Improvement is slow.

COLOR BLINDNESS

This is a hereditary defect of cones affecting the perception of one or more of the primary colours-red, green and blue. Males are more affected than females. The commonest defect is red-green blindness, in which, shades of red and green are not perceived. The diagnosis can be confirmed by using special charts or by making the patient compare the shades of wool of various colours.

Main points	:	Baihui	(GV-20)
		Tongziliao	(GB-1)
		Fengchi	(GB-20)
		Zanzhu	(UB-2)
		Sizhukong	(TW-23)
Supplementary points	:	Hegu	(LI-4)
		Taichong	(Liv-3)
		Yiming	(Ex-7)
Ear points	:	Eye	
		Eye I	
		Eye II	
		Liver	
		Shenmen	
		Subcortex	
Scalp needling	:	Visual area (both sides)	

Stimulation

Mild stimulation should be given 20 to 30 minutes daily for 10 days. Course may be repeated after a rest of 5 to 7 days.

Remarks

Results are satisfactory.

PHOTOPHOBIA

In photophobia the patient is unable to open his eyes in the presence of light because of irritation of the eyes due to various causes like: Conjunctivitis due to any cause, foreign body embedded in fornices of the conjunctiva, foreign body of the cornea, abrasion or ulcers of the cornea, exposure conjunctivitis due to ultraviolet light or bright light of the welding arcs, hypopyon (pus in the anterior chamber), perforating injuries of the eyeball, acute congestive glaucoma.

Main points

Group I	:	Baihui	(GV-20)
		Tongziliao	(GB-1)
		Fengchi	(GB-20)
		Taiyang	(Ex-2)
Group II	:	Jingming	(UB-1)
		Yintang	(Ex-1)
		Qiuhou	(Ex-4)
		Sibai	(St-2)
Supplementary points	:	Hegu	(LI-4)
		Quchi	(LI-11)
		Guangming	(GB-37)
		Taichong	(Liv-3)
Ear points	:	Eye	
		Eye I	
		Eye II	
		Liver	
		Shenmen	

Stimulation

Moderate stimulation by hand should be given daily for 20 to 30 minutes for 10 to 15 days.

Remarks

1. Results are excellent.
2. Further exposure to irritants should be prevented.

OPTIC ATROPHY

Atrophy of the optic nerve may occur because of syphilis, neurotoxins like tobacco or methylated spirit, glaucoma, tuberculosis, leprosy, pressure atrophy due to space occupying lesions pressing on the optic nerve, and malnutrition.

Main points

Group I	:	Baihui	(GV-20)
		Jingming	(UB-1)
		Chengqi	(St-1)
		Yintang	(Ex-1)
		Yiming	(Ex-7)
Group II	:	Yuyao	(Ex-3)
		Qiuhou	(Ex-4)
		Tongziliao	(GB-1)
		Yangbai	(GB-14)
		Zanzhu	(UB-2)
Supplementary points	:	Hegu	(LI-4)
		Yanglao	(SI-6)
		Neiguan	(Sp-6)

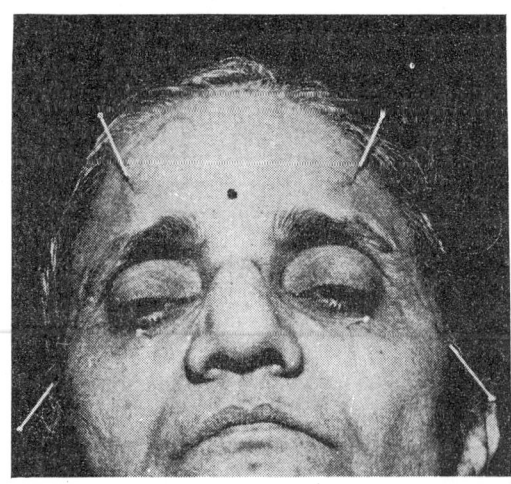

Optic atrophy

                  Taichong   (Liv-3)
                  Ganshu   (UB-18)
                  Shenshu   (UB-23)
                  Guangming (GB-37)

Ear points   : Ear
                  Eye I
                  Eye II
                  Liver
                  Shenmen
                  Endocrine
                  Subcortex

Scalp needling : Visual area

Stimulation

Moderate stimulation can be given on any of the points of above group on alternate days for 10 days and course may be repeated after a rest of 7 days.

Remarks

Improvement is slow and long-term therapy is needed.

DISEASES OF THE EAR

TINNITUS

Tinnitus is a sensation of noise in the ears or the head. It usually accompanies hearing loss or other disorders of the external, middle or internal ear. It is presumed to be due to irritation of the nerve endings in the cochlea by degenerative, vascular or vasomotor disease. The noise is much louder and more disturbing at night when the masking effect of the environmental sounds is not present.

Main points	:	Yifeng	(TW-17)
		Ermen	(TW-21)
		Tinggong	(SI-19)
		Tinghui	(GB-2)
		Fengchi	(GB-20)
		Yiming	(Ex-7)
Supplementary points	:	Baihui	(GV-20)
		Hegu	(LI-4)
		Zhongzhu	(TW-3)
		Xingjian	(Liv-2)
		Fenglong	(St-40)
		Shenshu	(UB-23)
		Taixi	(K-3)
Ear points	:	Internal ear	
		Shenmen	
		Subcortex	

		Sympathetic	
		Kidney	
Scalp needling	:	Vertigo-auditory area	

Point injection

A dose 0.5 to 1 ml of vitamin B complex can be injected alternate day in any of the following points:

Yifeng	(TW-17)
Fengchi	(GB-20)

Stimulation

Mild stimulation can be given 20 to 30 minutes daily for 10 days. Course may be repeated after a rest of 5 to 7 days.

Remarks

Results are excellent.

VERTIGO

Vertigo literally means "sense of turning" either of one's body (subjective) or of the surroundings (objective). The symptom is quite often described as dizziness or giddiness—words which are also used to describe symptoms such as unsteadiness, light headedness, weakness, faintness and blurring of vision. These symptoms usually indicate a psychoneurotic disorder and should not be confused with "true" vertigo. Vertigo may occur due to diseases of the cerebral cortex (aura of epilepsy), ocular muscles (paralysis), cerebellum (tumour), brainstem (vascular lesions), auditory nerve (accoustic neuroma) and the labyrinthine vestibular apparatus (aural vertigo).

Aural or labyrinthine vertigo is the commonest variety of vertigo. It is paroxysmal, has an abrupt onset, and is frequently associated with tinnitus and deafness. Vertigo is generally accompanied by nausea, vomiting, headache, nystagmus and ataxia.

Main points	:	Baihui	(GV-20)
		Tinghui	(GB-2)
		Fengchi	(GB-20)
		Yifeng	(TW-17)
		Ermen	(TW-21)
		Tinggong	(SI-19)
		Touwei	(St-8)
		Yiming	(Ex-7)
Supplementary points	:	Hegu	(LI-4)
		Neiguan	(P-6)
		Shenmen	(H-7)
		Yemen	(TW-2)
		Zusanli	(St-36)
		Taixi	(K-3)
Ear points	:	Internal ear	
		Kidney	
		Shenmen	
		Sympathetic	

Scalp needling   :   Vertigo-auditory area (both sides)

Stimulation

Mild to moderate stimulation should be given daily for 20 to 30 minutes for 10 to 15 days. Course may be repeated after a rest of 5 to 7 days.

Remarks
1. Results are excellent.
2. Complete rest should be advised during the acute phase.
3. The underlying cause should be properly investigated and treated with modern medicine.

MENIERE'S DISEASE

The condition is characterised by recurrent aural vertigo with tinnitus and deafness. There is dilatation of the endolymphatic system leading to degeneration of the vestibular and cochlear hair cells. It usually affects persons in the 5th decade of life. Tinnitus is more severe initially, but as the disease progresses and the degree of deafness increases, vertigo and tinnitus become less prominent.

The condition has to be differentiated from benign positional vertigo in which there is no deafness, middle ear disease, toxic labyrinthitis due to drugs like quinine, streptomycin and salicylates, motion sickness and vestibular neuronitis.

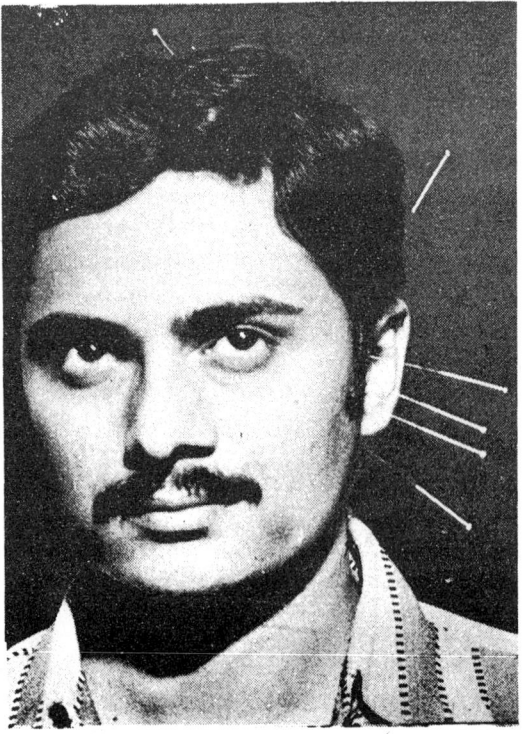

Meniere's Disease

Main points	: Baihui
	Tinghui
	Shuaigu
	Fengchi
	Yangbai
	Yifeng
	Ermen
	Tinggong
Supplementary points	: Dazhui
	Shenmen
	Hegu
	Quchi
	Zhongzhu
	Waiguan
	Foot Qiaoyin
	Zusanli
	Taixi
Ear points	: Shenmen
	Sympathetic
	Internal ear
	Kidney
Scalp needling	: Auditory area (both sides)

Stimulation

Mild electrical stimulation for 20 to 30 min daily for 10 days. Course may be repeated after 5 to 7 days.

Remarks
Results are excellent.

CHRONIC SUPPURATIVE OTITIS MEDIA

This condition is characterised by loss of hearing and ear discharge. It is usually associated with perforation of the tympanic membrane. Mastoiditis may develop as a complication. In such cases the perforation is marginal and the diagnosis can be confirmed by X-ray which shows loss of mastoid air cells. Meningitis or cerebral abscess may complicate the disease.

Main points	: Yifeng	(TW-17)
	Ermen	(TW-21)
	Tinggong	(SI-19)
	Tinghui	(GB-2)
Supplimentary points	: Baihui	(GV-20)
	Danzhui	(GV-14)
	Hegu	(LI-4)
	Quchi	(LI-11)
	Zhongzhu	(TW-3)
	Foot Qiaoyin	(GB-44)
	Zusanli	(St-36)
	Sanyinjiao	(Sp-6)
	Xuehai	(Sp-10)
	Taixi	(K-3)
Ear points	: Internal ear	
	Kidney	
	Shenmen	

Stimulation
Mild electrical stimulation can be given for 20 to 30 minutes daily for 10 days. Course may be repeated after a rest of 5 to 7 days.

Point injection
A dose of 20000 units of penicillin can be injected into Yifeng (TW-17).

Remarks
Results are satisfactory.

DEAF-MUTISM

If an individual is born deaf, he cannot learn to talk unless trained specially. Such individuals are called deaf mute. Though they cannot understand or speak words, their hearing is not completely absent and a response to sounds and music is observed and phonation in the form of grunting and producing peculiar noises is present. The basic defect is in the cortical centres for speech. Acquired deaf-mutism is a manifestation of hysteria. Congenital deaf-mutes should be differentiated from mentally retarded children, because in the former the intelligence is normal.

Deafness

Main points	:	Yifeng	(TW-17)
		Ermen	(TW-21)
		Tinggong	(SI-19)
		Tinghui	(GB-2)
		Shuaigu	(GB-8)
		Yiming	(Ex-7)
		Xiaguan	(St-7)
Supplementary points	:	Baihui	(GV-20)
		Yemen	(TW-2)
		Zhongzhu	(TW-3)
		Waiguan	(TW-5)
		Yanglao	(SI-6)
		Xiaxi	(GB-43)
		Foot-Linqi	(GB-41)

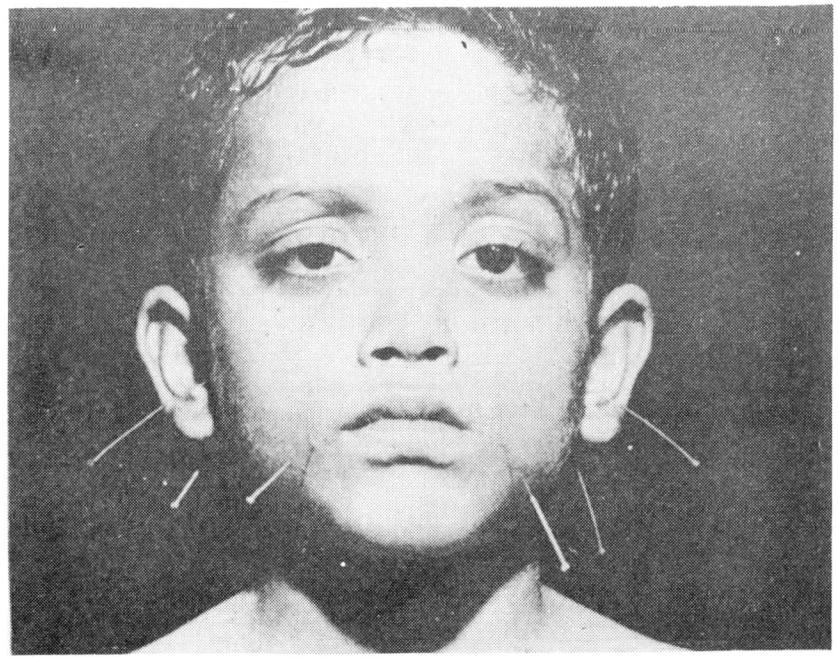

Deaf-mutism

Mutism

Main points	:	Dicang	(St-4)
		Lianquan	(CV-23)
		Chengjiang	(CV-24)
		Neck Futu	(LI-18)
		Tianrong	(SI-17)

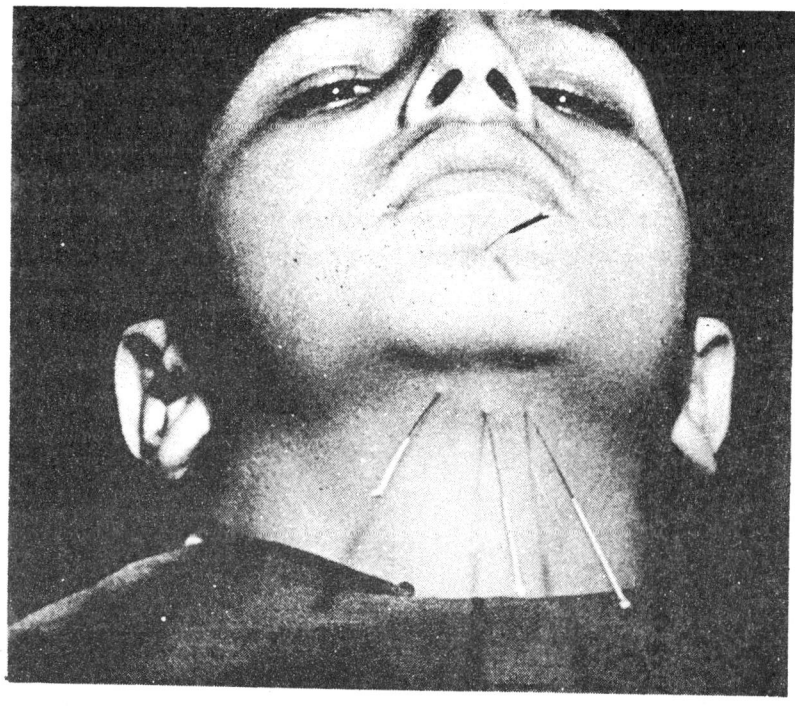

Mutism

Supplementary points	: Tongli	(H-5)
	Yinxi	(H-6)
	Hegu	(LI-4)
	Yamen	(GV-15)
	Baihui	(GV-20)
Ear points	: Internal ear	
	Kidney	
	Urinary bladder	
	Back of head	
	Shenmen	
Scalp needling	: Auditory area	
	Language area 2	
	Language area 3	

Stimulation

Mild electrical stimulation for 20 to 30 minutes daily for 10 days; course of therapy should be repeated after a rest of 5 to 7 days.

Long-term acupuncture therapy is advised in cases of deafness. Generally, deafness should be treated first and then muteness.

Point injection	: Yifeng	(TW-17)
	Ermen	(TW-21)
	Tinghui	(GB-2)

A dose of 0.5 ml of vitamin B_{12} can be injected in any of the points on alternate days.

Press needle therapy

Round body press needle can be applied on the internal ear area of the ear during the rest in between the courses.

Remarks

1. Speech therapy should also be advised.
2. Minimum 30 sittings of acupuncture are required to obtain significant results.
3. Points for deafness can also be used for any variety of acquired deafness. Response in such cases is faster.

DISEASES OF THE NOSE

RHINITIS

Rhinitis is a common disorder characterised by nasal congestion, a profuse watery nasal discharge, sneezing and lacrymation. It may occur as a part of upper respiratory infection, when it is accompanied by fever and sorethroat, or it may be an allergic manifestation.

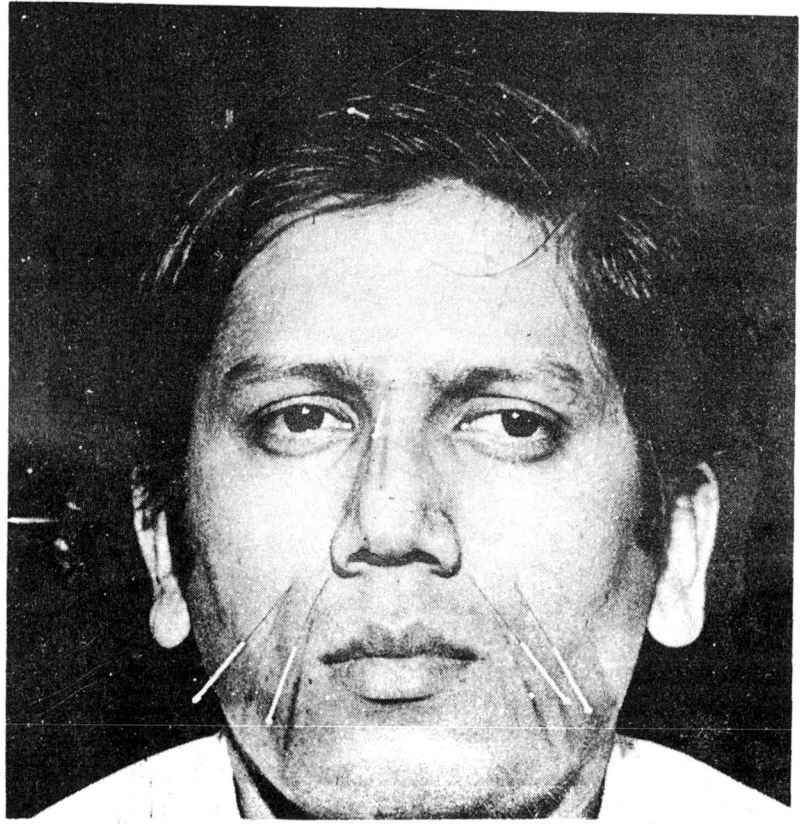

Allergic rhinitis

Allergic rhinitis (hay fever) is recurrent, seasonal, and associated with eosinophilia. Nasal polyps are commonly associated.

Main points	:	Yintang	(Ex-1)
		Juliao	(St-3)
		Nose Heliao	(LI-19)
		Yingxiang	(LI-20)
Supplementary	:	Hegu	(LI-4)
points		Quchi	(LI-11)
		Lieque	(L-7)
		Sanyinjiao	(Sp-6)
		Xuehai	(Sp-10)
		Zusanli	(St-36)
		Fenglong	(St-40)
Ear points	:	Nose area	
		Spleen	
		Lung	
		Internal secretion	
		Adrenal gland	
		Shenmen	

Stimulation

Mild electrical stimulation can be given for 20 to 30 minutes daily for 10 days and course of the therapy can be repeated after a rest of 5 to 7 days.

Remarks

1. Satisfactory results are obtained with acupuncture therapy.
2. L. K. Ding (Hong Kong) has tried needling on sphenopalatine ganglion in cases of chronic allergic rhinitis. He gave hand stimulation to the needles after inserting into sphenopalatine ganglion for 20 to 30 minutes daily for 10 days. He has observed good results with this method.

EPISTAXIS

Bleeding from the nose is a common symptom and is often alarming because the sight of blood itself causes anxiety. Bleeding is usually trivial and has no obvious cause. Such bleeding occurs from the little's area. Epistaxis may occasionally be the symptomatic expression of hypertension or bleeding disorders or it may be of traumatic origin.

Main points	:	Yintang	(Ex-1)
		Renzhong	(GV-26)
		Nose Heliao	(LI-19)
		Yingxiang	(LI-20)
		Shangxing	(GV-23)
Supplementary points	:	Baihui	(GV-20)
		Hegu	(LI-4)

Lieque   (L-7)
Sanyinjiao   (Sp-6)
Zusanli   (St-36)

Stimulation

Moderate stimulation by hand can be given.

Remarks

Results are good.

DISEASES OF THE ORAL CAVITY

TOOTHACHE

The only structure of the tooth which is sensitive to pain is its pulp which is normally protected by enamel. Dental caries, probably the most common disease in man, is the basic cause of chronic toothache. Enamel is destroyed by the effect of acid which is produced by the action of micro-organisms on a sugar substrate deposited on the tooth in the form of a plaque. When the pulp is exposed due to the destruction of the enamel, the tooth becomes sensitive to hot or cold food or drinks. Throbbing pain is suggestive of periapical abscess due to the spread of infection from pulp to the surrounding parts.

Upper toothache

Main points	:	Juliao	(St-3)
		Dicang	(St-4)
		Xiaguan	(St-7)
		Yingxiang	(LI-20)
		Quanliao	(SI-18)

Lower toothache

Main points	:	Daying	(St-5)
		Jiache	(St-6)
		Guanyuan	(CV-14)
		Sishencong	(Ex-6)
Supplementary points	:	Hegu	(LI-4)
(for both)		Quchi	(LI-11)
		Tongli	(H-5)
		Yifeng	(TW-17)
		Neiting	(St-44)
Ear points	:	Maxillary area	
		Mandibular area	
		Shenmen	
Scalp needling	:	Lower two fifths of sensory area (both sides)	

Stimulation

Moderate electrical stimulation should be given for 30 minutes daily for 5 to 7 days.

Remarks
1. Oral hygiene should be maintained.
2. The underlying infection should be treated with modern medicine.

APHTHOUS ULCERS

This is the most common variety of recurrent oral ulcers. The precise aetiology is not known but psychogenic, hereditary, hormonal and autoimmune factors have been implicated. Patient may experience soreness in the mouth for a day or two before the ulcers appear. The ulcers vary in size, shape and number, and are situated on the mucosa of lips, cheeks, tongue, and sometimes palate and pharynx. Surrounding mucosa is inflamed. The ulcers are extremely painful and make eating, swallowing, and sometimes even talking, difficult. Weight loss due to reduced intake may occur.

Main points		Renzhong	(GV-26)
		Yinjiao	(GV-28)
		Chengjiang	(CV-24)
		Jiachengjiang	(Ex-5)
		Dicang	(St-4)
Supplementary points	:	Baihui	(GV-20)
		Hegu	(LI-4)
		Quchi	(LI-11)
		Dazhui	(GV-14)
		Sanyinjiao	(Sp-6)
		Zusanli	(St-36)
Ear points	:	Mouth area	
		Fasiomandibular area	
		Tongue area	
		Adrenal gland	
		Internal secretion	

Stimulation
Mild stimulation should be given for 20-30 minutes daily for 10 days.

Remarks
1. Results are good.
2. High doses of vitamin B complex should also be administered.

24

GASTROINTESTINAL DISEASES

INDIGESTION

The term is used to denote any type of distress associated with the intake of food. When a patient describes his symptom as indigestion its meaning may be as varied as fullness in abdomen, abdominal pain, heartburn. belching, distension and flatulence. The diagnostic significance of all this descriptive terminology is virtually same. In a case of indigestion it is necessary to enquire about the location and duration of discomfort, relation to ingestion of food and specific food intolerance.

One of the common causes of indigestion is peptic ulcer. Acute gastritis, which may follow dietary indiscretion or an alcoholic binge, may cause burning sensation in the epigastrium and nausea. Symptoms similar to those of peptic ulcer may characterise chronic gastritis due to hyperacidity, and also due to hypoacidity. Gastric analysis will confirm the diagnosis. Upper abdominal discomfort, anorexia, nausea, intolerance to meal and hypoacidity are suggestive of carcinoma of the stomach.

Chronic colitis is characterised by disordered bowel habits, flatulence and tenderness over the colon which may be palpable. Chronic cholecystitis, viral hepatitis and cirrhosis of liver are discussed elsewhere. Indigestion may at times be a feature of systemic disease like cardiac failure, uraemia, tuberculosis and neoplasia. Even when all these conditions are excluded, some cases would remain in whom no demonstrable organic disease can be found. Such cases of functional indigestion have a psychic background. The symptoms are more at night, have no relation to meals, and are not accompanied by nausea or vomiting and tenderness or rigidity. The person has erructations, aerophagy, and collection of gas in the stomach and splenic flexure. The trapped gas may produce discomfort resembling that due to ischaemic heart disease.

Main points	:	Qihai	(CV-6)
		Zhongwan	(CV-12)
		Tianshu	(St-25)
		Pishu	(UB-20)

Supplementary points	: Baihui	(GV-20)
	Neiguan	(P-6)
	Zusanli	(St-36)
	Sanyinjiao	(Sp-6)
Ear points	: Stomach	
	Small intestine	
	Spleen	
	Shenmen	
Scalp needling	: Gastric area	

Stimulation

Mild to moderate stimulation daily 20 to 30 minutes for 10 to 15 days. Course may be repeated after a rest of 5 to 7 days.

Remarks

Results are good.

PAIN IN ABDOMEN

Pain in abdomen may be acute or chronic. Chronic abdominal pain is discussed along with indigestion. Acute abdominal pain may be the result of inflammation of the parietal peritoneum, obstruction to a hollow viscera, or vascular occlusion, or it may occur with some metabolic conditions or as a referred pain.

Inflammation of the peritoneum is characterised by pain which increases on movement, tenderness and rigidity. Such inflammation may occur due to perforation of peptic or intestinal ulcer or inflammation of abdominal viscera, e.g. acute pancreatitis. Perforation of gastric or intestinal ulcer is associated with gas under the diaphragm which obliterates the liver dullness and can be seen on a skiagram. Serum amylase is raised in acute pancreatitis. Pain due to intestinal biliary or ureteric obstruction is colicky. In intestinal obstruction, it is situated in the periumbilical region, and is accompanied by vomiting and absolute constipation. Skiagram of abdomen shows fluid levels. Biliary and ureteric obstruction are discussed elsewhere.

Vascular occlusion usually involves the superior mesenteric artery and is often atherosclerotic in origin. The pain is prominent after meals and there is evidence of vascular disease elsewhere in the body.

Referred pain in abdomen occurs in diseases of the thoracic viscera (pneumonia, myocardial infarction) spine (osteoarthritis) and genitalia (torsion of a testicle). Metabolic disorders which produce abdominal pain are diabetic ketoacidosis and prophyria.

EPIGASTRIC PAIN

Main points	: Zhongwan	(CV-12)
	Shangwan	(CV-13)
	Tianshu	(St-25)

Supplementary points	:	Baihui	(GV-20)
		Hegu	(LI-4)
		Neiguan	(P-6)
		Sanyinjiao	(Sp-6)
		Zusanli	(St-36)
		Neiting	(St-44)

PAIN IN UMBILICAL REGION

Main points	:	Tianshu	(St-25)
		Daheng	(Sp-15)
		Huangshu	(K-16)
		Zhongwan	(CV-12)
		Yanglingquan	(GB-34)
Supplementary points	:	Baihui	(GV-20)
		Hegu	(LI-4)
		Liangqiu	(St-34)
		Shangjuxu	(St-37)
		Neiting	(St-44)
		Sanyinjiao	(SP-6)
		Yanglingquan	(GB-34)

PAIN IN HYPOGASTRIUM

Main points	:	Guanyuan	(CV-4)
		Qihai	(CV-6)
		Daheng	(Sp-15)
		Guilai	(St-29)
Supplementary points	:	Baihui	(GV-20)
		Hegu	(LI-4)
		Liangqiu	(St-34)
		Zusanli	(St-36)
		Taichong	(Liv-3)
		Yanglingquan	(GB-34)

Stimulation

Mild electrical stimulation should be given for 20 to 30 minutes daily for 10 days. Course may be repeated after a rest of 5 to 7 days.

Remarks
1. Results are good as far as relief from pain is concerned.
2. The underlying cause should be investigated and treated accordingly.

PEPTIC ULCER

Ulceration of the gastrointestional tract due to the combined action of acid and pepsin (peptic ulcer) is commoly seen in stomach or duodenum but may occasionally involve oesophagus also. The precise aetiology is not known but heredity, stress and food habits are important factors. The effect of stress is probably mediated through the vagus nerve or the hypothalamus-pituitary-adrenocortical axis. Less often, drugs (aspirin, phenylbutazone), alcohol, smoking, vitamin deficiencies and hyperparathyroidism may be responsible for peptic ulcers.

The predominant feature is pain which may be burning in nature or dull aching with a sense of discomfort only. In gastric ulcer the pain is epigastric, starts after meals and is accompanied by vomiting and weightloss. In duodenal ulcer the pain is in epigastrium or right hypochondrium, relieved by meals (hunger pain) and not accompanied by vomiting. Some local tenderness may be present. Gastric analysis shows hypochlorhydria in most of the cases of gastric ulcer and hyperchlorhydria in duodenal ulcer. Barium meal may confirm the diagnosis. The important complications include perforation, haemorrhage, pyloric stenosis and malignant transformation.

Main points	:	Zhongwan	(CV-12)
		Tianshu	(St-25)
		Huangshu	(K-16)
		Daheng	(Sp-15)
		Weishu	(UB-21)
		Qimen	(Liv-14)
Supplementary points	:	Baihui	(GV-20)
		Hegu	(LI-4)
		Neiguan	(P-6)
		Liangqiu	(St-34)
		Zusanli	(St-36)
		Neiting	(St-44)
Ear points	:	Stomach	
		Spleen	
		Shenmen	
		Subcortex	
Scalp needling	:	Gastric area	

Stimulation

1. Mild electric stimulation should be given for 20 to 30 minutes daily for 10 days. Course may be repeated after the rest of 7 days.

2. Indirect moxibustion should be done on Zhongwan (CV-12), Shenjue (CV-8) and Geshu (UB-17)

3. Point injection : Injection novocain 0.5 to 1 ml to 1% or injection atropine 0.2 ml on Zusanli (St-36) both sides.

Remarks

1. Bland diet should be advised.

2. Physical and mental rest as well as abstinence from tobacco and alcohol are essential for quicker healing of the ulcer.

3. Results are excellent.

ACUTE APPENDICITIS

This is an acute inflammation of the vermiform appendix. Typically the patient has central abdominal pain and cramping due to distention of the appendix. This is associated with nausea, anorexia and vomiting. Within a few hours the pain shifts to the right iliac region due to the involvement of the peritoneal coat. Tenderness and rigidity in the right iliac region, fever, tachycardia and leucocytosis are the other features. Depending upon the position of the appendix (retrocaecal, pelvic, etc.), the site of pain and tenderness may vary. If not treated within 48 hours, an appendicular lump is formed due to adhesion of the coils of intestines and momentum to the inflamed appendix. When an appendicular lump forms the prognosis worsens.

Main points	:	Zhongji	(CV-3)
		Zhongwan	(CV-12)
		Tianshu	(St-25)
		Daheng	(Sp-15)
		Guilai	(St-29)
Supplementary points	:	Hegu	(LI-4)
		Quchi	(LI-11)
		Liangqiu	(St-34)
		Zusanli	(St-36)
		Lanwei	(Ex-33)
Ear points	:	Appendix area	
		Shenmen	
		Subcortex	
Scalp needling	:	Gastric area	

Stimulation
1. Mild electrical stimulation 20 to 30 minutes for 2 to 3 time a day can be given.
2. Point injection 0.1 to 0.2 ml atropine can be injected on Lanwei (Ex-33) both sides.

Remarks
1. Emergency surgical treatment should be advised when the pain continues for more than 24 hours, body temperature remains above 38°C, and there is leucocytosis over 15000/cu.mm.
2. Treatment can be continued for 2 to 3 days more after relief of symptoms.
3. Broad spectrum antibiotic should be prescribed for 7 to 10 days.

DIARRHOEA

Diarrhoea may be acute or chronic. Acute diarrhoea with passage of watery or blood mixed stools is usually a manifestation of gastrointestinal infection (cholera, gastroenteritis, dysentery) but may also occur due to indigestion of preformed toxins (food poisoning), poisonous chemicals, or drugs (purgatives, parasympthomimetic drugs). Acute diarrhoea may occasionally characterise colitis, regional enteritis or acute radiation sickness.

Chronic diarrhoea often poses a perplexing problem and needs careful historical and physical evaluation of the case and various investigations It may occur due to systemic disorders

like hyperthyroidism, tuberculosis and lymphosarcoma. When chronic diarrhoea is characterised by blood in stools, fever, malaise and weight loss, it is suggestive of chronic inflammatory conditions involving the small or large bowel, such as amoebic colitis, chronic bacillary
dysentery, ulcerative colitis, tuberculosis of the intestines, and regional enteritis. When
unaccompanied by fever, or blood in stool but characterised by weight loss and signs of
nutritional deficiency, chronic diarrhoea is a feature of malabsorption syndrome. The faecal
fat content in high (steatorrhoea).

Main points	:	Changqiang	(GV-1)
		Huiyin	(CV-1)
		Zhongwan	(CV-12)
		Tianshu	(St-25)
		Daheng	(Sp-15)
		Dachangshu	(UB-25)
Supplementary points	:	Baihui	(GV-20)
		Zusanli	(St-36)
		Tiaokou	(St-38)
		Gongsun	(Sp-4)
		Sanyinjiao	(Sp-6)
		Sanyangluo	(TW-8)
Ear points	:	Large intestine	
		Stomach	
		Shenmen	
		Subcortex	

Stimulation

1. Mild electrical stimulation for 20 to 30 minutes for 2 to 3 day can be given.
2. Indirect moxibustion in Shenjue (CV-8) also shows good result.

Remarks

1. Acute diarrhoea responds promptly to acupuncture therapy.
2. Cases of chronic diarrhoea should be thoroughly investigated and appropriate treatment should be given.
3. Due to the homeostatic effect of acupuncture, chronic diarrhoea also responds well.

CONSTIPATION

It is not possible to formulate a precise definition for constipation because of marked
Individual variation in the frequency of passage of stools. Constipation may be said to be a
condition characterised by infrequent passage of hard stools. Acute onset of severe constipation in a person who hitherto had apparently normal bowel habits signifies either a
mechanical obstruction to the bowels (carcinoma, faecal impaction, etc.) or a disturbance of
the neural, vascular or muscular integrity of the gut. Such disturbances result from severe
infections, cerebrovascular diseases, diseases of spinal cord, leading to paraplegia.
Hirschsprung's disease, mesenteric artery thrombosis, hypothyroidism, hyperparathyroidism,
major psychosis, parkinsonism and drugs like opium alkaloids.

More common than these organic causes are the functional ones. A long history of inter-mittent bouts of constipation accompanied by abdominal distress relieved by defecation and passage of hard stools of small size is characteristic of irritable colon syndrome. This is a manifestation of anxiety. Another variety of functional chronic constipation is dyschezia in which the rectal sensation is suppressed and desire to defecate lost. It may begin in pregnancy or because of faulty training in childhood or due to failure to respond to call to stool, sudden change to low roughage diet or sedentary life habits. Patients resort to purga-tives or enema and when the use of these is discontinued, the condition is aggravated.

Constipation gives rise to a psychological sensation of abdominal discomfort, headache and a sense of general ill health due to the widely held misbelief that bowels must be opened daily.

Main points	:	Zhongwan	(CV-12)
		Tianshu	(St-25)
		Daheng	(Sp-15)
		Pishu	(UB-20)
Supplementary points	:	Zhigou	(TW-6)
		Baihui	(GV-20)
		Zusanli	(St-36)
Ear points	:	Stomach	
		Spleen	
		Large intestine	
		Rectum	
		Sympathetic area	

Stimulation

Mild electrical stimulation can be given for 20 to 30 minutes daily for 10 days and the course may be repeated after the rest of 5 to 7 days.

Remarks

Because of the homeostatic effect of acupuncture on intestinal motility, constipation also responds well to the treatment.

PILES   (HAEMORRHOIDS)

Haemorrhoids are dilated veins occurring in relation to the anus and originating in the subepithelial plexus formed by radicles of superior, middle and inferior rectal veins. They may be internal, under the mucous membrane, or internoexternal, under the mucous membrane and skin. They usually occur independently but may occur secondary to carcinoma of rectum, portal hypertension, pregnancy and urethral obstruction. Haemorrhoids may be asymptomatic or may present with bleeding, prolapse, pain, or anaemia. When the haemo-rrhoids protrude during defecation but reduce spontaneously they are called first degree, when they have to be reduced manually they are called second degree, and when they cannot be reduced and remain protruded all the time they are called third degree haemorrhoids. The complications include profuse haemorrhage, strangulation, thrombosis, ulceration, gangrene, suppuration and pyelophlebitis.

Main points	:	Changqiang	(GV-1)
		Jizhong	(GV-6)
		Huiyin	(CV-1)
		Qihaishu	(UB-24)
Supplementary points	:	Baihui	(GV-20)
		Renzhong	(GV-26)
		Yanglingquan	(GB-34)
Ear points	:	Rectum	
		Large intestine	
		Sympathetic	
		Shenmen	

Stimulation

Moderate stimulation should be given for 20 to 30 minutes daily for 10 days. Course may be repeated after a rest of 5 to 7 days.

Remarks

Good results can be achieved in first and second degree haemorrhoids.

CHRONIC CHOLECYSTITIS AND GALLSTONES

Chronic cholecystitis is conventionally described as a disease of four F's—fat, flatulent, female of forty. But the diagnosis should not preferably be made unless gallstones are found on radiologic examination. Flatulent dyspepsia may be caused by many conditions like gastritis, hiatus hernia, irritable colon syndrome, and ischaemic heart disease, which should be carefully excluded before chronic cholecystitis is diagnosed.

Precipitation of biliary constituents—cholesterol, calcium and bile pigments—in the gall bladder or bile duct leads to gallstones. Obstruction of the bile duct may give rise to biliary colic—colicky pain in the right hypochondrium with referred pain in the right shoulder. It is accompanied by vomiting, fever, slight icterus and rigidity in the right hypochondrium. Complications of gallstones include acute cholecystitis, obstructive jaundice, stricture of the bile duct, cholangitis, acute pancreatitis, perforation of the gall bladder and biliary peritonitis, and carcinoma of the gall bladder. Only 20 per cent of the gallstones are radio-opaque. The remaining can be demonstrated only by cholecystography.

Main points	:	Zhongwan	(CV-12)
		Liangmen	(St-21)
		Zhangmen	(Liv-13)
		Riyue	(GB-24)
		Ganshu	(UB-18)
		Danshu	(UB-19)
Supplementary points	:	Baihui	(GV-20)
		Hegu	(LI-4)
		Quchi	(LI-11)
		Jianjing	(GB-21)
		Yanglingquan	(GB-34)

		Zusanli	(St-36)
		Neiting	(St-44)
		Dannang	(Ex-35)
Ear points	:	Liver	
		Gall bladder	
		Shenmen	
		Subcortex	
Scalp needling	:	Gastric area	

Stimulation

1. Strong stimulation should be given for 15 to 20 minutes daily for 10 to 15 days. Course may be repeated after a rest of 5 to 7 days.

2. Indirect moxibustion over Zhongwan (CV-12), supplementary points and Dannang (Ex-35) should be done for 5 to 10 minutes daily.

Remarks

1. Results are good in cases of chronic cholecystitis with or without gallstones.

2. That acupuncture is capable of expelling stones from the gall bladdar has been seen by the author during his visit to People's Republic of China.

VIRAL HEPATITIS

This is the most common of all the varieties of hepatitis that are caused by various viruses, microorganisms and drugs. Viral hepatitis is characterised by jaundice, enlarged tender liver, anorexia, nausea, vomiting and a low grade fever. Jaundice is not a constant feature and is absent in a large proportion of cases which are termed anicteric hepatitis.

The hepatitis virus is of two types, A and B, while A is responsible for infectious hepatitis, B causes serum hepatitis. Minor differences in the clinical features of these two varieties of hepatitis exist. While infectious hepatitis is transmitted by faecal oral route, serum hepatitis is transmitted by injection of contaminated serum or blood or even by the use of syringes or needles which have been contaminated by patient's blood. Serum hepatitis has a longer incubation period, longer course and a higher rate of complications and mortality. The complications include intrahepatic cholestasis, acute hepatic necrosis, aplastic anaemia, acute polyneuritis, delayed convalescence, relapse and postnecrotic cirrhosis.

Main points	:	Geshu	(UB-17)
		Ganshu	(UB-18)
		Danshu	(UB-19)
		Liangmen	(St-21)
		Qimen	(Liv-14)
		Riyue	(GB-24)
Supplementary points	:	Baihui	(GV-20)
		Quchi	(LI-11)
		Taichong	(Liv-3)
		Liangqiu	(St-34)
		Zusanli	(St-36)

		Dazhui	(GV-14)
		Yanglingquan	(GB-34)
Points for anorexia	:	Tianshu	(St-25)
		Sanyinjiao	(Sp-6)
		Zusanli	(St-36)
Ear points	:	Liver	
		Hepatitis point	
		Shenmen	
Scalp needling	:	Hepatocystic area	
		Gastric area	

Stimulation

1. Mild electrical stimulation for 20 to 30 minutes daily for 10 days.

Point injection

Dose of 0.5 to 1 ml of vitamin B_1 can be injected on Geshu (UB-17) both sides on alternate days.

Remarks

1. Serum hepatitis may be transmitted by contamination of acupuncture needles. There-fore, needles used on patients of viral hepatitis should not be re-used for other patients.
2. Prognosis depends upon initial levels, of serum bilirubin, S.G.O.T. and S.G.P.T.

CIRRHOSIS OF LIVER

Cirrhosis of the liver is a chronic disorder of multiple aetiology in which the liver shows diffused cellular damage, fibrosis and formation of degenerative nodules. These structural changes in the liver are responsible for various clinical features and complications of cirrhosis. Progressive loss of the liver cells leads to jaundice, ascites, oedema, dysfunction of central nervous system and cachexia. Fibrosis causes distortion of the intrahepatic vasculature leading to portal venous hypertension which is responsible for oesophageal varices, engorged veins on abdominal wall and splenomegaly. Degenerative nodules compress the venous and lymphatic radicles, adding to the portal hypertension and ascites.

Cirrhosis is divided into three varieties.

1. Micronodular : Liver is often large and uniformly granular. It is usually caused by by chronic alcoholism (portal cirrhosis) and biliary obstruction (biliary cirrhosis).
2. Macronodular : Liver is often shrunken and coarsely nodular. This variety follows viral hepatitis (postnecrotic cirrhosis, cryptogenic cirrhosis).
3. Mixed : This includes Indian childhood cirrhosis which is due to some unknown toxin.

The complications of cirrhosis are life threatening and include haemorrhage from oesopha-geal varices, progressive liver cell failure, hepatic encephalopathy and hepatoma.

Main points	:	Zhangmen	(Liv-13)
		Qimen	(Liv-14)
		Liangmen	(ST-21)

		Reyue	(GB-24)
		Geshu	(UB-17)
		Ganshu	(UB-18)
Supplementary points	:	Taichong	(Liv-3)
		Yanglingquan	(GB-34)
		Zusanli	(ST-36)
		Baihui	(GV-20)
Ear points	:	Liver area	
		Gall bladder	
		Hepatitis point	
		Shenmen	
Scalp needling	:	Hepatocystic area	
		Gastric area	

Stimulation

Mild electrical stimulation can be given for 20 to 30 minutes daily for 10 days. Course may be repeated after a rest of 5 to 7 days.

Remarks

1. Long term therapy is advised.
2. High protein diet and vitamin supplements are necessary.
3. Results are good.

25
RESPIRATORY DISEASES

UPPER RESPIRATORY TRACT INFECTION

Upper respiratory tract infection is often of viral or streptococcal origin. Different parts of the upper respiratory passages may be involved giving rise to rhinitis, sinusitis, tonsilitis, pharyngitis and laryngitis. The symptoms are as described below.

1. *Rhinitis* : Sneezing, running or blocked nose, headache conjunctival congestion.
2. *Sinusitis* : This is discussed in the next chapter.
3. *Tonsilitis and pharyngitis* : Sorethroat, dryness of throat, congested mucosa, tonsils are enlarged, fever, cervical lymph nodes may be enlarged, commonly associated with rhinitis.
4. *Laryngitis* : Change in voice, laryngoscopy shows erythama of vocal cords.

Main points	: Shanzhong	(CV-17)
	Tiantu	(CV-22)
	Lianquan	(CV-23)
	Chengjiang	(CV-24)
	Yingxiang	(LI-20)
	Feishu	(UB-13)
	Dingchuan	(Ex-17)
Supplementary points	: Baihui	(GV-20)
	Hegu	(LI-4)
	Quchi	(LI-11)
	Neiguan	(P-6)
	Lieque	(L-7)
	Fenglong	(St-40)
	Sanyinjiao	(Sp-6)
Ear points	: Lung	
	Large intestine	
	Internal secretion	
	Shenmen	

Subcortex
According to the part affected

Points according to symptoms

Nasal obstruction:

Yintang	(Ex-1)
Yingxiang	(LI-20)
Houxi	(SI-3)

Headache and common cold:

Baihui	(GV-20)
Xinhui	(GV-22)
Hegu	(LI-4)

High fever:

Dazhui	(GV-14)
Hegu	(LI-4)
Quchi	(LI-11)
Fenglong	(St-40)
Hot point in the ear	

Sore throat:

Tianrong	(SI-17)
Lianquan	(CV-23)

Stimulation

Mild stimulation daily for 20 to 30 minutes for 5 to 7 days.

Remarks

Acupuncture is beneficial in preventing recurrent attacks of upper respiratory tract infection.

SINUSITIS

Acute sinusitis is a bacterial infection of paranasal sinuses which usually follows acute upper respiratory tract infection, nasal allergy or dental abscess or extraction, or is superimposed on existing chronic sinusitis. The condition is characterised by pain, tenderness, redness and swelling over the involved sinus. Nasal mucosa is congested and purulent nasal discharge is present. The pain of sinusitis is maximum in the morning when the patient wakes up and gradually diminishes as the upright posture facilitates drainage. Pain increases on stooping. In maxillary sinusitis pain is referred to teeth and eyes, while in frontal sinusitis it is felt in the roof of the orbit. Pain is located between and behind the eyes in ethmoid sinusitis. The involved sinuses appear hazy on X-ray and transillumination. Recurrent acute sinusitis may lead to chronic sinusitis or complications like orbital cellulitis, osteomyelitis of the skull bones, meningitis, brain abscess and bronchiectasis.

Frontal sinusitis

Main points	:	Yangbai	(GB-14)
		Yintang	(Ex-1)
		Yuyao	(Ex-3)

Supplementary points	:	Hegu	(LI-4)
		Quchi	(LI-11)
		Sanyinjiao	(Sp-6)
		Xuehai	(Sp-10)
		Dazhui	(GV-14)
		Baihui	(GV-20)

Maxillary sinusitis

Main points	:	Juliao	(ST-3)
		Nose Heliao	(LI-19)
		Yingxiang	(LI-20) opposite side
		Quanliao	(SI-18)
		Tinghui	(GB-2)
Supplementary points	:	Baihui	(GV-20)
		Hegu	(LI-4)
		Quchi	(LI-11)
		Sanyinjiao	(Sp-6)
		Xuehai	(Sp-10)
		Zusanli	(St-36)
Ear points	:	Nose area	
		Adrenal gland	
		Internal secretion	
		Shenmen	
		Forehead	

Stimulation

Moderate stimulation should be given for 20 to 30 minutes daily for 10 days and the course may be repeated after a rest of 5 to 7 days.

Remarks

1. Immediate symptomatic relief is obtained.
2. For sustained relief long-term acupuncture therapy is advised.
3. In the acute stage, appropriate antibiotic should also be administered.

BRONCHITIS

Chronic bronchitis is defined as a condition characterised by cough with expectoration occurring on most of the days for at least 3 months in the year for at least 2 years. When the sputum is mucoid, the condition is called simple chronic bronchitis. At this stage, no objective signs are found. The condition may be complicated by infection, giving rise to chronic mucopurulent bronchitis, or by persistent widespread narrowing of the airways, giving rise to chronic obstructive bronchitis. In complicated cases expiratory wheezing is present and the sputum is mucopurulent. Pulmonary hypertension may develop and give rise to right ventricular hypertrophy and later on, failure. Skiagram of the chest shows prominent bronchovascular markings.

The disease usually manifests after 40 years of life and is caused by persistent heavy smoking, atmospheric pollution or occupations involving exposure to dust or fumes. Acute bronchitis may supervene on chronic bronchitis or occur in children due to viral infection.

Acute Bronchitis

Main points	: Shanzhong	(CV-17)
	Feishu	(UB-13)
	Dingchuan	(Ex-17)
Supplementary points	: Hegu	(LI-4)
	Quchi	(LI-11)
	Dazhui	(GV-14)
	Baihui	(GV-20)
	Chize	(L-5)
	Lieque	(L-7)

Chronic Bronchitis

Main points	: Shanzhong	(CV-17)
	Rugen	(St-18)
	Feishu	(UB-13)
	Dazhui	(GV-14)
	Dingchuan	(Ex-17)
Supplementary points	: Lieque	(L-7)
	Taiyuan	(L-9)
	Hegu	(LI-4)
	Quchi	(LI-11)

Points according to symptoms

Haemoptysis	: Shanzhong	(CV-17)
	Lieque	(L-7)
	Neiguan	(P-6)
Chest pain	: Shanzhong	(CV-17)
	Geshu	(UB-17)
	Hegu	(LI-4)
	Kongzui	(L-6)
Excessive sputum	: Fenglong	(St-40)
	Taixi	(K-3)
Ear points	: Lung	
	Large intestine	
	Internal secretion	
	Shenmen	
	Dingchuan	
Scalp needling	: Thoracic area	
	Gastric area	

Stimulation

1. Mild electrical stimulation for 20 to 30 minutes daily for 10 days. Course may be repeated after the rest of 5 to 7 days.

2.   Seven star needle tapping on the Hauto's points on alternate days.
3.   Indirect moxibustion over the body points for 5 to 10 minutes daily.
4.   Cupping on Shanzhong (CV-17), (UB-13) Feishu can also be done on alternate days.

Remarks
1.   Either cupping or needling can be done in children during acute bronchitis.
2.   Prognosis is quite satisfactory.
3.   Good results are obtained in children during acute bronchitis with cupping alone.
4.   Complications and progression of chronic bronchitis can be prevented with acupuncture.
5.   Smoking must be discouraged.

PULMONARY TUBERCULOSIS

Pulmonary tuberculosis is a chronic infection caused by *Mycobacterium tuberculosis*. The organism gains entry to the lungs by droplet spread. Because of the development of immunity and hypersensitivity the pathological and clinical features of first infection and subsequent infections differ. The former is called primary tuberculosis, and the latter postprimary.

Primary tuberculosis occurs mostly in children. The lesion is in the periphery of middle or lower lobe with enlargement of hilar lymphnodes. Healing is spontaneous and the condition is asymptomatic. However, in some cases symptoms are produced if there is a spread of the disease causing tuberculous pneumonia or milliary tuberculosis, or if the enlarged hilar lymphnodes press on a bronchus to produce atelectasis.

Postprimary tuberclosis is due to reinfection or activation of a dormant focus of infection. The lesions are in the apex of the lungs. The symptoms are cough with expectoration, haemoptysis, dyspnoea, fever, night sweats, anorexia, and weightloss. The signs vary according to the pathological changes produced. Such changes are infiltration, cavitation, fibrosis, pleural effusion, pneumothorax or milliary tuberculosis, X-ray is helpful in the diagnosis, and presence of acid-fast bacilli (AFB) in the sputum is confirmatory.

Main points	:	Shanzhong	(CV-17)
		Feishu	(UB-13)
		Dingchuan	(Ex-17)
Supplementary points	:	Hegu	(LI-4)
		Quchi	(LI-11)
		Dazhui	(GV-14)
		Baihui	(GV-20)
		Fenglong	(St-40)
		Sanyinjiao	(Sp-6)
Ear points		Lung	
		Large intestine	
		Shenmen	
		Dingchuan	

Stimulation
1.   Mild electrical stimulation can be given for 20 to 30 minutes daily for two weeks. Course of the therapy can be repeated after a rest of 5 to 7 days.

2. Point injection of streptomycin 0.2 g in any of the body points can also be given on alternate days.

Remarks
1. Acupuncture provides early symptomatic relief.
2. Appropriate antituberculous drugs must be given simultaneously.

BRONCHIAL ASTHMA

Bronchial asthma is characterised by attacks of widespread narrowing of peripheral airways resulting into breathlessness and wheezing. The condition is predisposed by hereditary factors. A nonspecific hyperirritability of tracheobronchial tree is genetically transmitted. The factors which precipitate an attack are exposure to allergens, exercise and infection. Allergens which precipitate an episode of asthma are mostly inhalants (e.g. pollen, dust, insect debris, animal hair, etc.) but may enter the body by other routes.

Asthma is of two types—extrinsic and intrinsic. Extrinsic asthma begins in childhood, is mostly seasonal, is truely intermittent and a family or personal history of other allergic conditions like rhinitis or urticaria is present. Intrinsic asthma begins in middle age, attack lasts for days or months and family history of allergy is absent. Prognosis in the latter is not as good as in the former.

An episode of asthma begins abruptly with breathlessness, cough and wheezing. It generally lasts for a few hours or a day. When the episode lasts for more than 48 hours the conditions is called status asthmaticus. Asthma has to be differentiated from other conditions causing sudden dyspnoea or wheezing. A foreign body in the respiratory passages produces inspiratory dyspnoea. In acute left ventricular failure evidence of heart disease and basal crepitations are present. Chronic bronchitis has already been discussed. Tropical eosinophilia is characterised by an absolute eosinophil count of more than 1500 per cu. mm.

Main points	: Shanzhong	(CV-17)
	Tiantu	(CV-22)
	Rugen	(St-18)
	Feishu	(UB-13)
	Dingchuan	(Ex-17)
Supplementary points	: Dazhui	(GV-14)
	Baihui	(GV-20)
	Hegu	(LI-4)
	Lieque	(L-7)
	Neiguan	(P-6)
	Sanyinjiao	(Sp-6)
	Xuehai	(Sp-10)
	Taixi	(K-3)
	Fenglong	(St-40)
Ear points	: Lung	
	Heart	
	Dingchuan	
	Shenmen	
	Internal secretion	

Scalp needling   :   Thoracic cavity area
                              Gastric area

Status asthmaticus

Main points   :   Tiantu   (CV-22)
                              Kongzui   (L-6)
                              Taixi   (K-3)
                              Xuehai   (Sp-10)
                              Yanglao   (SI-6)

Stimulation

Mild electrical stimulation for 20 to 30 minutes daily for 3 to 4 weeks. Course may be repeated after seeing the response.

Remarks

1. Long-term acupuncture therapy is needed.
2. Continuous use of press needle on the ear point is beneficial in status asthmaticus.
3. Good results are obtained even in cases of intrinsic asthma.
4. Excellent results have been achieved by Anton Jayasuriya (Sri Lanka) with the use of aforementioned points.

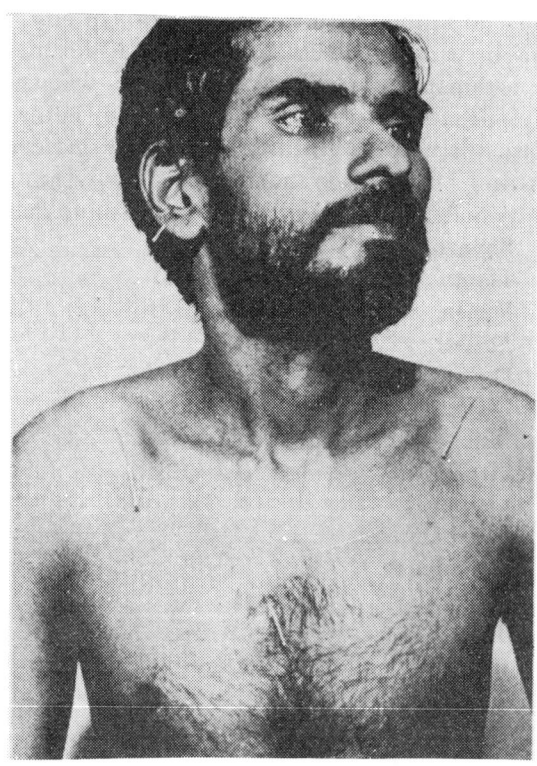

Bronchial asthma

26
CARDIOVASCULAR DISEASES

CARDIAC NEURORIS

Though this is not a cardiac disease, it is described here because it is often confused with angina pectoris. The persons involved are those who are unduly anxious about their heart, probably because of a family history of ischaemic heart disease. The chest pain is in the left inframammary region and usually occurs in the evening when the patient is fatigued, as opposed to the pain of angina pectoris which is substernal and related to exercise rather than fatigue. Other features of anxiety are present.

Main points	:	Shanzhong	(CV-17)
		Rugen	(St-18)
		Xinshu	(UB-15)
Supplementary points	:	Baihui	(GV-20)
		Hegu	(LI-4)
		Shenmen	(H-7)
		Neiguan	(P-6)
		Neiting	(St-44)
Ear points	:	Shenmen	
		Subcortex	
		Heart	
		Small intestine	
		Lung	

Stimulation

Mild stimulation should be given for 10 days. Course may be repeated after a rest of 5 to 7 days.

Remarks

Results are excellent.

ANGINA PECTORIS

Angina pectoris is one end of the clinical spectrum produced by disparity in the myocardial oxygen demand and its supply by coronary arteries. The most common cause of such disparity is coronary atherosclerosis though less often it is produced by conditions like syphilitic coronary ostial stenosis, anaemia and aortic stenosis.

The pain of angina pectoris is situated in the substernal or precordial region and radiates to the left shoulder, left arm, neck, jaw, epigastrium, back and rarely the right side. It is precipitated by exercise and emotional stress and relieved by rest and nitrites. The pain lasts only for a few minutes but is very intense. Rarely, the pain may occur at rest (angina decubitus).

The diagnosis is confirmed by electrocardiography. The characteristic change is S-T segment depression. In about half of the cases electrocardiographic abnormality is seen only during pain. In such cases exercise stress testing is employed for the diagnosis. Even this may be negative in about 10 per cent cases.

Initial attacks of angina pectoris, an increase in their frequency and angina decubitus may precede myocardial infarction and are considered as preinfarction angina.

Main points	:	Shanzhong	(CV-17)
		Rugen	(St-18)
		Xinshu	(UB15)
Supplementary points	:	Baihui	(GV-20)
		Neiguan	(P-6)
		Shenmen	(H-7)
		Taiyuan	(L-9)
		Hegu	(LI-4)
		Neiting	(St-44)
		Fuliu	(K-7)
Ear points	:	Heart	
		Small intestine	
		Subcortex	
		Shenmen	

Stimulation

Mild stimulation 20 to 30 minutes daily for 10 days. Course may be repeated after a rest of 5 to 7 days.

Remarks

1. Results are good.
2. Smoking and use of tobacco in any form should be strictly prohibited.
3. Weight reduction is necessary in overweight patients (see obesity).

MYOCARDIAL INFARCTION

Myocardial infarction is another end of the clinical spectrum of which one extreme is angina pectoris. Thrombosis on, haemorrhage into, or rupture of an atheromatous plaque in the coronary artery causes myocardial infarction or sudden death.

The situation and radiation of the pain of myocardial infarction are similar to those of angina pectoris, but the pain usually begins at rest and lasts for many hours, and is not relieved by nitrites. Intense, piercing or squeezing in nature, it is often accompanied by vomiting, excessive perspiration, dyspnoea and a sense of impending death. Only one of these symptoms may be present and pain absent in about 20 per cent of the cases. The characteristic electrocardiographic findings and/or raised levels of SGOT, LDH and CPK confirm the diagnosis.

A significant fact regarding myocardial infarction is high mortality (15 to 20 per cent). A more significant fact is that the death occurs early in the course of the disease—65 per cent deaths occurs in first 6 hours and 85 per cent in first 24 hours. The life threatening arrhythmias like asystole and ventricular fibrillation can, to a great extent, be prevented by the prompt treatment of arrhythmias like heart blocks and ventricular extrasystoles which precede them. Other cases of death include cardiac failure, pulmonary oedema, and cardiogenic shock. The mortality in presence of cardiogenic shock is 90 per cent.

Main points	: Shanzhong	(CV-17)
	Rugen	(St-18)
	Xinshu	(UB-15)
Supplementary points	: Baihui	(GV-20)
	Shaohai	(H-3)
	Shenmen	(H-7)
	Neiguan	(P-6)
	Hegu	(LI-4)
	Neiting	(St-44)
Ear points	Heart	
	Small intestine	
	Shenmen	
	Adrenalis	

Stimulation
1. Mild electrical stimulation can be given for 20 to 30 minutes daily for 10 days.
2. Course may be repeated after seeing the response.
3. Press needle on the ear points. Heart and Shenmen is also advised.

Remarks
1. In absence of complications, prognosis is good.
2. Arrhythmias should be treated on modern medical lines.
3. Cardiogenic shock should be treated as discussed in the relevant chapter.

PALPITATION

An uncomfortable awareness of the heart beat is called palpitation, but when the patient uses this word to describe his symptoms its meaning may be varied and different. In many of these instances it indicates anxiety. Indeed, in most of the cases, palpitation is an expression of anxiety rather than an organic heart disease.

Palpitation due to heart disease may occur in the presence of very slow or very rapid rate or due to an increase in the stroke volume. Thus, arrhythmias like complete heart block and paroxysmal atrial tachycardia can produce palpitation. Palpitation due to paroxysmal atrial tachycardia has an abrupt onset and a similar abrupt termination. Extrasystoles may be felt as occasional thumps in the chest. Aortic regurgitation and thyrotoxicosis may give rise to palpitation due to an increase in the stroke volume. All these conditions can be diagnosed by a careful examination of the pulse and blood pressure.

Anaemia and hypertension are uncommon causes of palpitation.

Main points	:	Shanzhong	(CV-17)
		Xinshu	(UB-15)
		Rugen	(St-18)
Supplementary points	:	Baihui	(GV-20)
		Shenmen	(H-7)
		Neiguan	(P-6)
		Yinlingquan	(Sp-9)
		Taichong	(Liv-3)
Ear points	:	Heart	
		Shenmen	
		Subcortex	
		Sympathetic	

If palpitation is associated with insomnia, Anmian I (Ex-8) and Anmian II (Ex-9) can also be added in the above group.

Stimulation

Mild stimulation is advised for 20 to 30 minutes daily for 10 days, course may be repeated after a rest of 5 to 7 days.

Remarks

Results are good.

HYPERTENSION

A persistent elevation of the diastolic blood pressure above an arbitrary level of 90 mm of mercury is defined as hypertension. It is usually associated with changes in the retinal blood vessels which can be seen on ophthalmoscopic examination. Hypertension is usually asymptomatic till it is diagnosed after which symptoms may occur due to anxiety. In occasional cases headache, palpitation and giddiness may be present, while in some the symptoms are produced by complications.

In 90 per cent cases no definite cause can be found to account for the elevated blood pressure. These cases are labelled as essential hypertension. Psychological stress and heredity are thought to play some part in the genesis of essential hypertension.

The remaining 10 per cent cases, where a definite cause for hypertension can be found, are due to renal diseases (chronic pyelonephritis, polycystic kidneys), endocrine diseases (Cushing's syndrome, Conn's syndrome, pheochromocytoma), cardiovascular diseases (coarctation of aorta), neurological diseases (brain tumours), drugs (corticosteroids, oral contraceptives), and toxaemia of pregnancy. These are the cases of secondary hypertension, and should be suspected in young persons and in the presence of severe hypertension (diastolic pressure over 130 mm Hg), accelerated hypertension, inequality of pulse, abdominal bruit and abnormal urine picture.

Hypertension is classified as benign and malignant. The latter has a rapidly progressive, downhill course : Uncontrolled hypertension may lead to various complications such as cerebral haemorrhage, retinal haemorrhages, left ventricular failure and renal failure.

Main points	:	Baihui	(GV-20)
		Yinxi	(H-6)
		Shenmen	(H-7)
		Taiyuan	(L-9)
		Neiguan	(P-6)
Supplementary points	:	Quchi	(LI-11)
		Zusanii	(St-36)
		Taichong	(Liv-3)
		Sanyinjiao	(Sp-6)
		Taixi	(K-3)
		Ganshu	(GB-18)
		Shenshu	(UB-23)
Ear points	:	Shenmen	
		Subcortex	
		Sympathetic	
		Adrenal	
		Blood pressure depression point	

Points according to symptoms

Headache and insomnia :	Baihui	(GV-20)
	Fengchi	(GB-20)
	Touwei	(St-8)
	Hegu	(LI-4)
	Neiting	(St-44)
Tinnitus and Vertigo :	Baihui	(GV-20)
	Sishencong	(Ex-6)
	Yifeng	(TW-17)
	Ermen	(TW-21)
	Tinggong	(SI-19)
	Tinghui	(GB-2)

Stimulation

Mild electrical stimulation can be given for 10 days and the course may be repeated after a rest of 5 to 7 days.

Remarks

1. If the blood pressure is more than 200/120 mm Hg, modern medicines should be used to bring down the blood pressure below this level.
2. Electrical stimulation is contraindicated if blood pressure is more than 200/120 mm Hg.
3. Taichong (Liv-3) is physiological danger point, patient should be constantly observed when this point is used.

4.   Secondary hypertension should be ruled out by proper investigations.

5.   Results are encouraging in mild to moderate hypertension.

BURGER'S DISEASE

Also known as thromboangitis obliterance, this condition is characterised by inflammation and thrombosis of the peripheral arteries and veins particularly affecting the legs. The changes are followed by gangrene of the affected limbs. The upper limbs and viscera are rarely involved. The disease predominantly affects the males. A definite relationship with smoking is present.

Main points	:	Weizhong	(UB-40)
		Chengshan	(UB-57)
		Huantiao	(GB-30)
		Yanglingquan	(GB-34)
		Zusanli	(St-36)
		Neiting	(St-44)
Supplementary points	:	Baihui	(GV-20)
		Sanyinjiao	(Sp-6)
		Ququan	(Liv-8)
		Taiyuan	(L-9)
		Fenglong	(St-40)
Ear points		Shenmen	
		Subcortex	
		Lung	
		Heart	
Scalp needling	:	Foot sensory motor area	
		Sensory area upper one-fifth both sides.	

Points according to symptoms.

a.   Pain in upper   :   Hegu   (LI-4)
     extremity   Taiyuan   (L-9)
                           Baihui   (GV-20)

     Pain in lower   :   Zusanli   (St-36)
     extremity   Neiting   (St-44)

b.   Numbness and coldness :

     Upper extremity :   Laogong   (P-8)
                          Shenmen   (H-7)

     Lower extremity :   Yongquan   (K-1)
                          Taixi   (K-3)
                          Femurwuli   (Liv-10)

Stimulation

Mild electrical stimulation should be given for 20 to 30 minutes daily for 15 days and course may be repeated after a rest of 5 to 7 days.

Injection of 0.5 to 1 ml of 1 per cent procain can also be given in the Yinlingquan (Sp-9).

Remarks

1. Smoking should be strictly forbidden.
2. If gangrene has occurred, surgery is indicated.
3. Prompt symptomatic relief is obtained with acupuncture.

27

UROLOGICAL DISEASES

RENAL COLIC

Renal colic, more aptly termed as ureteric colic, is an agonising pain passing from loin to groin, coming on suddenly, causing the patient to draw up his knees and roll about. It is often accompanied by vomiting and profuse sweating. The condition is mostly caused by a ureteric calculus or by a calculus impacted in the pelviureteric junction. On rare occasions renal colic may be produced by crystalluria or a blood clot. Different varieties of renal stones are known but colic is often caused by oxalate stones which are small as to travel down the ureter and have an irregular surface. Renal colic is often associated with fever and haematuria.

Main points	:	Yaoyangguan	(GV-3)
		Mingmen	(GV-4)
		Shenshu	(UB-23)
		Qugu	(CV-2)
		Zhongji	(CV-3)
		Guanyuan	(CV-4)
Supplementary points	:	Baihui	(GV-20)
		Sanyinjiao	(Sp-6)
		Taixi	(K-3)
		Shuiquan	(K-5)
		Weizhong	(UB-40)
		Jinmen	(UB-63)
		Hegu	(LI-4)
Ear points	:	Kidney	
		Urinary bladder	
		Urethera	
		Sympathetic	
		Subcortex	
		Shenmen	

Stimulation
1. Strong electrical stimulation for 20 to 30 minutes daily with adjustable wave for 2 to 3 times daily until the desired result is oberved.
2. Strong hand stimulation should be given Hegu (LI-4) during the acute pain.
3. Dose of 0.5 to 1 ml of 1 per cent procaine can be injected on Shenshu (UB-23) and Sanyinjiao (Sp-6).

Remarks
After relief from the acute pain, proper laboratory investigations should be carried out to diagnose the underlying cause.
1. Immediate relief from colic is obtained.
2. Author has seen expulsion of renal stones by acupucture therapy during his visit to Peoples Republic of China.

INCONTINENCE OF URINE

In voluntary passage of urine due to loss of voluntary control over the urethral sphincters is called incontinence. It is of following varieties:
1. Enuresis—This is discussed separately.
2. Stress incontinence—Leakage of urine on coughing or sneezing due to weakness of the sphincters. Common in women after childbearing.
3. Overflow incontinence—Urine involuntarily overflows from a bladder that is distended. This is usually neurogenic, due to injury to the spinal cord.
4. Total incontinence—There is continuous dribbling of urine due to constant relaxation of the sphincters. This is also neurogenic, due to injury to the cauda equina.

Main points

Group I	: Shenshu	(UB-23)
	Dachangshu	(UB-25)
	Yaoyangguen	(GV-3)
Group II	: Qugu	(CV-2)
	Guanyuan	(CV-4)
	Guilai	(St-29)
Supplementary points	: Taixi	(K-3)
	Sanyinjiao	(Sp-6)
	Weizhong	(UB-40)
	Yanglingquan	(GB-34)
Ear points	: Sympathetic	
	Shenmen	
	Kidney	
	Urinary bladder	
Scalp needling	: Foot sensaro-motor area	
	Genital area	

Stimulation
1. Mild electrical stimulation should be given for 20 to 30 minutes daily till the desired result is observed.

   2.   Moxibustion should be given on Qugu (CV-2) and Guanyuan (CV-4).

Remarks
1. Results are excellent in stress incontinence.
2. When incontinence is of neurogenic origin, long-term acupuncture therapy is needed.

RETENTION OF URINE

Retention of urine, associated with ditension of the bladder, which can be felt as a tender lump in the hypogastrium, must be differentiated from anuria in which the bladder is empty. Retention of urine may be acute or chronic. Chronic retention leads to overflow incontinence which has been discussed in the previous chapter. The common causes of acute retention of urine are senile enlargement of the prostate, urethral stricture, meatal stenosis, phimosis and postoperative reflex spasm of urinary sphincters. Drugs like atropine, other anti-cholinergic drugs, antihistaminics, and antihypertensives may cause retention of urine, particularly in the older individuals. Retention may be a feature of hysteria.

Main points			
Group I	:	Qugu	(CV-2)
		Zhongji	(CV-3)
		Guanyuan	(CV-4)
Group II	:	Shenshu	(UB-23)
		Dachangshu	(UB-25)
		Pangguangshu	(UB-28)
Supplementary points	:	Baihui	(GV-20)
		Taixi	(K-3)
		Sanyinjiao	(Sp-6)
		Yinlingquan	(Sp-9)
		Weizhong	(UB-40)
Scalp needling	:	Genital area (both sides)	

Stimulation
1. Mild electrical stimulation should be given for 20 to 30 minutes daily till the desired result is observed.
2. Moxibustion should be given on Guanyuan (CV-4), Shimen (CV-5) and Sanyinjiao (Sp-6).
3. Press needle on the kidney and bladder area.

Remarks
1. Underlying cause of retention of urine should be investigated and treatment should be planned accordingly.
2. Results are good.

ANURIA

The normal urine output is 1500 ml per day or approximately 60 ml per hour. When the urine output falls below 15 ml per hour the condition is called oliguria, and when below 3 to

4 ml per hour, it is called anuria. Retention of urine in the bladder must be carefully ruled out before the diagnosis of anuria is made. Anuria is an acute event usually caused by prerenal or renal conditions. Anuria due to prerenal (systemic) conditions is a result of redued kidney perfusion due to redution in blood volume or perfusion pressure. The conditions which give rise to these changes include shock, severe dehydration and addisonian crisis (acute adrenal cortical insufficiency). Anuria of renal aetiology is found in acute glomerulonephritis, malignant hypertension, eclampsia, burns, transfusion reaction, crush syndrome, and due to nephrotoxic agents like heavy metals and snake venom. All these conditions produce acute tubular necrosis.

Besides reduction of urine output, other chief metabolic defects include uraemia, hyperpotassaemia and acidosis. The patient manifests with acidotic breathing (deep, rapid respiration) impairment of consciousness, and sometimes hypertension, pulmonary oedema, and convulsions. During recovery, the patient passes through the stage of diuresis in which there is excessive urinary loss of water, sodium and potassium.

Main points	:	Qugu	(CV-2)
		Zhongji	(CV-3)
		Guanyuan	(CV-4)
		Shenshu	(UB-23)
		Guilai	(St-29)
Supplementary points	:	Baihui	(GV-20)
		Taixi	(K-3)
		Shuiquan	(K-5)
		Sanyinjiao	(Sp-6)
		Yinlingquan	(Sp-9)
		Zusanli	(St-36)
Ear points	:	Sympathetic	
		Shenmen	
		Bladder	
		Kidney	

Stimulation
1. Mild electrical stimulation can be given 20 to 30 minutes daily. Course may be repeated after a rest of 5 to 7 days.
2. 7 star needle tapping along the Hauto's point on lumbosacral region daily.

Remarks
1. The underlying cause should be investigated and treated.
2. Fluid and electrolyte balance should be maintained.
3. Low protein, low potassium diet should be prescribed.
4. Acupuncture shortens the phase of anuria and hastens the recovery.

OEDEMA

Oedema is defined as excessive collection of fluid in the extracellular (interstitial) spaces. It may be localised or generalised. Generalised massive oedema is called anasarca. It may be associated with ascites and hydrothorax. Oedema occurs when there is a decrease in the osmotic pressure of plasma (hypoproteinaemia) or an increase in the venous pressure (venous obstruction, cardic failure).

The causes of oedema are as follows :

1. Nephrotic syndrome Associated with gross albuminuria and hypoproteinaemia, and marked puffiness of face, specially in the morning.
2. Acute nephritis—Slight oedema, albuminuria, haematuria, hypertension.
3. Hypoproteinaemia—A feature of malnutrition. Signs of vitamin deficiency coexist.
4. Severe anaemia.
5. Cirrhosis of liver.
6. Cardiac failure—Dyspnoea, evidence of heart disease, engorged neck veins, congested tender liver.
7. Pericardial effusion—Engorged veins with no pulsations. X-ray chest is confirmatory.
8. Beri beri—Oedema, neuropathy, right ventricular failure.
9. Epidemic dropsy—Due to ingestion of oil derived from *Argemona mexicana* which contaminates mustard seed.
10. Venous thrombosis—Oedema confined to a limb.
11. Lymphoedema—Due to lymphatic obstruction, oedema confined to a limb, non-pitting in late stages, usually filarial.
12. Angioneurotic oedema—Tendency to urticaria, short lived.
13. Cyclic oedema—Occurs in females at the time of menstrual flow.

Main points	:	Baihui	(GV-20)
		Pishu	(UB-20)
		Shenshu	(UB-23)
		Shimen	(CV-5)
		Shuifen	(CV-9)
		Taixi	(K-3)
		Yinlingquan	(Sp-9)
		Shushi	
Ear points	:	Ascits point	
		Liver	
		Shenmen	
		Subcortex	
		According to part affected	

Stimulation

Mild electrical stimulation should be given for 20 to 30 minutes daily for 10 days. Course may be repeated after a rest of 5 to 7 days.

Remarks

1. Underlying cause of disease should be properly investigated.
2. Medical treatment should be combined with the acupuncture.
3. High protein, salt-restricted diet should be advised.

28

OBSTETRIC AND GYNAECOLOGICAL DISEASES

MORNING SICKNESS

About three-fourths of women complain of nausea and vomiting during first trimester of pregnancy. These symptoms generally begin just after the first missed period and are more severe in the morning. Morning sickness is a normal accompaniment of pregnancy, but when the severity of vomiting is more or when vomiting persists beyond the first trimester, the woman is at risk. This situation is called hyperemesis gravidium and needs urgent treatment.

Main points	: Baihui	(GV-20)
	Qihai	(CV-6)
	Zhongwan	(CV-12)
	Neiguan	(P-6)
	Zusanli	(St-36)
	Sanyinjiao	(Sp-6)
Ear points	: Liver	
	Stomach	
	Adernal	
	Shenmen	
	Sympathetic	

Stimulation

Mild hand stimulation should be given for 15 to 20 minutes for 2 to 3 times a day for 10 days and the course may be repeated after a rest of 5 to 7 days.

Remarks

1. Electrical stimulation is contraindicated as it may lead to abortion.
2. Prognosis is good.

MALPOSITIONS OF THE FOETUS

The normal presentation at the time of labour is vertex. Malpresentations (malpositions) include face, breech, shoulder and oblique presentations which may produce difficulty in labour. Such malpositions are due to maternal and foetal factors which do not allow engagement of the head. These factors include premature and postmature labour, hydramnios, placenta previa, multiple pregnancies, foetal anomalies and gross cephalopelvic disproportion.

Main point	: Zhiyin	(UB-67)

Stimulation

Indirect moxibustion with moxaroll on Zhiyin (UB-67) after 30 minutes daily once a day until the foetal position is corrected.

Remarks

The foetal position can often be corrected by acupuncture.

INFERTILITY

Infertility or sterility may be primary or secondary. Primary sterility may be due to a fault in either the female or the male partner. The defects in the female include hormonal imbalance, anovulatory cycles, blockade of the fallopian tubes or structural defects of uterus or vagina. The male infertility may be due to azoospermia or impotence. The term secondary sterility is used when a female who has borne children earlier ceases to be capable of being pregnant. This is usually an aftereffect of uterine infection acquired during the previous childbirths.

Main points	:	Guanyuan	(CV-4)
		Qihai	(CV-6)
		Weibao	(Ex-15)
		Tsukung	
Supplementary points	:	Baihui	(GV-20)
		Hegu	(LI-4)
		Quchi	(LI-11)
		Taodao	(GV-13)
		Dazhui	(GV-14)
		Sanyinjiao	(Sp-6)
		Taixi	(K-3)
		Ququan	(Liv-8)
		Zusanli	(St-36)

Stimulation

Mild electrical stimulation can be given for 20 to 30 minutes daily for 10 days. Course may be repeated after the rest of 5 to 7 days.

Remarks

1. A longer course of treatment should be advised.
2. Proper investigations should be carried out to diagnose the underlying cause.
3. Medical treatment may be combined with acupuncture.
4. The role of acupuncture is not yet established in cases of infertility.

AMENORRHOEA

Absence of menstruation may be primary in which menstruation never started, or secondary in which there is a cessation of menstruation. Amenorrhoea may be due to hormonal disturbances, psychiatric conditions, or genetic abnormalities of the female genital tract.

Physiological causes of amenorrhoea include pregnancy and menopause.

Main points	:	Guanyuan	(CV-4)
		Qihai	(CV-6)
		Guilai	(St-29)
		Qichong	(St-30)
		Geshu	(UB-17)
		Ganshu	(UB-18)
		Shenshu	(UB-23)
Supplementary points	:	Baihui	(GV-20)
		Hegu	(LI-4)
		Quchi	(LI-11)
		Sanyinjiao	(Sp-6)
		Diji	(Sp-8)
		Shuiquan	(K-5)
Ear points	:	Ovary	
		Uterus	
		Kidney	
		Liver	
		Internal secretion	
		Shenmen	
		Subcortex	
Scalp needling	:	Genital area (both sides)	

Stimulation

Moderate stimulations should be given for 10 days. Course may be repeated after the rest of 5 to 7 days.

Remarks

1. The cause of the disease should be investigated properly and treatment can be combined with modern medicine.
2. Results are good.

IRREGULARITIES OF MENSTRUATION

These include the following conditions:

1. Menorrhagia—Excessive bleeding with normal length of cycles.
2. Polymenorrhoea—Normal bleeding with shorter cycles.
3. Meterorrhagia—Irregular flow at times other than the normal menstrual period.
4. Oligomenorrhoea—Scanty bleeding or longer cycles. The significance of this is similar to that of amenorrhoea.

5.   Amenorrhoea—This has already been discussed.

Menstrual irregularities may be caused by local conditions such as uterine polyp or fibroid, hormonal imbalance due to administration of oestrogens or hypothyroidism and psychiatric diseases.

Main points	:	Qugu	(CV-2)
		Guanyuan	(CV-4)
		Guilai	(St-29)
		Mingmen	(GV-4)
		Shenshu	(UB-23)
Supplementary points	:	Baihui	(GV-20)
		Sanyinjiao	(Sp-6)
		Xuehai	(Sp-10)
		Xingjian	(Liv-2)
		Zusanli	(St-36)
		Neiguan	(P-6)
		Jianjing	(GB-21)
Ear points	:	Ovary	
		Uterus	
		Kidney	
		Internal secretion	
		Shenmen	
Scalp needling	:	Genital area (both sides)	

Stimulation

Mild electrical stimulation can be given 20 to 30 minutes daily for 10 days. Course may be repeated after a rest of 5 to 7 days.

Indirect moxibustion can be done over Qugu (CV-2) and Guanyuan (CV-4)

Remarks

Results are excellent.

DYSMENORRHOEA

Literally, dysmenorrhoea means painful menstruation. This condition is of two varieties—congestive and spasmodic. Congestive dysmenorrhoea is usually associated with inflammatory diseases of the uterus. The pain begins a few days before menstruation and is dull in nature. Spasmodic dysmenorrhoea generally affects the spinsters. The pain is colicky and starts with menstruation. When no obvious cause for dysmenorrhoea can be detected, the conditions is called primary dysmenorrhoea. This is of psychogenic origin.

Main points	:	Zhongji	(CV-3)
		Guanyuan	(CV-4)
		Zhongwan	(CV-12)
		Guilai	(St-29)
		Shenshu	(UB-23)
Supplementary points	:	Baihui	(GV-20)
		Sanyinjiao	(Sp-6)

		Diji	(Sp-8)
		Yinlingquan	(Sp-9)
		Zusanli	(St-36)
Ear points	:	Ovary	
		Shenmen	
		Internal secretion	
		Sympathetic	
		Uterus	
Scalp needling	:	Genital area	

Stimulation

1. Mild electrical stimulation should be given for 20 to 30 minutes daily 7 days before the date of menstruation. Course may be continued upto 3 to 4 days after the menstruation.
2. Indirect moxibustion be applied on Qugu (CV-2) and Guanyuan (CV-4).

Remarks

1. If menstrual cycles are regular, treatment should be started three days before the menstruation.
2. Minimum three courses of the treatment should be advised to the patient.
3. Treatment should be given once a week in between the periods.

LEUCORRHOEA

Discharge of mucous from the vagina is a normal event. When the discharge is excessive or foul smelling, it is termed leucorrhoea. This condition, which is often a cause of great concern to the sufferer is usually produced by some infection of the uterine cervix or of vagina. Excessive oestrogen secretion may be responsible for some cases.

		Qugu	(CV-3)
Main points	:	Qugu	(CV-3)
		Guanyuan	(CV-4)
		Shimen	(CV-5)
		Guilai	(St-29)
		Daimai	(GB-26)
Supplementary points	:	Quchi	(LI-11)
		Qimen	(Liv-14)
		Baihui	(GV-20)
		Sanyinjiao	(Sp-6)
		Yinlingquan	(Sp-9)
		Xingjian	(Liv-2)
		Zusanli	(St-36)
Ear points		Ovary	
		Uterus	
		Internal secretion	
		Shenmen	
Scalp needling	:	Genital area (both sides)	

Stimulation

1. Mild electrical stimulation can be given 20 to 30 minutes daily for 10 days. Course may be repeated after a rest of 5 to 7 days.
2. Indirect moxibustion can be applied on Guanyuan (CV-4), Zhongji (CV-3) and Shenjue (CV-8).

Remarks

1. Local infection should be treated with appropriate antibiotics.
2. An underlying malignancy should be ruled out.
3. Results are good.

PROLAPSE OF UTERUS

Uterus is supported by various ligamentous and muscular structures which are likely to get damaged during childbirth. Prolapse of uterus is caused by slackness of these structures by multiple pregnancies and childbirths. The uterus comes down and pulls the urinary bladder and the rectum along with it. This is called cystocoele and rectocoele respectively. Depending upon the severity, prolapse is described in three grades:

Grade   I   :   External os above introitus.
Grade   II :   External os at the level of introitus.
Grade   III :   External os protruding beyond introitus.

Main points	:	Huiyin	(CV-1)
		Guanyuan	(CV-4)
		Qihai	(CV-6)
		Changqiang	(GV-1)
		Weibao	(Ex-15)
		Ciliao	(UB-32)
		Xialiao	(UB-34)
Supplementary points	:	Baihui	(GV-20)
		Yanglingquan	(GB-34)
		Taichong	(Liv-3)
		Ququan	(Liv-8)
		Yinlingquan	(Sp-9)
		Zusanli	(St-36)
		Sanyinjiao	(Sp-6)
Ear points	:	Uterus	
		Kidney	
		Subcortex	
		Shenmen	
Scalp needling	:	Genital area on both sides	

Stimulation

1. Mild electrical stimulation for 20 to 30 minutes daily for 10 days. Course may be repeated after a rest of 5 to 7 days.
2. Indirect moxibustion can be applied over Qihai (CV-6) and Sanyinjiao (Sp-6) points.

Remarks
1. Exercises to tone the muscles of the pelvic floor should be advised.
2. Good results are observed in 1st and 2nd degree of prolapse.

MANAGEMENT OF NORMAL DELIVERY

Delivery or labour is a process by which the products of conception are normally delivered. The beginning of labour is marked by regular uterine contractions (pains) which become increasingly more frequent, forceful and prolonged with the passage of time. There are three stages of normal delivery.

Stage I : From the onset of labour pains to the full dilatation of cervix. Average duration is 15 hours for primi gravida and 8 hours for multipara.

Stage II : From full dilatation of cervix to the delivery of foetus. Average duration is 1 to 2 hours.

Stage III : From the delivery of foetus upto 1 hour after the expulsion of placenta.

Pain during labour is due to traction upon the supports of uterus, pressure upon structures surrounding the vagina, dilatation of the cervix and lower birth canal, accumulation of catabolites in myometrium, and fear, tension and anxiety. Excessive anxiety may result into uterine inertia.

Main points : Baihui (GV-20)
Hegu (LI-4) (both sides)
Sanyinjiao (Sp-6)
Neima

Technique : 1. During first stage, needles should be passed to all of above points.

Needling : Points of lower extremity should be passed in opposite leg of doctor's working.
Electrical stimulation should start on lower extremity points only. Dense and disperse or discontinued type of electricity should be used.

2nd stage : Strong hand stimulation to Hegu (LI-4) should be given.

3rd stage : Moxa on Kunlun (UB-60) can be given.

Remarks

Following observations have been made by Dr. Wilfred Pererra of Sri Lanka.
1. Acupuncture should be combined with all the routine measures taken for the normal delivery.
2. Acupuncture gives a painless delivery.
3. Exertion to the mother during labour is considerably less.
4. Post-partum haemorrhage is less common.
5. Due to the reduction in the duration of labour by acupuncture, chance of injury to the foetal head, if any, is reduced and consequently the mental development in such babies is higher than the routinely delivered babies.

29

METABOLIC DISEASES

OBESITY

Obesity results when the intake of calories in the form of food exceeds their consumption in the form of physical activity. The excess of calories are stored in the form of fat in the adipose tissue. The most common cause of disparity between the intake and the consumption of the calories is a reduction in the physical activities which occurs around the age of 40 to 60 years. Social customs, food faddism and psychological factors (e.g. failure to achieve) are also responsible for intake of more calories than required.

Disease states are sometimes responsible for obesity. Obesity is a feature of various endocrine diseases like Cushing's syndrome, hypogonadism, myxoedema, Sheehan's syndrome and hyperinsulinism. Diseases involving the hypothalamus (brain tumours, encephalitis) may disturb the feeding centre and cause obesity.

The ill effects of obesity include predisposition to diabetes mellitus, hypertension and coronary artery disease, and occurance of pickwickian syndrome (hypoventilation and pulmonary heart disease due to rigid chest wall)

Main points	:	Zhongwan	(CV-12)
		Rugen	(St-18)
		Liangmen	(St-21)
		Tianshu	(St-25)
		Daheng	(Sp-15)
Supplementary points	:	Baihui	(GV-20)
		Shenmen	(H-7)
		Neiguan	(P-6)
		Zusanli	(St-36)
		Yanglingquan	(GB-34)
		Sanyinjiao	(Sp-6)
Ear points	:	Stomach	
		Large intestine	
		Internal secretion	

Heart
Shenmen
Subcortex

Stimulation

Mild electrical stimulation should be given for 20 to 30 minutes daily for 2 weeks and course should be repeated after a rest of 2 weeks.

Tapping with seven star needle should be done on Hauto's point in lumbosacral region on alternate days.

Remarks
1. Fat and carbohydrate-free diet should also be advised with acupuncture.
2. Motivation of the patient is very essential.
3. Author has got very good results in cases of obesity with acupuncture in combination with Yogic exercises like Surya Namaskar, Vajrasan, etc.
4. Results are very good.

DIABETES MELLITUS

Diabetes mellitus is a metabolic disorder characterised by hyperglycaemia, glycosuria, tendency to ketosis and a liability to develop complications due to vascular degeneration. It is caused by a relative lack of insulin and/or an excess of glucagon. The aetiology is incompletely understood but heredity and obesity are important factors. Diabetes sometimes occurs due to destruction of pancrease by chronic pancreatitis (pancreatic diabetes).

Depending upon the onset and course, two types are known—juvenile diabetes and maturity onset diabetes. Juvenile diabetes occurs below the age of 30 years, has an acute onset, a tendency to develop ketosis and lower insulin requirements. The patient is thin built and shows a poor response to oral antidiabetic drugs. Maturity onset diabetes occurs after the age of 30 years with gradual onset. The patient is obese and resistant to ketosis. The response to oral antidiabetic drugs is satisfactory and insulin requirements are high.

In many cases patient is asymptomatic when diabetes is diagnosed by urine or blood tests. In some cases symptoms like polyuria, polydypepsia, polyphagia and weightloss are present while some cases present with symptoms due to complications.

Complications are rare if the condition is adequately controlled. Uncontrolled diabetics are prone to various complications like ketosis and coma, neuropathy, coronary artery disease, cerebrovascular disease, peripheral vascular disease and gangrene, retinopathy, nephropathy, skin infection, pulmonary tuberculosis, delayed wound healing, abortions, and postmaturity. It has been observed that vascular complications progress in spite of the adequate control of hyperglycaemia.

Main points	:	Baihui	(GV-20)
		Feishu	(UB-13)
		Pishu	(UB-20)
		Shenshu	(UB-23)
		Zusanli	(St-36)
		Taixi	(K-3)
		Yishu	

Supplementary points   :   Shousanli   (LI-10)
                              Quchi   (LI-11)
                              Geshu   (UB-17)
                              Weishu   (UB-21)
                              Guanyuan   (CV-4)
                              Zhongwan   (CV-12)
                              Zhangmen   (Liv-13)
                              Huata's points

Following homeostatic point can also be added in the above group :

                              Dazhui   (GV-14)
                              Sanyinjiao   (Sp-6)
                              Taichong   (Liv-3)
                              Qihai   (CV-6)

Ear points   :   Liver
                              Gall bladder
                              Pancreas
                              Shenmen
                              Sympathetic

Points according to symptoms

Polydypsia   :   Shousanli   (LI-10)
                              Quchi   (LI-11)
                              Geshu   (UB-17)
Ear points   :   Internal secretion, lung
Polyphagia   :   Weishu   (UB-21)
                              Zhongwan   (CV-12)
Ear points   :   Internal secretion, stomach
Polyuria   :   Guanyuan   (CV-4)
                              Shuiquan   (K-5)
                              Fuliu   (K-7)
Ear points   :   Internal secretion, kidney, urinary bladders

Stimulation

1. Mild to moderate stimulation should be given daily for one month.
2. Next course of acupuncture therapy should be advised to the patient according to the system.
3. Press needle on the ear point should be given to get a constant stimulation.
4. Tapping on Hauto's point is also advised.

Remarks

1. Mild to moderate cases of diabetes may be treated with acupuncture alone.
2. In severe cases of diabetes, acupuncture should be combined with modern medicine.
3. Proper dietary advice should also be given to patient.
4. Author has observed good results in cases of diabetes when acupuncture was combined with Yogic Asans.

30

SKIN DISEASES

ECZEMA

Eczema is not a specific disease but a characteristic inflammatory response of the skin to a variety of endogenous and exogenous agents. The inflammatory response consists of erythema and vasiculation in the acute stage and lichenification (increase in the thickness of skin folds) in the chronic stage. Various clinical types of eczema are known.

1. Atopic dermatitis: Intensely itchy lesions on face and flexures, onset during infancy, astháma and vasomotor rhinitis are frequently associated.
2. Neurodermatitis: Generalised or localised eczema at the site of repeated trauma or scratching.
3. Nummular eczema: Coin-shaped lesions on extensor aspect of the extremities and trunk.
4. Pompholyx : Vesicles and bullae on palms and soles.
5. Seborrheic dermatitis: Greasy scaling patches on scalp, eyebrows and nasolabial area.
6. Stasis dermatitis: Caused by venous insufficiency, e.g. varicose veins, venous thrombosis; lesions on legs and feet.
7. Contact dermatitis: Site and configuration depend upon the causal agents include cosmetics, perfumes, hair dyes, synthetic clothing, artificial jewellery, plastics, rubber gloves, footware, watch straps, coal tar derivatives, photographic chemicals, pesticides and certain drugs.
8. Photoallergic contact dermatitis: On parts exposed to sunlight, skin sensitising substances include tar and drugs like sulphonamides, phenothiazines and chloroquine.
9. Endogenous eczema: Generalised, secondary to ingestion of substances to which skin has become sensitised by local application (e.g. antibiotics).
10. Infantile eczema: Initial stage of seborrheic dermatitis or atopic dermatitis seen in infancy.

Main points	:	Baihui	(GV-20)
		Dazhui	(GV-14)
		Huagai	(CV-20)

Hegu	(LI-4)
Quchi	(LI-11)
Sanyinjiao	(Sp-6)
Xuehai	(Sp-10)
Zusanli	(St-36)

Ear points   :   Shenmen
Subcortex
Lung
Liver
Adrenal gland

Stimulation

1. Mild stimulation can be given daily for 20 to 30 minutes for 10 to 15 days. Course may be repeated after a rest of 5 to 7 days.
2. Cupping with tapping around the affected part is also advised.
3. Indirect moxibustion can also be done on any of the body points prescribed above.

Remarks

1. Acupuncture shows good result in cases of chronic eczema.
2. In the presence of secondary infection suitable antibiotics should also be advised with acupuncture.

PSORIASIS

Psoriasis is characterised by sharply demarcated areas of skin with abnormal scaling. The fundamental abnormality is a biochemical fault in epidermal cell formation with resultant rapid turnover of cells. The fault is inherited. Precipitating factors are infection, unfavourable environment, emotional stress, and trauma to the skin. The affected skin is reddened and scaly. Lesions are more extensive on the extensor aspect of the limbs and the trunk. Nails show pitting.

Main points :	Dazhui	(GV-14)
	Baihui	(GV-20)
	Hegu	(LI-4)
	Quchi	(LI-11)
	Chize	(L-5)
	Lieque	(L-7)
	Quze	(P-3)
	Sanyinjiao	(Sp-6)
	Xuehai	(Sp-10)
	Zusanli	(St-36)

Ear points   :   Shenmen
Subcortex
Lung
Adrenal gland
Internal secretion

Stimulation

Mild electrical stimulation for 20 to 30 minutes daily for 10 to 15 days. Course may be repeated after a rest of 5 to 7 days.

Remarks

1. In the refractory cases intravenous bleeding from Chize (L-5) and Quze (P-3) has shown a good response.
2. Press needle on the ear points is also advised to get a continuous stimulation.
3. Longer remissions can be achieved with acupuncture.

ACNE VULGARIS

Commonly spoken of as pimples, acne is characterised by hyperkeratosis, blockade of orifices, and inflammation of the sebacious glands leading to papules and pustules. These lesions are present on face, back, chest and shoulders. Scarring occurs after the rupture of the pustules. Acne is a common problem of adolescence and occurs due to androgen oestrogen imbalance. It can occur at any age with the administration of corticosteroids or oral contraceptives and in cases of Cushing's syndrome :

Main points	: Shanzhong	(CV-17)
	Rugen	(St-18)
	Jiachengjiang	(Ex-5)
Supplementary points	: Hegu	(LI-4)
	Lieque	(L-7)
	Shenmen	(H-7)
	Taodao	(GV-13)
	Dazhui	(GV-14)
	Sanyinjiao	(Sp-6)
Ear points	: Shenmen	
	Subcortex	
	Lung	
	Large intestine	
	Spleen	
	Internal secretion	
	Fasciomandibular area	

Stimulation

Mild electrical stimulation for 20 to 30 minutes daily for 10 days and the course may be repeated after 5 to 7 days.

Remarks

1. Patient should be advised a low fat diet.
2. Face should be thoroughly rubbed and washed at least 2 to 3 times a day.
3. Results are excellent.

VITILIGO

Skin owes its colour to melanin, pigment which is synthesised by malonocytes under the influence of malanocyte stimulating hormone (MSH) of anterior pituitary. In vitiligo, patches of skin show absence of melanin. These patches are depigmented. The condition is inherited. Hypopigmented patches are also seen in acquired leucoderma (occurring at the site of scars or eczema) tinea versicolor and tuberculoid leprosy. In these conditions the patches are never completely depigmented.

Main points	:	Hegu	(LI-4)
		Quchi	(LI-11)
		Baihui	(GV-20)
		Taixi	(K-3)
		Sanyinjiao	(Sp)
		· Zusanli	(St-36)
Ear points	:	Lung	
		Large intestine	
		Shenmen	
		Internal secretson	

Stimulation
1. Mild stimulation for 20 to 30 minutes daily is advised.
2. Tapping with 7 star needle on the affected area should be done daily.
3. Cupping can also be done after tapping on the affected area.

Remarks
1. Long-term therapy is needed.
2. Results are satisfactory.

ALOPECIA

A partial or total loss of hair is termed alopecia. When the involvement is patchy it is called alopecia areata. It may involve the hair margin or the beard area and is possibly of psychogenic origin. In alopecia totalis there is a total loss of hair from the scalp and in alopecia universalis, from all over the body. Alopecia areata has to be differentiated from tinea capitis and cicatricial alopecia due to scarring.

Diffuse alopecia may accompany hypothyroidism, leprosy and administration of cytotoxic drugs.

Main points	:	Lieque	(L-7)
		Hegu	(LI-4)
		Quchi	(LI-11)
		Dazhui	(GV-14)
		Baihui	(GV-20)
		Taixi	(K-3)
		Sanyinjiao	(Sp-6)
		Zusanli	(St-36)

Stimulation
1. Mild electrical stimulation can be given to the body point for 20 to 30 minutes daily for 15 days. Course may be repeated after a rest of 5 to 7 days.
2. Tapping with 7 star needling on the meridians crossing the affected area is also advised.

Remarks
1. Long-term therapy is required.
2. Results are good in alopecia areata.

31
MEDICAL EMERGENCIES

COMA

"Everyone knew what conciousness was until he attempted to define it"
—William James

Since it is difficult to define consciousness, it is also difficult to define unconsciousness and to differentiate between minor degree of unconsciousness and sleep. The impairment of consciousness may vary from confusion, stuper semicoma to coma. During coma there is no response to external stimuli like pain, the reflexes are sluggish, the plantars are sluggish or extensor, the pupils are dilated, and respiration is slow.

Coma is a manifestation of innumerable conditions, both neurologic and non-neurologic (systemic). Coma without localising neurological deficit, without signs of meningeal irritation and with normal cerebro-spinal fluid (CSF) picture indicates a systemic illness. Such an illness may be poisoning with opium, barbiturates or alcohol, diabetic coma, hepatic coma, uraemia, hypoglycaemia, hypoxia, shock, severe infection, heat stroke, and eclampsia. Similar picture may occur in epilepsy, cerebral concussion and hypertensive encephalopathy.

Coma associated with abnormal CSF picture occurs in subarachnoid haemorrhage, meningitis and encephalitis. Presence of localising neurological signs is suggestive of cerebral diseases such as cerebrovascular disease, head injury, cerebral abscess and cerebral tumour.

Whatever be the cause of coma, the most important aspect of its management is attention to the respiration.

Main points	:	Renzhong (GV-26)
		Yongquan (K-1)
		Neiguan (P-6)
		Yintang (Ex-1)
		Shenmen (H-7)
		Quchi (LI-11)
		Jing well points
Ear points	:	Heart
		Lung
		Liver
		Subcortex
		Adrenal gland

Stimulation
1. Strong hand stimulation should be given to all the points prescribed above.
2. Moxibustion should be given to Fengchi (GB-20) and Shenjue (CV-8).

Remarks
1. Proper investigations should be carried out to diagnose the underlying cause of coma and relevant treatment should be given.
2. Level of consciousness improves with acupuncture.

SHOCK

Shock is a condition in which there is a widespread, serious decrease in the blood supply to the tissue resulting into impairment of cellular function. Such decrease in the blood supply may occur due to reduction of the blood volume (hypovolaemic shock), reduction of the cardiac output (cardiogenic shock), pooling of blood due to dilation of capacitance vessels (e.g. anaphylactic shock), or a combination of these mechanisms (e.g. septic shock). Clinically, shock is characterised by a fall of blood pressure, tachycardia, perspiration, cold and clammy skin, clouding of consciousness, oliguria, tachypnea and peripheral cyanosis.

Hypovolaemic shock is the commonest variety and often results from haemorrhage due to injury or from pathological sites like peptic ulcer. Internal haemorrhage is quite often concealed and shock may be its first manifestation. Hypovolaemia also occurs due to excessive vomiting or diarrhoea, diabetic ketosis, and fluid loss in cases of burns and intestinal obstruction. Reduction of the cardiac output resulting into shock occurs in some cases of myocardial infarction (cardiogenic shock) and when there is a mechanical obstruction to the blood flow due to massive pulmonary embolism or pericardial effusion. Intense peripheral vasodilation results into shock. This happens in cases of anaphylactic shock secondary to bee sting, scopion sting or injection of certain drugs (pencillin, ATS) to which the patient is allergic.

A decrease in the vasomotor tone due to hypoxia, general and spinal anaesthesia, and certain drugs (e.g. reserpine) may produce shock (neuropathic shock).

Septic shock, due to gram-negative septicaemia, is the only type which is associated with high body temperature.

Main points	:	Renzhong	(GV-26)
		Yongquan	(K-1)
		Sanyinjiao	(Sp-6)
		Neiguan	(P-6)
		Shenjue	(CV-8)
		Zusanli	(St-36)
		Shenmen	(H-7)
		Jingwell points	
Ear points	:	Adrenal gland	
		Subcortex	
		Heart	
		Thyroid gland	
		Lung	
		Liver	
		Sympathetic	

Stimulation
1. Strong stimulation to all the points prescribed above.
2. Bleeding with a three-edged needle from Jingwell points.

Remarks
1. Additional point should be selected according to the cause.
2. Needle should be stimulated constantly.
3. General principles of the treatment of shock, e.g. bed-rest, raising the foot end of the bed, administration of intravenous fluids.

HIGH FEVER

Though one of the common symptoms, fever sometimes becomes a cause of concern if the body temperature is high (more than 103°F) or if it remains undiagnosed for a long period of time, as it is not uncommon.   High fever not only increases protein catabolism but also exerts deleterious effects on central nervous and haemopoietic systems.   The commonest cause of high fever is infection.   In such cases fever is associated with constitutional symptoms like malaise, headache, nausea, anorexia and prostration.   Other conditions that cause high fever include inflammatory, neoplastic and vascular diseases of central nervous system, particularly involving hypothalamus and pons, heat stroke, thyroid crisis.

Main points	:	Dazhui	(GV-14)
		Quchi	(LI-11)
		Hegu	(LI-4)
Supplementary points	:	Hegu	(LI-4)
		Jianshi	(P-5)
		Shenmen	(H-7)
Ear points	:	Subcortex	
		Hot point	

Points according to symptoms
High fever with no sweating :

| | Hegu | (LI-4) |
| | Dazhui | (GV-14) |

High fever with excessive sweating :

	Dazhui	(GV-14)
	Jianshi	(P-5)
	Fuliu	(K-7)

High fever with headache and bodyache :

	Hegu	(LI-4)
	Quchi	(LI-11)
	Neiting	(St-44)
	Dazhui	(GV-14)

Stimulation
1. Moderate stimulation should be given by hand.   Needle can be kept for 45 minutes to 1 hour until response is observed.

2. Stimulation may be repeated 4 to 6 hourly until patient is relieved from high fever.
3. Use of moxa is also advised on any of the above points for 5 to 10 minutes.
4. Dose of 0.5 to 1 ml of analgin can also be injected in either Hegu (LI-4) or Quchi (LI-11).

Remarks

Author has observed good response with acupuncture in hyperpyrexia due to meningitis and viral encephalitis also.

HEAT STROKE

Heat stroke is a condition in which a sudden rise of body temperature above 105°F occurs due to cessation of sweating consequent to some neurological malfunctioning after exposure to high environmental temperature. Chances of heat stroke are higher if the atmospheric humidity is also high.

The patient may present with headache, exhaustion or delirium but at times becomes comatose without any preceding symptoms. The skin is hot a: ‹ dry. A temperature above 108° F is likely to cause permanent neurological damage and death.

Conditions which predispose to heat stroke are : chronic infections (malaria, tuberculosis), dehydration, chronic systemic diseases (e.g. diabetes, chronic renal failure, chronic alcoholism) and reduced fluid intake.

Main points	:	Dazhui	(GV-14)
		Renzhong	(GV-26)
		Yongquan	(K-1)
		Taixi	(K-3)
		Sanyinjiao	(Sp-6)
		Shenmen	(H-7)
		Weizhong	(UB-40)
		Hegu	(LI-4)
		Quchi	(LI-II)
		Jingwell points	
Ear points	:	Shenmen	
		Subcortex	
		Sympathetic	
		Heart	
		Adrenal gland	

Points according to symptoms

Heart cramps	:	Hegu	(LI-4)
		Quchi	(LI-11)
		Chengshan	(UB-57)
		Yanglingquan	(GB-34)
		Taichong	(Liv-3)

Stimulation

1. Strong stimulation is advised.

2. Bleeding from Jing well points can also be done.

3. Acupressure can also be tried on the following points :

Hegu	(LI-4)
Neiguan	(P 6)
Shenmen	(H-7)

Remarks

General principles of treatment should also be employed with acupuncture to get a quick response.

TETANUS

Tetanus is an acute, often fatal, disease caused by the action of the exotoxin of Clostridium tetani on anterior horn cells resulting into generalised rigidity and spasms. The organism is an anaerobe and multiplies and liberates toxin in closed infected wounds.

The initial symptoms are difficulty in swallowing and stiffness in the jaw, abdomen or back. These are associated with risus sardonicus, lock jaw, neck rigidity, and board like abdominal rigidity. Reflex spasms usually occur within 24 to 72 hours of the first symptom. This interval is called the onset time. Frequency and severity of the spasms vary. They may be precipitated by trivial sensory stimuli like light, sound and changing the drawsheet. Spasms are maximum by the third day and start diminishing on 10th day.

Prognosis is worse with a shorter incubation period, shorter onset time, occurrence of fever in first 48 hours and in neonates (tetanus neonatorum). Causes of death are asphyxia due to spasm of laryngeal or respiratory muscles, bronchopneumonia and pulmonary oedema. The overall mortality is 6 per cent.

Main points	:	Baihui	(GV-20)	
		Hegu	(LI-4)	
		Yanglao	(SI-6)	
		Zhizheng	(SI-7)	
		Shenmen	(H-7)	
		Neiguan	(P-6)	
		Neiting	(St-44)	
		Geshu	(UB-17)	Specific point for paralysis of diaphragm muscles.
		Pishu	(UB-20)	
Ear points		Shenmen		
		Subcortex		
		Crus of the helix		
		Lung		
		Heart		
		Internal secretion		

Points according to symptoms

A. Generalised spasms :	Hegu	(LI-4)
	Neiguan	(P-6)
	Huatuojiaji	(Ex-21)
	Yanglingquan	(GB-34)
	Qihai	(CV-6)

B.	Laryngeal spasm	:	Quchi	(LI-11)
			Fengmen	(UB-12)
			Liangquan	(CV-23)
C.	Stiffness of the	:	Dazhui	(GV-14)
	neck		Fengchi	(GB-20)
			Houxi	(SI-3)
			Lieque	(L-7)
			Dashu	(UB-11)
D.	Lock Jaw	:	Ermen	(TW-21)
			Quanliao	(SI-18)
			Tinggong	(SI-19)
			Xiaguan	(St-7)
			Tinghui	(GB-2)
			Hegu	(LI-4)
			Yanglingquan	(GB-34)

Stimulation
1. Strong hand stimulation is always advised in cases of tetanus.
2. Moxibustion also can be done over Geshu (UB-17).

Remarks
1. ATS in appropriate doses should be administered.
2. Muscle relexants may be needed to control the spasms.
3. Acupuncture decreases the frequency and severity of spasms and is thus capable of preventing death due to laryngeal or respiratory muscle spasm.

32

MISCELLANEOUS DISEASES

ANAEMIA

A reduction of haemoglobin level below normal is defined as anaemia. The normal haemoglobin levels for adult males are 14 to 16 gm and for adult females 12 to 14 gm per 100 ml of blood. Anaemia manifests in the form of pallor. Symptoms are produced only if anaemia develops rapidly or if it is severe. They include breathlessness, palpitation, headache giddiness and tiredness.

Anaemia is caused by various conditions described below :

1. Deficiency of haemopoietic factors, particularly iron, folic acid, and vitamin B_{12}. Deficiency anaemia is more common in women, especially during pregnancy. Iron deficiency anaemia may complicate chronic blood loss due to piles, peptic ulcer, hookworm infestation or menorrhagia. It is characterised by koilonychia.

2. Aplastic anaemia occurs due to bonemarrow depression which may be caused by various drugs (e.g. amidopyrine, phenylbutazone).

3. Haemolytic anaemia is caused by excessive RBC destruction. This may occur due to defective RBCs (haemoglobinopathies such as sickle cell anaemia, and enzyme deficiencies such as that of G6 PD), or factors in serum (drug induced haemolytic anaemia, autoimmune haemolytic anaemia). Haemolytic anaemia is characterised by jaundice and reticulocytosis.

4. Myeloblastic anaemia occurs due to infiltration of the marrow by leukaemia, carcinoma, etc.

5. Miscellaneous conditions, e.g. chronic infection, uraemia, hepatic failure.

Main points : Hegu (LI-4)
Quchi (LI-11)
Jiuwei (CV-15)
Qimen (Liv-14)
Geshu (UB-17)
Xuanzhong (GB-39)

Supplementary points	: Zusanli	(St-36)
	Sanyinjiao	(Sp-6)
	Qihai	(CV-6)
	Baihui	(GV-20)
Ear points	: Shenmen	
	Subcortex	
	Liver	
	Spleen	

Stimulation

1. Mild electrical stimulation can be given for 15 days and the course may be repeated after a rest of 5 to 7 days.
2. Indirect moxibustion can be done on the following points:

        Geshu   (UB-17)

        Xuanzhong   (GB-39)

Remarks

1. The case should be thoroughly investigated and relevant treatment should be given.
2. Deficiency of iron, folic acid and vitamin B_{12} is particularly responsible for most of the cases of anaemia in India. Iron and vitamin supplements should be administered in such cases.
3. Results are satisfactory even in cases of refractory anaemia.

ALLERGY

Defence mechanism of the body consist of immunoglobulins (antibodies) and sensitised lymphocytes (cell-mediated immunity, CMI) which react with the foreign substances (antigens) to which the body is exposed. These reactions are normally beneficial to the host, but may sometimes becomes detrimental and are then termed allergy or hypersensitivity. The manifestation of hypersensitivity are due to the production of various chemical mediators like histamin and serotonine. Depending upon the interval between exposure to the allergen and the onset of symptoms hypersensitivity reactions are classified into immediate, subacute and delayed.

Immediate hypersensitivity or anaphylaxis may be localised or generalised depending upon the route of exposure and the rate of absorption of the allergen. Generalised anaphylactic the form of respiratory distress, wheezing, urticaria and shock. This generally happens following exposure to the injected radio-opaque media and insect stings.

Localised anaphylactic reactions may occur at different sites. On the skin the manifestation is urticaria, wheels with erythematous margins and blanched centre. Urticarial patches may colaease to produce angioneurotic oedema which is generally localised to one limb. When the eyes are affected, conjunctivitis is produced. When the allergen is inhaled (e.g. pollen, house dust) it may give rise to allergic rhinitis and bronchiolitis. The latter manifests in the form of bronchospasm. When the allergen is ingested (e.g. shellfish, egg) gastroenteritis may result.

Subacute hypersensitivity reactions consist of arthus reaction and serum sickness. Delayed hypersensitivity is commonly seen in the form of contact dermatitis. This is an abnormality of CMI and follows skin contact with various allergens. It is dealt along with eczema.

Main points	:	Dazhui	(GV-14)
		Baihui	(GV-20)
		Quchi	(LI-11)
		Sanyinjiao	(Sp-6)
		Xuehai	(Sp-10)
		Taichong	(Liv-3)
Supplementary points	:	Xingjian	(Liv-2)
		Jimai	(Liv-12)
		Zhangmen	(Liv-13)
		Dadu	(Sp-2)
		Taixi	(K-3)
		Lieque	(L-7)
Ear points	:	Sympathetic	
		Subcortex	
		Internal secretion	
		Adrenal	
		Lung	
		Large intestine	

Stimulation

1. Mild stimulation for 20 to 30 minutes daily can be given for 10 days and the course may be repeated after a rest of 5 to 7 days.
2. Tapping with 7 star needles over Huato's points is also advised.

Remarks

1. In refractory and chronic cases Hegu (LI-4) can also be used.
2. The main action of acupuncture is to modify the reticuloendothelial activity.
3. Prognosis is quite satisfactory.

ACUPUNCTURE
ANAESTHESIA

33

INTRODUCTION TO
ACUPUNCTURE ANAESTHESIA

HISTORY

Acupuncture anaesthesia is the principle form of anaesthesia at the Peking Worker, Peasant and Soldier Hospital. First application of the acupuncture anaesthesia was made in a surgical procedure in 1958 in Sian city (Shensi Province of China). It was the case of a breast abscess and an incision drainage was done. As a matter of fact, this was not the birth of acupuncture anaesthesia. It was long before this event when the acupuncture analgesia was being practised by the medical workers to alleviate post-operative pain successfully. This procedure was first used in the dental operations and then encouraged by the results, applied it in the tonsillectomies, thyroidectomies and herniorrhaphies.

Since 1959, Chinese medical workers have been using acupuncture anaesthesia in head and neck surgery, pneumonectomies, amputations and abdominal operations. About 10,000 operations were performed between 1958 and 1966. From 1966 to 1972 about 4,00,000 operations were performed under acupuncture anaesthesia in China. Now, in modern China, it forms the anaesthesia of common choice in most of the surgical procedures.

Acupuncture anaesthesia is comparatively a recent development and not yet universally accepted by the anaesthetists world over. However, the importance of acupuncture anaesthesia in the surgical procedures is being greatly felt and the modern medical man is expected to revise his opinion on the subject in near future.

ADVANTAGES OF ACUPUNCTURE ANAESTHESIA

1. It is very safe, even in poor risk cases.
2. There are no dangerous side effects like those of drug toxicity and allergy.
3. There is no inhibition of the cardiac and respiratory functions, no fall of blood pressure and no alternation in the pulse rate. At times slight bradycardia may occur.
4. Hepatic and renal damage does not occur.
5. It is not expensive. Sophisticated equipment and costly drugs are not required.
6. It is simple and medical workers in distant rural areas can make use of it with success.
7. It is comfortable to the patient. He is not kept fasting. There is faster recovery without nausea and vomiting.

8. Intravenous fluids are usually not needed.
9. Patient can talk during operation.
10. Results of the operation are known on the operation table, for example in thyroidectomy injury to the recurrent laryngeal nerve can bo judgcd by asking the patient to talk.
11. There is no chancc of venous thrombosis and embolism.
12. No change in the skin temperature and electrical resistance of the anaesthesised area.
13. There is little or no haemorrhage.
14. Post-operative pain is much less.

DISADVANTAGES

1. Sometimes the anaesthesia is incomplete.
2. Acupuncture anaesthesia works better above the diaphragm than below the diaphragm.
3. It is unsuitable for emergencies because it takes 15 to 20 minutes for induction.
4. In cancer surgery there is some risk of spread of the cancer because of the needling in the vicinity of the disease.
5. Sometimes there is pulling reaction of the internal organs and muscular tensions, e.g. nausea, vomiting, distension of the viscera, pulling pain, etc.

INDICATIONS

1. Neurosurgery.
2. Thyroidectomy.
3. Laryngectomy.
4. Pulmonary and cardiac surgery.
5. Herniorrhaphy.
6. Paediatric surgery.
7. Surgery during shock.
8. Dental extractions.
9. Abdominal operations like appendicectomy, gastrectomy, gastric perforation, cholcystectomy, spleenectomy.
10. Obstetric and gynaecological operations like caessarean section, tubectomy, hysterectomy.
11. Eye operations.
12. Haemorrhoidectomy.
13. Orthopaedic operations.

CONTRAINDICATIONS

1. Severe injury to the brain with coma.
2. Uncooperative children.
3. Hysteria, neurosis, agitation and other psychological disorders.
4. Cardiac arrhythmias.
5. Obstruction of the respiratory tract.

MOST COMMONLY USED ACUPUNCTURE POINTS

1. Lung meridian

Yunmen	(L-2)
Chize	(L-5)
Kongzui	(L-6)
Lieque	(L-7)
Yuju	(L-10)

2. Large intestine meridian

Sanjian	(LI-3)
Hegu	(LI-4)
Quchi	(LI-11)
Jianyu	(LI-15)
Neck-Futu	(LI-18)
Yingxiang	(LI-20)

3. Stomach meridian

Chengqi	(St-1)
Juliao	(St-3)
Jiache	(St-6)
Xiaguan	(St-7)
Biguan	(St-31)
Zusanli	(St-36)
Xiajuxu	(St-39)
Fenglong	(St-40)
Xiangu	(St-43)
Neiting	(St-44)

4. Heart meridian

Qingling	(H-2)
Shaohai	(H-3)
Tongli	(H-5)

5. Spleen meridians

Taibai	(Sp-3)
Gongsun	(Sp-4)
Sanyinjiao	(Sp-6)
Yinlingquan	(Sp-9)
Xuehai	(Sp-10)
Fushe	(Sp-13)
Daheng	(Sp-15)

6. Small intestine meridian

Houxi	(SI-3)
Yanglao	(SI-6)
Jianzhen	(SI-9)
Jianzhongshu	(SI-15)
Quanliao	(SI-18)

7. Urinary bladder meridian

Zanzhu	(UB-2)
Ganshu	(UB-18)
Dachangshu	(UB-25)
Baihuanshu	(UB-30)
Shangliao	(UB-31)
Ciliao	(UB-32)
Zhongliao	(UB-33)
Chengshan	(UB-57)
Kunlun	(UB-60)
Jinggu	(UB-64)

8. Kidney meridian

Yongquan	(K-1)
Taixi	(K-3)
Dazhong	(K-4)
Zhaohai	(K-6)
Fuliu	(K-7)

9. Pericardium meridian

Ximen	(P-4)
Neiguan	(P-6)

10. Triple warmer meridian

Zhongznu	(TW-3)
Waiguan	(TW-5)
Zhigou	(TW-6)
Sanyangluo	(TW-8)
Yifeng	(TW-17

11. Gall bladder meridian

Tinghui	(GB-2)
Shuaigu	(GB-8)
Yangbai	(GB-14)
Fengchi	(GB-20)
Daimai	(GB-26)
Wushu	(GB-27)
Weidao	(GB-28)
Huantiao	(GB-30)
Yanglingquan	(GB-34)
Waiqiu	(GB-36)
Yangfu	(GB-38)
Xuanzhong	(GB-39)
Foot-Linqi	(GB-41)
Xiaxi	(GB-43)

12. Liver meridian

Taichong	(Liv-3)
Zhongdu	(Liv-6)
Zhangmen	(Liv-13)

13. Governing vessels meridian

Yaoshu	(GV-2)
Yaoyangguan	(GV-3)
Mingmen	(GV-4)
Jizhong	(GV-6)
Taodao	(GV-13)
Dazhui	(GV-14)
Baihui	(GV-20)
Renzhong	(GV-26)

14. Conceptional vessels meridian

Qugu	(CV-2)
Zhongji	(CV-3)
Qihai	(CV-6)
Zhongwan	(CV-12)
Jiuwei	(CV-15)
Chengjiang	(CV-24)

15. Extra-ordinary points

Taiyang	(Ex-2)
Huatuo Jiaji points	(Ex-21)
Lanwei	(Ex-33)
Dannang	(Ex-35)

ESSENTIAL PREANAESTHETIC PROCEDURES AND PREPARATION OF THE PATIENT

1. Patient must be explained about the exact experience he is going to have during the procedure so that he is mentally prepared for it and cooperates during the operation.
2. Patient must perform breathing exercises.
3. Blood examination, urine examination, and all other routine laboratory investigations must be done. Water and electrolyte imbalance must be corrected.
4. A close and detailed consultation between the surgeon and the anaesthetist is essential before the operation.
5. *Acupuncture test* : Before operation, some acupuncture points must be selected to perform trials for making out the "Techi" condition of the patient, and toleration for stimuli. This is called "acupuncture test". While eliciting "Techi" condition, patient is asked about the feeling of dullness, distension, heaviness, tenseness and test, besides "Techi" feeling and tolerance, patient's threshold to pain is also assessed, and a record of his response towards the needling is made so as to judge the force needed for manipulation of needles or electrical stimulation.

PREMEDICATION

1. Sedatives and analgesics in low dosages are administered; commonly used drugs are : phenergan, luminol, chlorpromazine, phenobabitol, demerol.
2. Anticholinergic drugs : atropine and scopolamine.

PROCEDURE

Points are selected, needles applied and stimulated. Following procedures are used for the stimulation.

1. Manual stimulation of the needles

The anaesthetist holds the needle between thumb, index and middle fingers. The rotating movements of the needle are controlled by the thumb while the thrust of the needle is guided by the index and middle fingers. The depth of thrust may vary from 0.5 to 1 t-sun and the amplitude of rotation varies from 180 to 360 degrees. The frequency of twirling varies between 100 to 160 movements per minute. This procedure requires the help of many workers.

2. Electrical acupuncture

In this technique, the needles are stimulated electrically. The stimulus used (clinically 4 to 6 volts of intensity are usually used) may vary from 6 to 18 volts. Sometimes 2000 Hertz may be used. To avoid point resistance the type of stimulation should be changed from time to time.

Electrical stimulation is required throughout the operation. Only a few persons are needed for carrying out the procedure.

Other procedures used for the purpose are as follows :

1. Finger massage of the point.
2. Injecting the point with distilled water.
3. Supplemental local anaesthesia along the line of incision can be given. Most commonly lidocaine is used for this purpose.

Induction time

15 to 20 minutes.

Selection of the points

Selection of the appropriate acupuncture points has evolved through a process of practical investigation, observation and experience. Following are the different ways for making a prescription :

1. Application of the different traditional and modern theories.
2. Selecting the points from experience and observations.
3. Compound acupuncture point prescription.

APPLICATION OF DIFFERENT TRADITIONAL AND MODERN THEORIES

(a) Body needle anaesthesia, according to the theory of "the meridian".
The points are selected from the meridians. The therapeutic properties of the points are taken into consideration and a group of points is chosen. For example.
(i) Analgesic points—Hegu (LI-4), Neiting (St-44).
(ii) Tranquillising points—Shenmen (H-7), Baihui (GV-20), Sishencong (Ex-6).
(iii) Homestatic points—Zusanli (S-t36), Sanyinjiao (Sp-6), Qihai (CV-6).
(iv) Distal points having the specific effect on the proximal area can also be chosen—Hegu (LI-4) for the face and front of the neck, Weizhong (UB-40) for the lower spine.

(b) Application of neurophysiological knowledge of acupuncture : Points can be chosen according to the innervation of the part of the body and segmental (dermatome or myotome) relation of the site of the operation to the point, e.g. Neck Futu (LI-18) in the thyroid operations.

(c) Ear needle anaesthesia : Whole body is represented in the ear. The point pertaining to the particular organ can be selected during the surgical procedure on the same. There are certain points on the ear endowed with some special effects like Shenmen, endocrine point and subcortex. These can also be selected depending upon the need. Ear point detector can be used for searching the points.

(d) Nose needle, hand needle, and foot needle : Nose, hand and foot have a number of points on them with special effects. Any one of them can be prescribed along with the other points or independently out of experience.

(e) Scalp needle anaesthesia : Various areas and centres of the brain are represented on the scalp in a very systematic way. The points on the opposite side are used for anaesthetising corresponding part of the body.

2. Selecting the points from experience and observations.

   (a) Use of incisional needles: Needling is done on the two extremes of the proposed site of incision. Abdomen, breast, neck and thorax are the most common fields for such needling.

   (b) Needling on Governing vessel line from tip of the upper lip to columella and on conceptional vissel line from lower lip to the chin. It is said that they cover all Yang and Yin meridians. (seen by one of the authors while visiting China).

   (e) Points with specific effect discovered by various scholars out of experience :

Zusanli	(St-36)	for gastrointestinal operation
Neiguan	(P-6)	for heart surgery
Sanyinjiao and Nema	(Sp-6)	for ceaserean section
Quanliao	(SI-18)	for craniotomy
Ciliao	(UB-32)	⎫
Yaoshu	(GV-2)	⎬ for abdominal hysterectony
Mingmen	(GV-4)	⎭

3. Compound acupuncture point prescription :

Points are selected from various groups describen above and used in combination. In the beging, it was a common practice to use many points at a time, but now it is generally agreed that only few points should be taken and they should not disturb the site of operation. The points with relative strong "Qi" specific effects on the operative field are also selected. The main points are used first.

34

POINTS PRESCRIPTIONS FOR ANAESTHESIA

DENTAL EXTRACTION

Main points

Upper jaw

Incisors	:	Piercing Renzhong (GV-26) through to Yingxiang (LI-20)
Canine	:	Renzhong (GV-26) through to Yingxiang (LI-20) and Quanliao (SI-18)
Premolar	:	Xiaguan (ST-7)
		Quanliao (SI-18)
Molar	:	Jiache (St-6)
		Quanliao (SI-18)

Lower jaw

Incisors	:	Chengjiang (CV-24)
		Jiache (St-6)
Canine	:	Chengjiang (CV-24)
		Daying (St-5)
		Jiache (St-6)
Premolar	:	Chengjiang (CV-24)
		Jiache (St-6)
Molar	:	Chengjiang (CV-24)
		Jiache (St-6)
		Xiaguan (St-7)

Supplementary points on both sides	:	Hegu (LI-4)
		Xiangu (St-43)
		Neiting (St-44)
Ear needle points	:	1. Area 1 and 4 of ear lobe
		2. Apex of tragus
		3. Shenmen

ABDOMINAL OPERATIONS

Appendicectomy

Main points	: Lanwei	(Ex-33)
	Nei-Ma Neiche Mastui (7 t-sun above medical malleolus)	
	Fengchi	(GB-20)
	Zusanli	(St-36)
	Daimai	(GB-26)
Ear needle points	: Appendix	
	Mouth	
	Shenmen	On both sides or right side
	Lung	
	. Large intestine	

Incisional needles on both the ends of the line of the incision.

GASTRIC PERFORATION

Main points	: 1. Zusanli	(St-36) both sides
	2. Shangjuxu	(St-37)
	3. Sanyinjiao	(Sp-6)
Ear points	: Stomach	
	Spleen	
	Shenmen	Both sides or left side
	Sympathetic	
	Lung	

Gastrectomy

Main points	: Taichong	(Liv-3) both sides
	Zhangmen	(Liv-13)
	Sanyinjiao	(Sp-6)
	or	
	Zusanli	(St-36)
	Shangjuxu	(St-37)

Incisional needles on both ends of incision.

Ears points	: Stomach	
	Spleen	
	Shenmen	
	Sympathetic	
	Lung	

Cholecystectomy

Main points	: Zusanli	(St-36)
	Sanyinjiao	(Sp-6)

Incisional needles on both ends of incision.

Compound prescription

Distal points	: Hegu	(LI-4)
	Neiguan	(P-6)

Ear points   :   Both sides
                            Piercing Shenmen through gall bladder area
                            Sympathetic
                            Lung

Splenectomy

Main points   :   Shangqiu   (Sp-5) both sides
                            Sanyinjiao   (Sp-6)
                            Zusanli   (St-36)
                            Taichong   (Liv-3)

Compound prescription :   Gongsun   (Sp-4) both sides

Ear points (both sides)

                            Spleen
                            Tripple warmer
                            Lung
                            Sympathetic
                            Shenmen

Operations on the kidney

Main points   :   Waiqiu   (GB-36) ⎫
                            Kunlun   (UB-60) ⎬ both sides
                            Taixi   (K-3)   ⎭

                            Mingmen   (GV-4) ⎫ both sides
                            Ciltao   (UB-32) ⎭

                            Xiangu   (St-43) ⎫
                            Taichong   (Liv-3) ⎬ both sides
                            Taibai   (Sp-3) ⎭

                            Hegu   (LI-4) ⎫
                            Waiguan   (TW-5) ⎪
                            Houxi   (SI-3) ⎬ both sides
                            Ximen   (P-4)   ⎭

Ear points   :   Kidney
                            Urinary bladder
                            Shenmen
                            Lung
                            Sympathetic
                            Spleen

OBSTETRIC AND GYNAECOLOGICAL PROCEDURES

Episiotomy

Main points   :   Sanyinjiao   (Sp-6)
                            Taichong   (Liv-3)

Ear points   :   External Genitalia
                            Shenmen

Delivery (Wilfred S. Parera, 1977)

Baihui	(GV-20)	
Hegu	(LI-4)	both sides strong manual stimulation
Neima		
Sanyinjiao	(Sp-6)	Electrical stimulation are one side only

When the labour pains start, the needles are placed on (GV-20) and other needles on the left side of the body.

Effect

There is quickening of uterine contractions and reduction in the intensity of labour pains. Thus there is painless delivery in a short time.

Caesarean section

Main points	:	Renzhong	(GV 26)
		Jizhong	(GV-6)
		Yaoqi	(Ex-20)
Supplementary points	:	Daling	(P-7)
		Hegu	(LI-4)
		Taichong	(Liv-3)
		Ququan	(Liv-8)
		Zusanli	(St-36)
		Kunlun	(UB-60)
		Shugu	(UB-65)
		Sanyinjiao	(Sp-6)
		Neima	

Incisional needles, on both extremes of the line of incision :

Ear points (both sides)

- Ovary
- Shenmen
- Lung
- Uterus
- Abdomen

Every 5 to 6 minutes the stimulation can be transferred, from Kunlun (UB-60) and Shugu (UB-65) to Sanyinjiao (Sp-6) and Zusanli (St-36) to Ququan (Liv-8).

Stimulation of both arms and legs is continued. When slight pain is felt after cutting the skin the stimulation from the points on the arm is changed to the points on the face.

Hysterectomy and Ovarian Cystectomy

Main points	:	Yaoshu	(GV-2)
		Mingmen	(GV-4)
		Daimai	(GB-26)
		Ciliao	(UB-32)
		Zhongliao	(UB-33)

Supplementary points	:	Nei-Ma	
		Zusanli	(St-36)
		Neiting	(St-44)
		Sanyinjiao	(Sp-6)
		Hegu	(LI-4)
		Huatuojiaji	(Ex-21)

Incisional needles on both extremes :

Ear points	:	Uterus	
		Shenmen	
		Lung ·	

Tubectomy

Main point	:	Daimai	(GB-26)
Supplementary points	:	Zhongdu	(Liv-6)
		Zusanli	(St-36)
Ear points	:	Ovary	
		Shenmen	
		Lung	
		Uterus	

OPTHALMIC SURGERY

Main points	:	Yintang	(Ex-1)
		Taiyang	(Ex-2)
		Yuyao	(Ex-3)
		Yangbai	(GB-14)
		Sibai	(St-2)
		Sizhukong	(TW-23)
Supplementary points	:	Hegu	(LI-4)
		Waiguan	(TW-5)
Ear points	:	Eye	
		Eye I	
		Eye II	
		Shenmen	
		Liver	

OPERATIONS ON THE THORAX

Acupuncture anaesthesia gives a satisfactory analgesia and in addition it has a regulating effect on the physiologic functions is relatively safe, simple and effective.

The problems during anaesthesia are :

1. Pain sensation of different degrees when cutting the periosteum and pleura.
2. Dyspnoea may sometimes occur on opening the chest.

If the patient is cooperative, these problems are minimised.

Main points	:	1.	Hegu	(LI-4)
		2.	Sanyangluo	(TW-8)
		3.	Waiguan	(TW-5)

4.	Binao	(LI-14)
5.	Neiguan	(P-6)
6.	Ximen	(P-4)
7.	Neiguan	(P-6)
8.	Jianliao	(TW-14)

Ear points : Shenmen
Lung
Thorax
Sympathetic
Heart
Dingchuan
Kidney
Chest

CARDIAC SURGERY

Main points : Hegu (LI-4) ⎫
Neiguan (P-6) ⎬ on both sides
Zhigou (TW-6) ⎭

Ear points : Shenmen ⎫
Lung ⎪
Thorax ⎬ left side only
Heart ⎭

TONSILLECTOMY

Main points : Jiache (St-6)
Tianchuang (SI-16)
NeckFutu (LI-18)

Supplementary points : Hegu (LI-4)
Zhigou (TW-6)
Neiting (St-44)

Ear points : Thorax
Pharynx and Larynx (both sides)
Tonsil
Shenmen
Sympathetic

LARYNGECTOMY

Main points : Hegu (LI-4)
Zhigou (TW-6)

Ear points : Adrenal gland
Pharynx
Larynx
Shenmen
Sympathetic
Lung
Kidney

THYROIDECTOMY

Main points	:	Yingchuang	(St-16)
		Neck-Futu	(LI-18)
		Jiache	(St-6)
Supplementary points	:	1. Hegu	(LI-4) both sides
		2. Neiguan	(P-6)
		3. Ximen	(P-4)
		4. Point of thyroid gland	[2 t-sun above Neiguan (P-6) both sides].
Ear points	:	Throat	
		Neck	
		Lung	
		Subcortex	
		Shenmen	

HAEMORRHOIDECTOMY

Main points	:	Baihuanshu	(UB-30)
		Yishe	(UB-49)
		Huiyin	(CV-1)
		Changqiang	(GV-1)
Ear points	:	1. Lower segment of the rectum	
		2. Lung (on both sides)	
		3. Shenmen	

REPAIR OF INGUINAL HERNIA

Main points	:	Zusanli	(St-36)
		Daimai	(GB-26)
		Weidao	(GB-28)
		Sanyinjiao	(Sp-6)
		Taichong	(Liv-3)
		Ganshu	(UB-18)
		Dachangshu	(UB-25)
		Daheng	(Sp-15)
		Wei-Ma	
Ear points	:	Sympathetic	
		Lung	
		Small intestine	
		Genital area	
Compound prescription	:	Zusanli	(St-36)
		Ear-Genital area	

OPERATION ON THE SKULL AND BRAIN

(Removal of tumours of cerebral hemisphere, sella turcica, and other intracranial and extracranial operations.)

Main points	:	Xiaohai	(SI-8)
		Quanliao	(SI-18)
		Foot-Linqi	(GB-41)
		Jiexi	(St-41)
		Xiangu	(St-43)
		Taichong	(Liv-3)
		Hegu	(LI-4)

ORTHOPAEDIC PROCEDURES

Operations on the vertebral column
1. Both sides	:	Hegu	(LI-4)
		Waiguan	(TW-5)
or			
2. Both sides		Hegu	(LI-4)
		Neiguan	(P-6)
Ear points	:	Shenmen sympathetic, thoracic	
		Lumbar vertebra	
		Lung	
		Kidney	

Fracture of Radius (Reduction)
Main points	:	Quchi	(LI-11)	⎫
		Waiguan	(TW-5)	⎬ opposite sides
		Shousanli	(LI-10)	
		Hegu	(LI-4)	⎭
Ear points	:	Elbow to wrist		
		Shenmen		
		Lung		

Internal fixation of the femur in fractures
Main points	:	1.	Zusanli	(St-36)
			Xiangu	(St-43)
			Weizhong	(UB-40)
			Fuyang	(UB-59)
			Waiqiu	(GB-36)
			Xuanzhong	(GB-39)
			Qiuxu	(GB-40)
			Sanyinjiao	(Sp-6)
		2.	Yanglingquan	(GB-34)
			Weizhong	(UB-40)
			Ligou	(Liv-5)
		3.	Yanglingquan	(GB-34)
			Waiqiu	(GB-36)
			Xuanzhong	(GB-39)
			Weizhong	(UB-40)
			Fenglong	(St-40)
			Zhongdu	(Liv-6)

Ear points	:	Buttock
		Shenmen
		Lung
		Sympathetic
		Kidney
		Adrenal gland

Amputations

Mid-thigh amputation		Huantiao	(GB-30)
Main points	:	Yishe	(UB-49)
		Huato's points	
Ear points	:	Knee joint	
		Hip joint	
		Shenmen	
		Lung	
Below knee amputation		Huantiao	(GB-30)
Main points	:	Yishe	(UB-49)
		Huato's points	
Ear points	:	Piercing knee	
		Ankle joint	
		Shenmen	
		Lung	

REFERENCES

1. Andrew Brondwein, Josue Corcos : "Acupuncture analgesia in dentistry," *Am. J. Acupuncture*, 5 (3), 241-247, July-Sept., 1975.
2. Ch' Angshan County People's Hospital, Peking: "Acupuncture anaesthesia in splenectomy," *Chin. Med. J.*, 2, 90, 1973.
3. Department of Anaesthesiology, Hsuan Wu Hospital, Peking, "Acupuncture anaesthesia in neurosurgery," *Chin. Med. J.*, 2, 67-70, 1973.
4. Department of Physiology, Anwei Medical College, "Effect of needling of the philtrum on haemorrhagic shock in cats," *Chin. Med. J.*, 2, 98-100, 1973.
5. Department of Surgery, Peking Children's Hospital, Peking, "Acupuncture anaesthesia in pediatric surgery," *Chin. Med. J.*, 2, 91-94, 1973.
6. Dong-Acu. District of Wan—Ding, Kwantung, "Observations on 232 operations performed under acupuncture anaesthesia," *Chin. Med. J.*, 5, 285-328, 1973.
7. Eye, Ear, Nose and Throat, Hospital of Shanghai First Medical College, "Laryngectomy under acupuncture anaesthesia," *Chin. Med. J.*, 2, 78-79, 1973.
8. Hiromary Ogata, Tadasu Matsumoto, Hidezi Tsukahara, *Am. J. Acupuncture*, 5 (4), Oct.-Dec. 1977.
9. Hua Shan Hospital, Shanghai First Medical College, Shanghai, Observations on analgesic effect on needling..chuanliao point in neurosurgery, *Chin. Med. J.*, 2, 71-73, 1973.
10. Kaname Kakizaki, Michio Tany, Eiichi Ishizuka, Seiya Kimura, "Caesarean section by acupuncture," *Am. J. Acupuncture*, 1, 108-111, July-Sept. 1973.
11. Shanghai First Tuberculosis Hospital, Shanghai, "Fulmonary resection under acupuncture anaesthesia," *Chin. Med. J.* 2,, 80-84, 1973.
12. Shanghai First People's Hospital, Shanghai, "Acupuncture anaesthesia in thyroidectomy," *Chin. Med. J.*, 2, 24-77, 1973.
13. Stanley L. Wiss, "Application of acupuncture analgesia in surgery and a physiological explanation of its basis, *Am. J. Acupuncture*, 3, 47-52, March 1975.
14. Thoracic Section, Acupuncture Anaesthesia Group of the Second Teaching Hospital of Human Medical College, Changsha, Human, "Acupuncture anaesthesia in cardiac surgery," *Chin. Med. J.*, 2, 89, 1973.

MAGNETOTHERAPY AND FUTURE OF ACUPUNCTURE

35

MAGNETOTHERAPY IN ACUPUNCTURE

We are now aware that acupuncture treatment works by stimulating various important points in the body by piercing specially made needles. There are various other ways also in stimulating the different points of the body, namely electrical stimuli, magnetic emanations, mechanical vibrations, injections, massages, etc. We shall discuss in this chapter the use of magnets in the treatment of different diseases.

PRINCIPLES OF MAGNETOTHERAPY

Properties of water change when it is brought in contact with magnetic fields. Blood is also similarly influenced and gets ionised. It flows more easily, improving circulation and avoiding clotting. Magnetic emanations exercise a positive effect on the haemoglobin of blood and remove excess of calcium, cholesterol, etc.

Magnetic emanations pass through the tissues and secondary currents are induced. These currents produce impacting heat which reduces pain and swellings.

Magnetic treatment works by reviving, reforming and promoting growth of cells, rejuvenating tissues and increasing the number of healthy blood corpuscles.

Functions of autonomic nerves are normalised and the internal organs controlled by them regain their proper functions. It is also beneficial for mental retardation and weak memory.

It helps to maintain homostasis of the body. One feels in full vigour and vitality after this treatment.

MODE OF APPLICATION OF MAGNETS

Each magnet has two poles—north and south. North pole retards the growth of germs and bacteria and is applied on boils, eczema or infections, etc. South pole relieves pain and reduces swellings, etc. Only one pole is applied on the diseased part or painful spot if the disease is localised in a small portion. If it extends to greater parts or whole body, both the poles are applied in the following manner:

Dr. H.L. Bansal, New Delhi.

For the ailments of the upper half of the body magnets are used under both the palms, and for the ailments of the lower half of the body magnets are applied under both the soles.

If the magnets are applied on the right and left sides, north pole is applied on the right side and south pole on the left side; if on the upper and lower sides, north pole on the upper side and south pole on the lower side; if on the front and back sides; north pole on the front side and south pole on the back side.

The pole to be applied is kept in constant contact with the relevant part of the body. Generally one sitting of 10 to 12 minutes either in the morning or in the evening is sufficient. But in severe cases another sitting with a gap of 10 to 12 hours may also be required.

ADVANTAGES OF MAGNETOTHERAPY

Magnetotherapy has some special advantages. It is easy, safe and simple, yet gives quick results in some cases. There is no adverse effect, reaction or shock. It is economical as the same magnets can be used on hundreds of patients for treating various ailments. If the magnets lose their effectiveness, they can be recharged to regain their lost strength. Magnetotherapy can be given alone or in combination with other methods of treatment, like acupuncture.

MAGNETISED WATER AND ITS DOSAGE

Water can be magnetised with the emanations of magnets. Magnetised water is especially useful for improving appetite and digestion and the kidney function. It also helps to dissolve and flush out stones from kidney and gallbladder. It can be prepared just overnight. Keep two glass tumblers or bottles, full of boiled and cooled water, on two strong magnets. After 12 to 24 hours, transfer the water of both the containers to a third vessel and mix it well. The mixed water is ready for use.

The dose of magnetised water for adults is two ounces (50 ml) at a time. Three such doses may be taken every day. A dose may be taken in the morning before breakfast and two doses may be taken after both the major meals. For children, the dosage may be reduced to one ounce. Magnetised water works as a medicine and should not be taken in excess quantities like simple water.

RESULTS OF MAGNETOTHERAPY

Very satisfactory results have been noticed in the following diseases : Arthritis, asthma, backache, bed-wetting, boiles, cervical spondylitis, diseases of bowel and uterus, eczema, flatulence, headache, injuries, pains of the body, rheumatism, scanty menstrual flow, toothache, sleeplessness, sprains, stiffness, swellings, etc.

ACUPRESSURE AND MAGNETOTHERAPY

Besides the use of needles, the practice of acupressure, that is acupuncture without needles, is also gaining popularity on account of its simpler approach. Various meridians passing through the hands and feet have connections with all the important organs of the body. Hence alleviation of pain or restoration of proper functioning of the inner organs can be easily manipulated by the application of magnets to hands and feet, as the effect of the application of magnets to the palms or soles goes to their other side also and influences all the meridians and their connected organs. Thus the correctness of the methods of application of magnets to palms and soles is verified and proved by the independent system of treatment by acupressure.

USE OF MAGNETS ON ACUPUNCTURE POINTS

The Chinese have described the acupuncture points as very small in size, but some western acupuncturists do not subscribe to this view and believe that a stimulus anywhere in the appropriate determatome will work. Both of them may achieve equal results if the oriental's acupuncture point lies within the area of hypersensitivity of the occidental. This shows that the area around an acupuncture point absorbs the effect of stimulation and the central acupuncture points or the lines of meridians are like the lines of force around a magnet and postulate the magnetic theory.

As there are more than a thousand acupuncture points in the human body, the points must be quite small and each of them must be located in a very small area. It is naturally difficult, therefore, to locate the exact points of acupuncture for piercing the needles. There are also great chances of wrong points being pricked as some of them are very closely placed.

UTILISATION OF ACUPUNCTURE POINTS IN MAGNETOTHERAPY

Physicians who are interested in carrying out treatment by utilising acupuncture points in the body may also try the application of magnets on or near the selected points. Further research work on the combination of magnetotherapy and acupuncture therapy is being carried by Dr. A. L. Agrawal at Acupuncture Research Centre, Raipur.

36

THE FUTURE OF ACUPUNCTURE IN THE THIRD WORLD

The questions which need to be answered are : Does acupuncture work ? Does western medicine work? In what areas do they work? Can the two forms of treatment work together, if so how and by whom?

Most important of all is whether the third world has any alternative but to develop acupuncture and traditional medicine, for western medicine continues to be increasingly costly and is taking up bigger share of each country's gross national product (GNP).

Unfortunately, the third world mainly believes in the western medicine as deeply as the west. This is why western medicine is so popular, although it works no better than the traditional medicine, and in fact generally it is less efficacious.

We hear about the scientific method as if an experiment in a test tube, or the plethora of statistics, is better than the thousands of years of experience in the use of the traditional medicine by the peoples of Africa, India, South America, China, Sri Lanka and others. This is not science but stupidity.

The third world has cultures continuing from the times immemorial which have served the people in good stead, have kept them well and still continue to do so.

Two years ago, in a seminar sponsored by the King's Fund, a most respected British organisation, Dr. Fry, a well-known lecturer on medical affairs, informed the meeting that during the recent strike by paramedical personnel in the U.K. the death rate had decreased by 3 per cent. This had previously also occurred under similar circumstances in Italy, Israel, the U.S.A. and other western countries. Does this mean that western medicine is abused by the common man, by the media and by the medical profession? Western medicine has lost sight of the simple and common illnesses which have become unimportant. Everything is geared towards the complicated, the difficult and the involved. Drugs are used for the simplest of conditions that smash at the body when it is only giving a small cry for help.

Let us look at the way the cost of health services has risen in the west which would happen if the western medicine was used extensively in the developing world. In 1949 the health

Dr. Sidney Rose-Neil, President, British Acupuncture Society, 34 Alderney Street, London (U.K.).

450

service in the United Kingdom cost £ 437,000,000 and used 3.92 per cent of the gross national product and cost £ 9 per head. In 1978 it cost £ 8,000,000,000 used 5.71 per cent of the gross national product and cost £ 141 per head. An increase of 650 per cent in 30 years in real terms.

The United Kingdom has little to show for this expenditure, expectancy has only risen about 3 years taken at birth and 1½ years taken at 45 years in the last 30 years and even this could be attributable to better living standards.

In 1976 over 350,000,000 prescriptions for medicines were made out under the National Health Service. An average prescription now costs over £ 1.50. A man in 1900 in the United Kingdom who reached the age of 70 had a life expectancy of 5 years. There is no evidence to show whose life is prolonged by the western medicine.

The United Kingdom government is quite concerned with the escalating costs of the health service. Cuts being made are resisted by every section of the medical profession which tells us how many more people will die if there were cuts. Neither the medical profession nor the government face the reality of the situation. However, the third world is in a position to do so.

The number of patients is not decreasing in the west. For malignant cancer in the United Kingdom in 1961 there were 229,000 cases and in 1974, 347,000 cases. For nervous diseases the number increased from 70,000 to 97,000. For heart diseases the increase was from 194,000 to 309,000 during the same period and for circulatory conditions from 210,000 to 265,000. For diseases of the urinary system the increase was from 69,000 to 91,000. For diseases of pregnancy and childbirth the ncrease was from 790,000 to 1,000,000. With diseases of the muscular skeletal system the increase was from 155,000 to 209,000. For the lesser complaints the increase was up from 981,000 to 1,550,000.

The cost of seeing a mentally handicapped patient in a hospital in the United Kingdom in 1976 as an outpatient was £ 128. Certainly you may add 50 per cent to these costs for 1979.

If the patient was mentally ill it cost £ 93. An orthopaedic first appointment for an outpatient cost £ 48. If the patient had tuberculosis the cost was £ 49. This was in 1976. If a new outpatient attended for the first time in 1976 a small hospital of up to 50 beds, it cost the state £ 16. If the hospital had 50 to 100 beds, it cost the state £ 24, if the hospital was over 100 beds the cost for every first appointment rose to £ 38. Add 50 percent to these astronomical costs for 1979 as compared with 1976. The costs of each subsequent attendance in a small hospital up to 50 beds was £ 6, in a 50 to 100 bed hospital £ 7, and in a large hospital over 100 beds it rose to £ 9.

If a drug works, why do we need to change it? Because it builds up side effects, the patients become addicted, drugs are prescribed in stronger doses.

Effects become worse than the disease. This happens not in a small minority but to an ever increasing percentage. Side effects have reached such proportions in western medicine that authorities estimate that one in three patients go to their doctor because of iatrogenic diseases, and one in five go into hospital for the same reason.

The World Health Organisation at the Thirtieth World Assembly in May 1977 adopted a resolution which expressed the need for the further development of traditional medicine throughout the world. It recognised that the traditional medicine has a holistic approach to health and that disease is a disequilibrium of man's total ecology and not caused by pathogenic agents. This cuts across widely accepted western ideas and highlights the lack of a western medical philosophy which still clings to the antiquated germ and virus theories of disease.

A World Health Organisation meeting on the promotion and development of traditional medicine was held in Geneva in December 1977. The objectives were to make suggestions for the collaboration among different systems of health in the third world. The meeting asked "What is the traditional medicine?". However, in 1976 the World Health Organisation Regional Office for Africa met in Brazzaville and had already arrived at a definition:

". . . the sum total of all the knowledge and practices, whether applicable or not, used in diagnosis, prevention and elimination of physical, mental or social imbalance and relying exclusively on practical experience and observation handed down from generation to generation, whether verbally or in writing. A solid amalgamation of dynamic medical know-how and ancestral experience."

Again the African Regional Office further adopted an excellent definition of the traditional healer:

". . . a person who is recognised by the community in which he lives as competent to provide health care by using vegetable, animal and mineral substances and certain other methods based on the social, cultural and religious background, as well as on the knowledge, attitudes and beliefs that are prevalent in the community regarding physical, mental and social well-being and the causation of disease and disability."

Practitioners of Ayurveda have defined life "as the union of body, senses, mind and soul. . . positive health as the blending of physical, mental, social, moral and spiritual welfare." This is medicine with a philosophy steeped in the life we lead and in our living environment.

The British Acupuncture Association has defined acupuncture briefly as:

"a branch of medicine founded upon the principle that health is dependent upon a proper balance of vital energy forces within the body and treatment for the purposes of therapy, prophylaxy, with a view to bringing about a balance of such energy forces by methods of the skin with needles in well defined areas according to well defined laws; and is a system of healing which combines the physical, the emotional and the spiritual being into one harmonious unity."

The World Health Organisation in 1978 passed a resolution which requested the Director General of the World Health Organisation to co-ordinate the efforts of governments "to develop and apply scientific criteria and methods for proof of safety and efficacy of medicinal plant products; to disseminate information on these matters among the member states; to designate regional research and training centres for the study of medicinal plants."

Acupuncture was not included in this particular resolution, for although every developing country has its own age-old traditional medicine, acupuncture is imported. However, the working parties at the World Health Organisation are aware of the needle for acupuncture to be used extensively in all third world countries. I have had several successful meetings with Dr. Bannerman, secretary of the Committee for the Development of Traditional Medicine, and with Dr. Ch'en Wen-Chieh, chairman of the same committee and also with Dr. Torfs from the Committee of Appropriate Medical Technology. They are unanimous in their desire to see acupuncture as part of all developing countries medicines. They are fully aware of its efficiency and its low cost.

Dr. Bannerman said at the Annual General Meeting of the International Federation of Practitioners of Natural Therapeutics in 1977 "For far too long, traditional systems of medicine and modern medicine have gone their goals identical—to improve the health of mankind and thereby the quality of life? Only the blinkered mind would assume that each has nothing to learn from the other."

Unfortunately, the divergence between the two systems of medicine has paralleled the division of the world between rich and poor. The privileged and the well-to-do living in large cities enjoy access to all the complex technology and the so-called life-saving equipment of western medicine. But hundreds of millions of people have no such access as the traditional healer, the herbalist and the traditional birth attendant are the agents of health care to whom they turn. On an average, there is no more than one auxillary health worker for 10,000 persons in the third world.

The promotion and development of traditional medicine fosters dignity and self-confidence in any community through self-reliance. What is more respectable than to take care of oneself within one's own means? The integrity and dignity of a people stems from self-respect and self-reliance.

The western doctor cannot escape his responsibility in relation to death by illness in the developing world. The western doctor does not basically accept that wrong eating habits are a major cause of disease. Because of these attitudes it has taken many years to appreciate that tinned milk must be wrong for children and mother's milk must be right. Add to this the west's blind belief that technology is always good and we now have the powdered milk distaste. Thousands, if not millions, of third world babies have died because of this almost unprecented calamity, which may turn out to the greatest human calamity of all times.

The War on Want Association in the United Kingdom has issued a report entitled "The baby killer scandal". Mr. Terry Locey, general secretary of the Association has explained that much of the illness arose from the water with which the milk powder was mixed. Mothers in many developing countries are unable to sterilise water completely and infection can be passed on to their babies. There is no dispute over the content of the milk powder but mothers do not always dilute it correctly and their babies suffer as a result of a weak or over-rich solution. The result of this, says the report, could be seen in clinics, hospitals, slums and graveyards—children whose bodies have wasted away until all that is left is a big head on top of a shrivelled body.

The Daily Telegraph of the 4th October states:

The findings of the report point to one thing—the baby milk industry should eliminate all forms of promotion in developing countries to both the public and the health profession. No one should be allowed to profit at the expense of sick and starving babies.

If the western medicine had a true philosophy as indeed traditional medicine has, it becomes obvious that human milk must be better than tinned milk, that whole-brown rice must be better than white rice, that all foods should be eaten unspoiled or else disease must develop. This is all part of the philosophy of all traditional medicines.

Dr. Mahler, Director General of the World Health Organisation said in November 1977:

"The training of health auxiliaries, traditional midwives and healers may seem very disagreeable to some policymakers, but if the solution is the right one to help people, we should have courage to insist that this is the best policy in the long run and is by no means as expedient acceptance of an inferior solution".

The Thirtieth World Health Assembly of the World Health Organisation on the 19th May 1977 urged governments to give adequate importance to the utilisation of their traditional systems of medicine with appropriate regulations as suited to their national health systems. Further, Dr. Mahler was urged to assist member states to organise educational and research activities and to award fellowships for training in research techniques related to traditional and indigenous systems of medicine.

On the 11th January 1979 the Tenth Meeting of the Committee of the World Health Organisation on Traditional Medicine requested Dr. Mahler to intensify his efforts to promote the involvement of member states in the further development of the programme and to assist governments to develop more realistic and flexible approaches to traditional medicine and also to allocate necessary financial and other resources.

All schools of medicine are modern if directed towards providing health care. The essential differences among various systems of medicine arise from the cultures of the peoples who practise the different systems.

The traditional medicine has always been an integral part of all cultures. This branch of medicine has tended to stagnate through not exploiting some of the useful discoveries of technology. But for the developing countries traditional medicine should be preferred to western medicine. Unfortunately western professional health personnel have regarded traditional medicine as of no importance. This is a serious fallacy as traditional medicine is neither static nor dead.

In cultural evolution, traditional medicine has preserved its role of providing health care in all communities. The World Health Organisation General Meeting held in 1978 recorded: "traditional medicine has intrinsic utility, it should be prompted and its potential developed for the wider use and benefit of mankind. It needs to be given due recognition and developed so as to improve its efficacy, safety, availability, and wider application at low cost. It is already the people's own health care system and is well accepted by them."

Traditional medicine has a holistic approach towards viewing man in his totality within a wide ecological spectrum and of emphasising the viewpoint that ill health is brought about by a disequilibrium of man in his total ecological system and not only by single pathogenic agents. In this context it should be remembered that acupuncture has been used for thousands of years with continuous success and has never been a system which considered disease to be caused by single pathogenic agents: rather the philosophy of acupuncture has always held that disease is caused by bodily unbalances.

Acupuncture is an art where practice has in the past outstripped its scientific evaluation. However, this is now changing and the evaluation of acupuncture in "western scientific terms" is well documented.

Until the west adopts a viable philosophy, integration with traditional medicine will remain difficult. This is further complicated by "administrative intransigence" as it is called by Dr. Mahler. The west is reluctant to demystify its medicine and accept as colleagues those from other schools. But this must end. The pressures are too great and the needs of the developing countries too important. Dr. Mahler has further said that western-type medicine is simply not working; it is too expensive, and the developing countries become dependent on imported drugs and the wrong kind of health personnel.

Western drugs consume 50 per cent of the developing world's health budget, an intolerable situation. Over half of the world's population does not have proper health care. The World Health Organisation has postulated a target that it is the duty of all governments to achieve comprehensive health cover for all people by the year 2000.

It is estimated that one-third of the children born in the developing world will die before they reach the age of 5. This is as high as 5,000,000 for the year 1979. Malnutrition has much to do with these problems and there is no separation between medical and social care.

How then does acupuncture fit into western medicine? In actual fact, however successful acupuncture may be, the western world does not depend upon it. Acupuncture can save western countries enormous amounts money every year and a great deal of human suffering —but the future of acupuncture does not lie with the western world but with the third world.

Western medicine saves lives which makes some of it essential, but most of it is unnecessary, and much of it is damaging. Acupuncture is not only safe, it also saves lives.

Highly skilled doctors who have undergone western training leave their own third world countries and work in the west. There is no way the third world can solve this problem under present conditions. A western doctor who is native of a developing country may have taken several years of training in the United Kingdom. He may then decide to stay on in the United Kingdom, and today there are so many third world doctors in the United Kingdom that the British Health Service would collapse without them.

Each third world western trained doctor who works in the west is a loss to his own country. However, even when the young doctor works in his own country, he prescribes western drugs and uses western methods. After all that is his training. It is difficult for him to make a break from his western training and accept that what has been going on for thousands of years in his own country is medically efficacious.

Many western doctors accept acupuncture but still use western drugs thinking they are getting the best of both worlds. But only acupuncture and indigenous medicine truly go hand in hand, their philosophies and practices as an art run parallel.

In China today over a million doctors practise acupuncture, in Japan sixty thousand, and throughout the East the total approaches three million. In Russia it is taught in several universities. In France and Germany it is used in many hospitals where this treatment can be obtained under the national health schemes.

There are over ten thousand practitioners in Europe. There is no country in the world where its efficacy is not being accepted and its use spreading. Acupuncture is not a panacea, and should be combined with other therapies for the treatment of degenerative illnesses. It may be said that acupuncture can benefit every condition, but not cure every individual case.

In the field of research a Japanese electronics engineer has developed apparatus which records the difference between the twelve radial Chinese acupuncture pulses. Professor Kim Bong Han, a Korean, has demonstrated photographically the existence of the acupuncture meridians as a separate physiological system. He also showed the meridians documented with histological, pathological and photographic evidence.

One of the most important recent innovations has been the introduction of electro-acupuncture. Here a meter records the reduced skin resistance over the acupuncture points. A photo-electric cell indicates to the practitioner when he is over these points. Treatment can then be applied prophylatically or therapeutically. Electro-acupuncture gives objective diagnostic readings, essential for research. The first objective evidence thus provided showed that the meridians and points existed as a demonstrable system.

New techniques are being introduced into practice continuously. For example, the head technique is one where needles are inserted into areas of the scalp. The Chinese have discovered a close connection between certain conditions and the state of the life energy around the areas of the skull.

Another new technique is the long-needle technique, for paralysis. Here, long needles are inserted, alongside the bone of the leg, up to fifty centimetres in length. This is a specialised technique and good results can be obtained with otherwise intransient cases. A further new and successful technique is the suturing of two acupuncture points with a dissolvable material, such as cat gut.

The new method of ear acupuncture is proving highly efficacious. Linked with ear acupuncture is a process known as stapling. Small needles are used in the ear and other parts of the body, and left in place for up to two weeks. They have been particularly helpful in alleviating withdrawal symptoms linked with all forms of addiction including drugs, tobacco and alcohol.

Acupuncture is an art where practice is far outstripping its scientific evaluation.

In China the use of acupuncture anaesthesia began in 1958, when it was used to relieve postoperative pain; success led to the idea of extending its use to replace anaesthetic drugs in surgical operations. That same year acupuncture anaesthesia was introduced successfully in tonsillectomy. The patients reported feeling no pain during operations. The technique was then extended to tooth extractions. One great advantage of this technique is that the patients are fully conscious throughout even a major operation, and they can cooperate and respond to the surgeon's directions and questions. Its range of application is quicker, and without side effects. Some patients, for whom anaesthesia by drugs is contra-indicated, can now undergo surgery safely by the use of acupuncture anaesthesia. Of great importance is the active role that the patient is enabled to take, under acupuncture anaesthetisation, favouring speed and success in the surgical operation, and rapid postoperative recovery.

Looking for explanations for the energy fields which are evidently manipulated in acupuncture is not new to the west. Luigi Galvani, the founder of electro-physiology, discussed these ideas over a century ago. Reichenbach, McDougall, Berman, Reich and many others have all been working indirectly towards the same goal.

Dr. Ann Wooley-Hart of London has been experimenting with skin differentials obtained during acupuncture treatment. She has shown that the potential alters during treatment, and regulates towards the norm.

Dr. Albert Krueger's paper "Are negative ions good for you?" (*New Scientist*, 14 June 1973) opened new theoretical possibilities and his explanations presented as to how negative and positive ions influence health fit in with concepts of acupuncture.

Professor Adolph Smith of Montreal University has postulated that the effects of acupuncture may be produced by the stimulation of ATP. Dr. Krueger (in the *New Scientist*) considered that ions stimulate ATP. If the acupuncture needles produce their effect by stimulating the ions, these could, in turn, stimulate ATP energy, thus substantiating Professor Smith's theory further.

Dr. Thelma Moss from the United States, has been using Kirlian Techniques, a form of high-frequency photography, developed by Kirlian is Russia in 1939. With this method energy emissions at the acupuncture points are photographed. This work has now been repeated almost endlessly by many research workers.

Professor Kozyrev from the USSR has shown that an energy, he names "time", is most dense at the receiving point, and stimulates in an anti-clockwise direction, and relaxes in a clockwise direction. This is exactly what the acupuncturist claims is part of the effect of his needles.

The very latest research is the work being conducted with endorphins. The experiments are very promising and may be the missing link and show how acupuncture suppresses pain.

I started and run in the United Kingdom what is perhaps the only clinic of traditional medicine in Europe. We have been open for 12 years and have 93 beds. We use most traditional methods of medicine, including herbal homeopathy, manipulation, massage, water treatments, special diets and, of course, acupuncture.

We treat those suffering from most chronic diseases; rheumatism, hypertension; ailmentary, circulatory, heart, skin and gynaecological conditions, to name just a few. Almost all our patients are medical failures and come to us after the western doctors and hospitals have failed.

We are dealing with western medical failures and nine out of ten of our patients leave the clinic with a new lease of life. We reduce their drug dependency and often are able to get them free from their western drugs entirely.

It costs about £ 90 a week to actually keep a patient at our clinic using traditional methods. This must be compared with £ 350 a week which it costs to keep someone in a hospital.

Sri Lanka is one of the first countries to integrate western medicine with its own herbals together with acupuncture. Traditional doctors who graduate in Sri Lanka are of no use to the western hospitals because their knowledge will not be sufficient in this respect for employment in the west. This is a good thing for the country.

The future of acupuncture in the third world is intimately interwoven with the very future of the health of the people of the developing world. If the aim of the World Health Organization is to be achieved for all peoples of the world by the year 2000, it can only happen if there is full acceptance of traditional medicine and acupuncture.

From the operational point of view, the most cogent reason for the radical development and promotion of traditional medicine is that it is the surest means to achieve total health care coverage of the world population, using acceptable, safe, and economically feasible methods.

You are the acupuncture doctors of the third world, you have a duty to your country as no other doctors have had before you to do everything in your power to expand the great art of acupuncture.

The future health of thousands of millions of people depend on how you use and develop our acupuncture. I believe the future of traditional medicine and acupuncture in the developing countries is the future of the very health of its people and indeed of the whole world.

INDEX

Abdomen 28
  Pain in 374
  Tonggu (Tungku) 188
  Yinjio (Yinchiao) 226
  Zhongzhu (Chungchu) 186
  Zigong 240
Acne vulgaris 415
Acupuncture
  Anaesthesia 427
  Basis for 11
  Contra-indications and complica-
  Tions of 102
  Contra-indications of 103
  Effects of 15
  Electric stimulator used for 65
  Foot 282
  Hand 280
  Magnetotherapy 447
  Needles 92
  Neurophysiological basis for 11
  Nose 278
  Nose, head and foot 278
  Recent points of 246
  Therapy 287
Acus 1
Acuscope 77
Acute conjuntivitis 356
Acute appendicitis 377
Addiction 296
Alarm points 107
Alcohol 297
Allergy 425
Alopecia 416
Amenorrhoea 405
Angina pectoris 392
Ankylosing spondylitis 346
Anmian-I 238
Anmian-II 238
Anorexia nervosa 296
Anterior chest wall 27
Antihelix 259
  Trunk 263
Anti-tragus 259
  Head region 263

Anuria 400
Anxiety neurosis and neuroasthenia
  291
Aphasia 332
Appendicectomy 437
Apthous ulcers 371
Area 274
  Auricule 259
  Facio-mandibular 262
  Motor area-1 273
  Sensory area-2 273
  Choreo-tremor controlled area-3
  274
  Vasomotor area-4 274
  Foot sensory motor area-5 274
  Verigo-auditory area-6 274
  Language area 2—7 275
  Language area 3—8 275
  Localisation of the brain projection
  273
  Usage area-9 275
  Visual area-10 275
  Equilibrium area-11 275
  Gastric area-12 276
  Thoracsiccavity area-13 276
  Genital area-14 276
  Hepatocystic area-15 276
Artemisia vulgaris 1
Auricular lobule 259, 261
Auriculo therapy 259

Back 26
Backache 347
Bafeng (Ba eight) 245
Baihuanshu (Paihuanshu) 175
Baihui (Paithui) 221
Baohuang (Paohuang) 179
Baxie (Pahsieh) 243
Bell's Palsy 312
Benshen (Penshen) 204
Bian 2
Biguan (Pikuan) 143
Bingfeng (Pingfeng) 163
Bizhong 281

Brain 24
Bronchial asthma 389
Bronchitis 386
Bulang (Pulang) 188
Burong (Pujung) 141

Caesarean section 439
Cardiac surgery 441
Carpal tunnel syndrome 342
Cataract 355
Cavum conchae (thoracic region)
  267
Cerebral palsy 327
Cervical
  Spondylosis 351
  Spondylarthrosis 351
Chang qiang (Chang Chiang) 216
Check area 262
Chen Chen 254
Chengjiang (Cheng Chiang) 228
Chengjin (Chengchin) 179
Cheng Guang (Cheng Kuang) 169
Chenggi (Chengchi) 136
Cheng ling 204
Chengman 141
Chenming 246
Chenshu (shoulder locus) 254
Chest Zigong (Tzukung) 228
Chichuan 250
Chieh Hehsueh (tuberculosis point)
  249
Chiehshi 256
Chienming 254
Chien San Chen (shoulder three
  needle) 254
Chich Jao (ulner radial) 254
Chihchuanchih 255
Chihping 255
Chihhsueh 248
Chiutienfeng 252
Chize (Chihtse) 121
Cholecystectomy 437
Chongmen (Chungmen) 153
Chong Yang (Chungyang) 146

Chronic cholecystitis and gallstones 380
  Suppurative otitis media 365
Chuangwei 253
Chuanhsi (anti asthma) 249
Chuche 249
Chuchuehshu 249
Chuehyin 248
Chungku 247
Chungkui 252
Chungkung 252
Chuoyu 250
Chupi 254
Ciliao (Tzuliao) 175
Cirrhosis of liver 382
Color blindness 360
Coma 418
Common needle (filliform needle) 92
Commonly used auriculars points 269
Constipation 378
Cranial surface of the auricle 268
Crus of helix 259, 265
Cupping 73
Cymba conchae 265

Dabao (Tapao) 154
Dadu (Tatu) 147
Daduan (Tatun) 212
Dahe (Taheh) 186
Daheng (Taheng) 153
Daju (Tachu) 142
Daling (Taling) 192
Daimai (Taimo) 206
Dangerous Points 111
Dannang 244
Danshu (Tanshu) 172
Darwin's theory of evolution 14
Dashu (Tachu) 170
Daying (Taying) 138
Dazhong (Tachung) 184
Dazhui (Tachui) 220
Deaf-Mutism 365
Deafness 366
Delivery 439
Detachment of retina 365
Diabetis mellitus 411
Diarrhoea 377
Dicang (Titsang) 138
Different methods of moxibustion 99
Diji (Tichi) 150
Dingchuan 240
Diseases
  Berger's 396

Cardiovascular 391
Dequervain's 341
Ear 362
Eye 354
Gastro-intestinal 373
Meniere's 364
Metabolic 410
Miscellaneous 424
Musculo-skeletal 337
Neurological 306
Nose 368
Obstetric and gyneacological 403
Oral cavity 370
Psychiatric 291
Respiratory 384
Urological 398
Disorders of speech 331
Distal points 112
Distribution and description of the auricular acupuncture points 261
Diwuhui (Tiwuhui) 210
Drug addiction 297
Dubi (Tupi) 144
Duiduan (Tuituan) 221
Dushu (Tushu) 172
Dysmenorrhoea 406

Ear-Heliao (Heliao) 199
Eczema 413
Electrostimulation 76
Embryological theory 14
Endorphine release theory 14
Epigastric pain 374
Epilepsy 333
Episiotomy 438
Epistaxis 369
Erbai 241
Erjian (Erhehieh) 127
Ermen (Erhmen) 199
Extra-ordinary points on the head and neck 236
  Lower extremity 243
  Trunk 239
  Upper extremity 241
Extra pyramidal disorders 328

Face 24
Fengfu 220
Feiching 257
Feishu 170
Feiyang 179
Femur-Futu (Futu) 143
  Juliao (Chuliao) 207
  Wuli (Wuli) 214
  Zhongdu (Chungtu) 208

Fengehi (Fengchih) 204
Fengkuan 252
Feng lung 145
Fengmen (Fengmen) 170
Fengshi (Fengshih) 207
Fengyen 252
Five elements, the concept of 8
Floating points (Ah-Shi points) 107
Foot drop 326
  Linqi (Tsulingchi) 209
  Qiaoyin (Tsuchiaoyin) 210
Frontal headache 307
Front of the neck 21
Frozen shoulder and shoulder hand syndrome 343
Fuai 153
Fubai (Fupai) 203
Fujie (Fuchieh) 153
Fuliu 185
Fushe 153
Fuyang 180

Ganshu (Kanshu) 172
Gaohuang (Kaohuang) 177
Gastrectomy 437
Gastric perforation 437
Gate control theory of pain 12
Geguan (Kekuan) 178
Geshu (Keshu) 172
Glaucoma 355
Gluteal Region 29
Golfer's elbow (pulled elbow) 343
Gongsun (Kungsun) 149
Guanchong (Kuangchung) 195
Guangming (Kuangming) 209
Guanmen (Kuanmen) 142
Guanyuan (Kuanyuan) 225
Guanyuanshu (Kuanyuanshu) 174
Guilai (Kuilai) 143

Haemorrhoidectomy 442
Hand stimulation 75
Hand-Wangu (Wanku) 162
Hanyan 202
Head 24
  and neck 246
  Linqi (Linchi) 204
  Qiaoyin (Chiaoyin) 203
  Wangu (Wanku) 203
Headache 306
  at vertex 308
Heat stroke 421
Heat stimulation 74
Heading 243
Hegu (Heku) 127

Helix 259, 265
Hemiplegia 316
Henfing 256
Henggu (Hengku) 186
Heyang (Hayang) 179
Hidden Subdermal Needles 94
High fever 420
High frequency vibration 79
Hip joint 341
Houchimen 250
Houding (Houting) 221
Houtinghui (back of listening conference) 246
Houxi (Houhsi) 162
Houyeh 253
Huagai (Huakai) 228
Huanghsu 186
Huangmen 178
Huantiao 207
Huaroumen (Huajoumen) 142
Huatuojiaji 241
Huiyin 225
Huizhong (Huitsung) 197
Hungyin (terrent sound) 248
Hunmen 178
Hsiachui 251
Hsiaochiao 255
Hsiaokukung 253
Hsihsia 255
Hsinshih 247
Hsuehy Atien 251
Husband-wife law 10
Hypertension 394
Hysterectomy and ovarian cystectomy 439
Hysteria 302

Impotence 293
Incontinence of urine 399
Indirect moxibustion 100
Infertility 404
Influential points 111
Insomnia 295
Inter-tragic incisure 259
Irregularities of menstruation 405

Jequan (Chichuan) 155
Jiache (Chiache) 138
Jiacheng Jiang 238
Jianjing (Chien Ching) 205
Jianli (Chienli) 226
Jianliao (Chiehliao) 198
Jianshi (Chienshih) 192
Jianwaishu (Chiehwaishu) 164
Jain Zhen (Chien Cheng) 163

Jian Zhong 241
Jian Zhongshu (Chienchungshu) 164
Jiaosun (Chuehsun) 199
Jiaoxin (Chiaohsin) 186
Jiexi (Chiehhai) 146
Jimai (Chime) 215
Jimen (Chimen) 153
Jinggu (Chingku) 180
Jinghi 239
Jingmen (Chingmen) 206
Jingming (Chingming) 167
Jingqu (Chingchu) 122
Jinjin Yuye 238
Jinmeh (Chimen) 180
Jing-Well points 107
Jinsuo 219
Jiuwei (Chiuwei) 227
Jizhong (Chichung) 219
Jueyinshu (Chuchyinshu) 171
Jugu (Chuku) 132
Jujue (Chuchueh) 227
Juliao (Chuliao) 137

Kanyen 256
Kongzui (Kungtsui) 121
Kufang 140
Kuiyang, Hsuxh (ulcer point) 250
Kunlun 180
Kyungrank system 15

Lanwei 243, 256
Laogong (Laokung) 192
Laryngectomy 441
Laser stimulator 79
Leucorrhoea 407
Liangman 141
Liangqiu (Liang Chiu) 143
Lanquan (Liehchuan) 228
Lidui (Litul) 146
Lieque (Liehchueh) 122
Lingdao (Lingtao) 157
Linghou 244
Linghsia 246
Lingou (Likou) 213
Ling Shu 2
Lingtai 219
Lingxu (Linghsu) 188
Living body and electricity 47
Lougu (Louku) 150
Lower limb 30, 255
Lung Suen (deaf point) 248
Luochen 253
(stiffness of neck) 254
Luoti 257

Luozhen 242
Luxi (Luhsi) 198

Magic gate 2
Magnetic stimulation 77
Malpositions of the foetus 403
Management of normal delivery 409
mandible 23
Medial Xiyan 243
Medical emergencies 418
Meichong 168
Meridians 13
  Belt vessel (Dia Mai) 230
  Conceptional vessel (the Ren meridians) 223
  Eight extra 107, 229
  Gall bladder 199
  Governing vessels (the Du channel) 216
  Heart 155
  Jin ankle vessel (Yinchiao Mai) 231
  Kidney 181
  Large intestine 124
  Liver 210
  Lung 117
  Pericardium 189
  Points 107
  Small intestine 159
  Spleen 42
  Stomach 134
  Systemic description of 117
  Tripel warmer 193
  Urinary bladder 165
  Vital vessel (Chongmai) 231
  Yang ankle vessel (Yangchiao Mai) 231
  Yang regulating vessel (Yangwei Mai) 234
  Yin regulating vessel (Yinwei Mai) 235
Methods of diagnosis 83
  Pulse diagnosis 87
Mexital retardation 301
Mid-day and mid-night law and organ clock 10
Migraine 308
Mingmen 218
Modern diagnostic methods 83
Morning sickness 403
Mother and son law 9
Motor gate theory 12
Moxibustion 73, 98
Muchihchieh Hengwen 252
Muchi Hehien 252

Muchilihengwen 255
Muchuang 204
Myalgia chest 352
Myocardial infarction 392
Myopia 354

Naohu 221
Naohui 198
Naokong (Naokung) 204
Naoshu 163
Neck-Futu (Futu) 133
Nei Ching 2
Neiguan (Neikuan) 192
Neijing 2
Neiting 146
Neiyangchih 256
Network of Jing Luo 7
Night blindness 357
Nocturnal enuresis 300
Nomenclature 105
Nose-Heliao (Heliao) 133
Nuehmen 253

Obesity 410
Obstetric and gynaecological proce-
 dures 256
Occipital headache 308
Oedema 401
Operation of the kidney 438
 on the thorex 438
 on the skull and brain 442
Opthalmic surgery 440
Optic atrophy 361
 Neuritis 358
Orbits 23
Orthopaedic procedures 443
Osteo arthritis of the cervical spine
 351

Pain in the region of mandibular
 branch 312
 Maxillary branch 311
 Ophthalmic branch 310
Palpitation 393
Paralysis of abdominal muscles 323
 Diaphragm 322
 Lower extremity 317, 322
 Upper extremity 321
Paraplegia 318
Parkinsonism 335
Peptic ulcer 375
Peripheral neuropathy 328
Photophobia 360
Physiology of the control of body
 function 32

Pianli (Pienli) 130
Pientao 247
Piken 250
Piles (haemorrhoids) 379
Piliu 246
Pishu 172
Piting 246
Planter fascitis 345
Pohu 177
Point injection therapy and embed-
 ding therepy 97
Points
 Back-Shu 107
 Bonfluent 115
 Extra-ordinary 236
 Five shu 114
 Luo-conneoting 111
 Mu-front 109
 Yuan (source) 110
Poliomyelitis 320
Postherpetic neuralgia 330
Preparation of the moxawool and its
 use 98
Press needle 93
Principles of yin and yang 7
Prolapse of uterus 408
Psoriasis 414
Ptosis 315
Pulmonary tuberculosis 388
Pulse diagnosis 86
Pungue 1
Pushen 180

Qi, the concept of 6
Qianding (Chienting) 221
Qiangjian (Chiang Chien) 221
Qiangu (Chienku) 161
Qichong (Chichung) 143
Qihai (Chihai) 226
Qihaishu (Shihaishu) 174
Qihu (Chihu) 140
Qimai (Chihmo) 198
Qimen (Chimen) 215
Qingling Yuan (Chinglen Yuan) 197
Qingling (Chingling) 155
Qishe (Chishe) 140
Qiuhou 238
Qiuxu (Chiuhsu) 209
Qixue (Chihsueh) 186
Quanliao (Chuanliao) 164
Qubin (Chupin) 203
Quchai (Chucha) 168
Quchi (Chuchi) 130
Quepen (Chuepen) 140
Qugu (Chuku) 225

Ququan (Chuchuan) 214
Quyuan (Chuyuan) 164
Quze (Chutse) 191

Rangu (Janku) 184
Renying (Jenying) 139
Renzhong (Jenchung) 222
Repair of inguinal hernia 442
Retention of urine 400
Rheumatoid arthritis 338
Rhinitis 359
Riyue (Jihyueh) 206
Rugen (Juken) 140
Rules for selection of the points 289
Ruzhong (Juchung) 140

Sanjian (Sanchien) 127
Sanjiaoshu (Sanchiaoshu) 173
Sanyangluo (Sanyanglo) 197
Sanyinjiao (Sanyinchiao) 149
Scalpneedling Therapy 271
Scapha 259, 265
Scapula 27
Schizophrenia 304
Sciatica 348
Sedation points 116
Self stimulation 75
Sequelae of poliomyelitis 323
Seven star needle (plum-blossom
 needle) 93
Shangguan (Shangkuan) 202
Shanglian (Shanglien) 130
Shanglianquan 239
Shangliao 175
Shanglienchuan 248
Shang Qiu (Shang Chiu) 149
Shangqu (Shangchu) 187
Shangwan 227
Shang Xing (Shanghsing) 222
Shang Yang 226
Shangyan Kuan 257
Shangying Hsiang 246
Shanjuxu (Shangchuhsu) 145
Shanken 246
Shanting 222
Shanzhong (Shanchung) 227
Shaochong (Shaochung) 158
Shaofu 158
Shaohai 157
Shaoshong 124
Shaoyangwei 255
Shaoze (Shaotse) 161
Shencang (Shentsang) 188
Shendao (Shentao) 219
Shenfeng 188

Shenji (kidney heat) 257
Shenjue (Shenchueh) 226
Shenmai (Shenmo) 180
Shenmen 158
Shenshu 173
Shentang 178
Shenzhu (Shenchu) 219
Shidou (Shihtou) 153
Shiguan (Shih Kuan) 188
Shihchi Chui Hsia 250, 251
Shihmieh 255
Shihtsang 248
Shimen (Shihmen) 225
Shiqizhui 241
Shixuan 243
Shock 419
Shouchumen 253
Shousanli (Sanli) 130
Shufu 189
Shugu 181
Shuhsi (inguinal point) 249
Shuidao (Shuitao) 143
Shuifen 226
Shuiquan (Shuichuan) 184
Shuitu 139
Sibai (Szupai) 137
Sidu (Szutu) 197
Sifeng 243
Siman (Szuman) 186
Sinusitis 385
Sishencong 238
Sizhukong (Ssuchu Kung) 199
Skin diseases 413
Smoking 298
Special sense organs 354
Splenectomy 438
Squint 314
Status asthmaticus 388
Sterilisation of the needles 94
Stimulation, types of 72
Suliao 222
Superior and inferior crus of antihelix 264
Supra-tragic incisure 259
(heart and external ear) 262
Surface anatomy 19
Su Wen 2
Systemetisation 3
Szuchiang 257

Taibai (Taipai) 147
Tai Chong (Tai Chung) 212
Taixi (Taihsi) 184
Tai Yang 286
Taiyi 142

Taiyinchiao 255
Taiyuan 123
Taku Kung 252
Taodao (taotao) 219
Te-chi (taking of vital energy) 94
Temporal headache 307
Tempromandibular arthritis 341
Tennis elbow 342
Tetanus 422
Thalamic neuron theory 12
Than Chong (Tienchung) 203
Thorex and abdomen 248
Thyroidectomy 442
Tianchi (Tienchin) 189
Tianchuang 164
Tiadding (Tieting) 132
Tianfu (Tienfu) 120
Tianjing (Tienching) 197
Tianliao (Tienliao) 198
Tianquan (Tienchuan) 191
Tianrong (Tienjung) 164
Tianshu (Tiens u) 142
Tiantu (Tientu) 228
Tianxi (Tienhsi) 153
Tianyou (Tienyu) 198
Tianzhog (Tientsung) 163
Tianzhu (Tienchu) 169
Tiayueh 251
Tics (habit spasms) 298
of the eye 299
of the face 299
of the neck 300
Tienchu 247
Tihe 238
Ting Chung (listening clever) 247
Tinggong (Tingkung) 165
Tingh Sueh (listening point) 247
Tinghui (Tinghui) 202
Tingmin 247
Tingtou 248
Tinnitus 362
Tituo 248
Tongli (Tungli) 158
Tonggu (Tungku) 181
Tongtian (Tungtien) 169
Tongziliao (Tungtzuliao) 202
Tonification points 115
Tonsillectomy 441
Toothache 369
Touwei 138
Traditional Chinese diagnostic methods 84
Pulse Positions 86
Law of Energy Flow 8
Tragus 259

Transcutaneous acupuncture 79
(Corresponds to nose and pharynx) 262
Treatment of neuroasthenia 292
Triangular fossa (detoid fossa) 265
needle (sanlingchen) 104
Trigeminal neuralgia 310
Tsuieu 251
Tsu Kung 249
Tsuyichung 256
Tubectomy 440

Upper limb 25, 252
Ultrasonic stimulator 81
Urological diseases 398

Vertigo 363
Viral hepatitis 381
Vishu (pancreas point) 251
Vitiligo 416

Weiguan (Waikuan) 196
Waihuaichien 255
Waiqiu (Waichiu) 209
Walling (Wailing) 142
Wanli 256
Weibao 240
Weicang (Weitsang) 178
Weidao (Weitao) 206
Wei Jesueh 251
Weiji (stomach heat) 257
Weipao 248, 249
Weishang 239
Weishu 173
Wenliu 130
Wrist drop 325
Wry Neck (torticollis) 350
Wuchu 168
Wuming 240, 249
Wushu 206
Wuyi 140

Xiabai (Hsiapai) 121
Xiaguan (Hsiakuan) 138
Xialian (Hsialien) 130
Xiangu (Hsienku) 146
Xiaochangshu (Hsiaochangshu) 174
Xiaoluo (Hsiaolo) 197
Xiawan (Hsiawan) 226
Xiaxi (Hsiahsi) 210
Xiguan (Hsikuan) 214
Xiaohai (Hsiaochai) 162
Xingjian (Hsingchien) 212
Ximen (Hsimen) 191

Xinhui (Hsinhui) 222
Xinshu (Hsinshu) 172
Xiong Xiang (Hsiung-Hsiang) 154
Xiyangguan (Hsiyangkuan) 208
Xuanji (Hsuanchi) 228
Xuanli (Shuanli) 203
Xuanlu (Hsuanlu) 203
Xuanshu (Hsuanshu) 218
Xuanzhong (Hsuanchung) 209
Xuechai (Hsuchhai) 252

Yamen 220
Yangbai (Yangpai) 204
Yangchi (Yangchih) 196
Yang fu 209
Yanggang (Yangkang) 178
Yanggu (Yangku) 162
Yangjiao (Yangchiao) 209
Yanglao 162
Yangling Kuan (Yanglingchuan) 208
Yangxi (Yanghsi) 128
Yaoqi 241
Yaoshu 216
Yaoyangguan (Yangkuan 216
Yaoyi 250
Yatong 243
Yatung (Tooth Point) 254
Yeling 253
Yellow Emperor's Classic of Internal

Medicine 2
Yemen 195
Yiching (pollution point) 249
Yifeng 198
Yiming 238
Yinbai (Yinpai) 147
Yinbao (Yinpao) 214
Yindu (Yintu) 188
Ying Chuang 140
Yinghsia 253
Ying Siang 247
Yingu (Yinku) 186
Yingxiang (Yingsiang) 133
Yinjiao (Yinchiao) 223
Yinkou 250
Yinlian (Yinlien) 214
Yinlingquan (Yinling Chuan) 151
Yinshang 256
Yinshi (Yinshih) 143
Yinxi (Yinhsi) 158
Yintang 236
Yishe 178
Yixi (Yishi) 178
Yongquan (Yungchuan) 183
Youmen (Yumen) 188
Yuanye (Yuanyeh) 206
Yuji (Yuchi) 123
Yunmen 120
Yutang 228

Yuyao 236
Yuzhen (Yuchen) 169
Yuzhong (Yuchung) 188

Zangzhu (Tsanchu) 168
Zengyin 239
Zhangmen (Changmen) 215
Zhaohai (Chaohai) 185
Zhejin (Chechin) 206
Zhengying (Chengying) 204
Zhibian (Chihpien) 179
Zhigou (Chinkou) 195
Zhishi (Chihshih) 179
Zhiyang (Chihyang) 219
Zhiyin (Chihyin) 181
Zhizheng (Chiheheng) 162
Zhongchong (Chungchung) 193
Zhongdu (Chungtu) 214
Zhongfeng (Chungfeng) 212
Zhongfu (Chungfu) 120
Zhongji (Chungchi) 225
Zhongliao (Chungliao) 175
Zhongquan 251
Zhongshu (Chungshu) 219
Zhongting (Chungting) 227
Zhongzhu (Chungchu) 196
Zhouliao (Chouliao) 131
Zhourong (Choujung) 186
Zusanli (Tsusanli) 145